Skin and Pregnancy

This text fills the gap between medical specialties in this topic, covering the dermatological diseases appearing during or affected by pregnancy; it also looks at safe drug usage and the cosmetic and aesthetic concerns of the pregnant woman. Most of the conditions discussed require a combined approach and treatment by the dermatologist and gynecologist and obstetrician, and this text establishes a united therapeutic approach for all practitioners.

T0303910

Skin and Pregnancy

A Comprehensive Guide for Clinical Practice

Edited by

Rashmi Sarkar MD, FAMS, IFAAD
Director Professor
Department of Dermatology
Lady Hardinge Medical College
and Associated KSCH and
SSK Hospital
New Delhi, India

Swati Agrawal MD, FICOG, FMAS
Professor
Department of Gynaecology
Lady Hardinge Medical College
New Delhi, India

Assistant Editor

Soumya Jagadeesan MD
Professor
Department of Dermatology
Amrita School of Medicine
Kochi, India

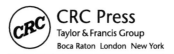

CRC Press
Taylor & Francis Group
Boca Raton London New York

CRC Press is an imprint of the
Taylor & Francis Group, an **informa** business

Designed cover image: Editors

First edition published 2025
by CRC Press
2385 NW Executive Center Drive, Suite 320, Boca Raton, FL 33431

and by CRC Press
4 Park Square, Milton Park, Abingdon, Oxon, OX14 4RN

CRC Press is an imprint of Taylor & Francis Group, LLC

Library of Congress Cataloging-in-Publication Data
[Insert LoC Data here when available]

ISBN: 978-1-032-58348-8 (hbk)
ISBN: 978-1-032-58347-1 (pbk)
ISBN: 978-1-003-44969-0 (ebk)

DOI: 10.1201/9781003449690

Typeset in Times
by Apex CoVantage, LLC

Contents

Contributors

Hossein Akbarialiabad
St George Hospital
University of NSW
Sydney, Australia

Pooja Arora
Atal Bihari Vajpayee Institute of Medical
    Sciences and Dr. Ram Manohar
    Lohia Hospital
New Delhi, India

Anuradha Kakkanatt Babu
Aster Medcity
Kochi, Kerala, India

Anmol Bhargava
GS Medical College & KEM Hospital
Mumbai, India

Yasmeen Jabeen Bhat
Government Medical College
J&K, India

Nisha Suyien Chandran
National University Hospital
Singapore

Julia Cheng
University of California
San Francisco, CA, USA

Kanika Chopra
Lady Hardinge Medical College
New Delhi, India

Arunima Dhabal
Jagannath Gupta Institute of
    Medical Sciences and Hospital
Kolkata, India

Emily Garelick
Philadelphia College of
    Osteopathic Medicine
Philadelphia, PA, USA

Taru Garg
Lady Hardinge Medical College
New Delhi, India

Prashantha GB
Department of Dermatology
Base Hospital
Lucknow, India

Renata Heck
Hospital de Clínicas de Porto Alegre
Porto Alegre, Brazil

Mark W Hocevar
Warren Alpert Medical School of
    Brown University
Providence, RI, USA

Anncilla Jose
Aster Medcity
Kochi, Kerala, India

Rajat Kandhari
Dr Kandhari's Skin and Dental Clinic
New Delhi, India

Radhika Krishna
Amrita Institute of Medical Sciences and
    Research Centre
Kochi, Kerala, India

Valencia Long
National University Hospital
Singapore

Apoorva Maheshwari
MedLinks Aesthetics
Delhi, India

Jenny E Murase
University of California and Palo Alto
    Foundation Medical Group
Mountain View, CA, USA

Dedee F Murrell
St George Hospital
University of NSW
Sydney, Australia

Soumya Narula
All India Institute of Medical Sciences
Bhopal, Madhya Pradesh, India

Prateek Nayak
Amrita Institute of Medical Sciences and
    Research Centre
Kochi, Kerala, India

Shekhar Neema
Base Hospital, an Affiliate of
    King George Medical University
Lucknow, India

Vinitha Varghese Panicker
Amrita Institute of Medical Sciences and
    Research Centre
Kochi, Kerala, India

Indrashis Podder
College of Medicine and Sagore Dutta Hospital
Kolkata, India

Shital Poojary
K.J. Somaiya Medical College
Mumbai, India

Sara D Ragi
Warren Alpert Medical School of
    Brown University
Providence, RI, USA

Noor S
Dr Kandhari's Skin and
    Dental Clinic
New Delhi, India

Kurat Sajad
Government Medical College
J&K, India

Shalini Warman
Tata Main Hospital
Jamshedpur, India

Vidya Yadav
Lady Hardinge Medical College
New Delhi, India

1 Normal Changes in the Skin during Pregnancy

Kanika Chopra and Swati Agrawal

1.1 INTRODUCTION

The pregnancy period is characterised by the occurrence of various endocrinological, immuno-logical, vascular and metabolic changes which influence skin and its appendages in various forms. Nearly 90% of pregnant women may develop skin-related changes. These changes can be a cause of distress to pregnant women. These changes can be physiological, aggravation of pre-existing skin changes or pregnancy-specific dermatoses. Most of the pregnancy-specific dermatoses in pregnancy can be managed conservatively, but a few may require early termination of pregnancy. It is impor-tant for the clinician to distinguish normal findings from abnormal to decide the course of manage-ment. The current chapter discusses normal physiological skin changes in pregnancy.

1.2 PHYSIOLOGICAL SKIN CHANGES IN PREGNANCY

The appearance of the skin is related to its pigmentation as well as the presence of vasculature, glands and connective tissues. During pregnancy, changes can be seen in the skin, hair and mucous membranes, as classified in Table 1.1.

1.3 PIGMENTARY CHANGES

Hyperpigmentation is one of the earliest signs of pregnancy and is more pronounced in dark-complected individuals. Estrogen and progesterone are known to cause melanocytic stimula-tion, leading to hyperpigmentation.[1] The placenta also produces bioactive sphingolipids, which induce melanogenesis by increasing enzymes, tyrosinase and tyrosinase-related proteins 1 and 2.[2] Hyperpigmentation during pregnancy can be seen in localised areas due to differences in the den-sity of melanocytes within the epidermis. Rarely, generalised hyperpigmentation is also seen when associated with hyperthyroidism. Clinically, hyperpigmentation can be seen in the following areas of the body:

- *Linea nigra*: Darkening of midline skin on abdomen starting from xiphoid process to pubic symphysis, as in Figure 1.1. It can also be associated with displacement of the umbi-licus to the right in certain cases, known as ligamentum teres sign.[2] This shift may persist postpartum until abdominal muscles regain their tone.

TABLE 1.1

Physiological Skin Changes during Pregnancy

- Pigmentary changes
- Vascular changes
- Hair and nail changes
- Glandular changes

DOI: 10.1201/9781003449690-1

- **Melasma**: Darkening of facial skin. Melasma is also known as chloasma or mask of pregnancy. It is found in 45–75% of pregnant patients.[3] Genetic predisposition, exposure to sunlight, hormonal factors related to pregnancy and certain skin prototypes may be risk factors for the development of melasma. Melasma may resolve over a period of 1-year postpartum but may persist in 10% of cases.[3] Clinically, melasma can be either centrofacial (hyperpigmentation involving cheeks, forehead, upper lips, nose and chin), seen in Figure 1.2; malar (darkening of cheeks and nose); or mandibular (involvement of the ramus of the mandible).

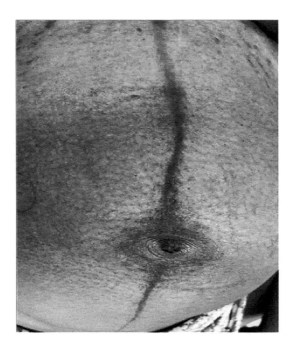

FIGURE 1.1   Linea nigra.

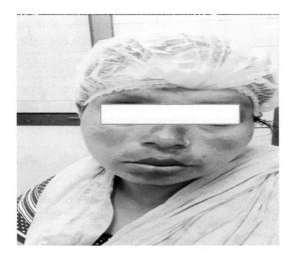

FIGURE 1.2   Melasma can be centrofacial (hyperpigmentation involving cheeks, upper lips, nose and chin).

- *Secondary areola:* Darkening of peri-areolar skin.

- Other areas like nipples, axillae, genitalia, perineum, anus, inner thigh and neck.

Changes can also be observed in pre-existing freckles and nevi.[2] They can become hyperpigmented and may grow in size or in number. Increased pigmentation can be due to an increase in the number of estrogen and progesterone receptors on the surface of nevi or freckles.

The prime management of hyperpigmentation in pregnant women is reassurance and avoiding exposure to the sun. Hyperpigmented skin lightens over a period of several months postpartum. However, if melasma persists after delivery and the woman is anxious cosmetically, it can be treated with topical agents like hydroquinone, tretinoin, vitamin C and kojic acid.[4] The success of treatment depends on the degree of melanin deposition.[5]

1.4   VASCULAR CHANGES

Vascular distension and instability along with proliferation of newer blood vessels lead to changes in the skin during pregnancy. Pituitary and adrenal glands and the placenta secrete various vascular growth factors, causing changes. Physiological hemodilution also happens. The various changes seen are:

- *Edema*: Edema develops due to increased vascular permeability, hormone-induced sodium retention or even compression of the inferior vena cava by the enlarging uterus.
- *Vascular spiders*: These are also known as spider angioma, spider nevi or spider telangiectasia. These can be seen in 66% of light-skinned and 11% of dark-skinned pregnant patients.[6] They develop in the second to fifth months of pregnancy as red lesions with branches extending out from central puncta. They are seen in areas such as the neck, face, upper chest and arm which are supplied by superior vena cava. The majority of these lesions (90%) regress within 3 months of delivery.[6,7]
- *Palmar erythema*: It is usually limited to either hypothenar or thenar eminence. It can be diffuse or mottled. It is seen in 66% of light-skinned and 33% of dark-skinned pregnant patients.[8]
- *Varicosities*: These can be seen in the lower extremities, anorectal region or vulva.[3,9]
    - *Lower extremities*: 50% of pregnant patients may experience dilatation of superficial veins of lower extremities, especially in the third trimester (Figure 1.3). It is due to high levels or estrogen and progesterone, along with other risk factors like prolonged standing.

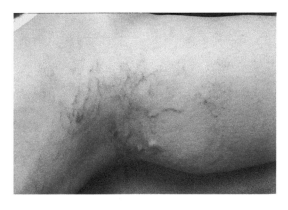

FIGURE 1.3   Varicosities as seen in lower extremeties, usually in third trimester of pregnancy.

- *Anorectal*: Increased vascularity is seen as hemorrhoids in the anorectal region. It is found in approximately 70% of pregnant patients. There is an increased risk of pain and bleeding due to hemorrhoids, especially in the third trimester.[10]
- *Vulvar varicosities*: The reasons behind development of varicosities in the vulvar region are increase in blood volume, increase in venous pressure in femoral or pelvic vessels from enlarging uterus, no valves in perineal vessels and relaxation of the muscular walls of blood vessels (Figure 1.4).
- ***Gingival hyperemia***: Gingival hyperemia can occur in 80% of pregnant women.[1,3] Increased incidence of gingivitis and even progression to periodontitis occur.[9,11] Gingivitis can develop due to pre-existing periodontal diseases or vitamin C deficiency. Periodontitis may occur due to decreased levels of matrix metalloproteinase levels subsequent to high progesterone levels. This may further increase the risk of dental caries.
- ***Nasal mucosal hyperemia***: Hyperemia of the nasal mucosa can develop, and women may complaint of rhinitis.
- ***Vasomotor instability***: Changes like episodic flushing, extremes of temperature sensation, purpura or urticaria can develop due to vasomotor instability.[9]
- ***Pyogenic granuloma***: Pyogenic granulomas are also known as lobular capillary hemangioma. These are benign and vascular tumors with a friable surface. These appear as small, soft, exophytic growth pink-red in color made of granulation tissue. These lesions are most commonly seen in oral mucous membranes such as in gingiva. Extra-gingival sites include lips and fingers.[12,13] Spontaneous resolution is seen following delivery but may take weeks to months.

1.5   CHANGES IN HAIR

Changes in hair are also seen during pregnancy due to increased activity of ovarian and placental androgen on the pilosebaceous unit. Increased estrogen levels lead to an increased duration of the anagen phase of hair. The percentage of anagen hair by the second trimester is 85–95%.[2] The scalp hair appears thicker and fuller. There can be new findings of facial hirsutism and acne in the third trimester, as can be seen in Figure 1.5. In the post-delivery phase, the telogen phase overpowers the anagen phase, and hair fall starts by 70–80 days postpartum, known as telogen effluvium.[2]

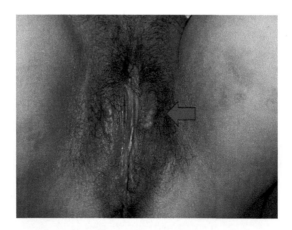

FIGURE 1.4   Vulvar varicosities.

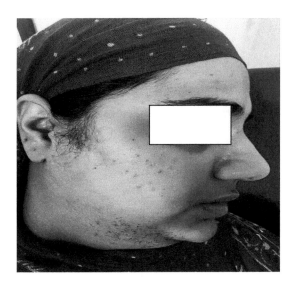

FIGURE 1.5   Facial hirsutism and acne as seen in the third trimester.

1.6   CHANGES IN NAILS

An increase in nail growth is observed during pregnancy. The nails become soft and brittle. Distal onycholysis and subungual hyperkeratosis are also seen. Melanonychia, hyperpigmentation of nail beds, may be seen in few cases.[6] The changes are usually benign, and only reassurance is required.

1.7   GLANDULAR CHANGES

Activity of the eccrine gland increases during pregnancy. This leads to hyperhidrosis, miliaria and dyshidrotic eczema. Sebaceous gland activity increases around the areola (Montgomery's gland or tubercles) and also acne.[6,8]

1.8   MISCELLANEOUS CHANGES

- **Striae gravidarum**: Striae gravidarum are commonly known as striae distensae or stretch marks. These are benign lesions, pink to violet in color, which start to develop in the sixth–seventh month of pregnancy, as shown in Figure 1.6. These may also be associated with pruritis. Stretch marks are commonly seen on the abdomen, breast, lower back, buttocks, thighs and upper arms. These are due to hormonal factors of pregnancy, intrinsic alteration in skin structure and increased tension on skin. Striae gravidarum never disappear and may remain as linear depressions with fine wrinkles. They can be of cosmetic worry to women, and some may go for treatment. Aloe oils, topical tretinoin and 308-nm excimer-pulsed dye laser have been used for the treatment of striae gravidarum, with limited success.
- **Skin tags**: Skin tags, also known as molluscus fibrosum gravidarum, develop on the face, neck, axilla, chest or groin region. These are inflammatory areas develop during the second half of pregnancy and may regress postpartum.[6]
- **Pruritis**: Another problem related to skin seen most commonly during pregnancy is pruritis. Pruritis in pregnancy can be either physiological or pathological (pregnancy-specific dermatosis or due to pre-existing skin disorders). Physiological pruritis most commonly affects the abdomen and is seen in 60% of pregnant patient.[14] Pregnancy-specific

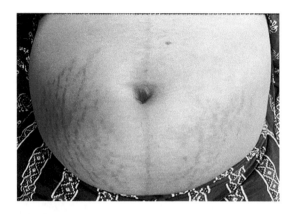

FIGURE 1.6   Striae gravidarum, which start to develop in the sixth to seventh month of pregnancy.

dermatosis of pregnancy includes intrahepatic cholestasis of pregnancy, polymorphic eruptions of pregnancy, atopic eruptions and pemphigoid gestationalis.
*   Other lesions like keloids, dermatofibromas or neurofibromas may increase in size during
    pregnancy.[1,3]

1.9   CONCLUSION

Changes occurring in the skin and related appendages during pregnancy are inevitable. A thorough knowledge about these changes is imperative in order to differentiate them from pathologies
which might be detrimental to the fetus and also for the clinician to be able to reassure and counsel the pregnant woman about their possible resolution during the postpartum period. However,
some changes like hyperpigmentation and varicosities may persist beyond puerperium, requiring
treatment.

REFERENCES

1. Kroumpouzos G, Cohen LM. Dermatoses of pregnancy. *J Am Acad Dermatol.* 2003; 45: 1–19.
2. Kar S, Krishnan A, Shivkumar PV. Pregnancy and skin. *J Obstet Gynecol India.* 2012; 62: 268–275.
3. Barankin B, Silver SG, Carrutheres A. The skin in pregnancy. *J Cutan Med Surg.* 2002; 6: 236–240.
4. Katsambas AD, Stratigos AJ. Depigmenting and bleaching agents: coping with hyperpigmentation. *Clin Dermatol.* 2001; 19: 483–488.
5. Muallem MM, Rubeiz NG. Physiological and biological skin changes in pregnancy. *Clin Dermatol.* 2006; 24: 80–83.
6. Elling SV, Powell FC. Physiological changes in the skin during pregnancy. *Clin Dermatol.* 1995; 15: 35.
7. Winton GB, Lewis CW. Dermatoses of pregnancy. *J Am Acad Dermatol.* 1982; 6: 977.
8. Martin AG, Leal-Khori S. Physiological skin changes associated with pregnancy. *Int J Dermatol.* 1992; 31: 375.
9. Kroumpouzos G, Cohen LM. Dermatoses of pregnancy. *J Am Acad Dermatol.* 2003; 45: 1–19.
10. Ferdinande K, Dorreman Y, Roelens K, et al. Anorectal symptoms during pregnancy and postpartum: a prospective cohort study. *Colorectal Dis.* 2018; 20: 1109.
11. Gungormus M, Akgul HM, Dagistanli S, et al. Generalised gingival hyperemia occurring during pregnancy. *J Int Med Res.* 2002; 30: 353.
12. Aldulaimi S, Saenz A. A bleeding oral mass in a pregnant woman. *JAMA.* 2017; 318: 293.
13. Arunmozhi U, Priya RS, Kadhiresan R, et al. A large pregnancy tumor of tongue: a case report. *J Clin Diagn Res.* 2016; 10: 2010.
14. Szczech J, Wiatrowski A, Hirnle L, et al. Prevalence and relevance of pruritis in pregnancy. *Biomed Res Int.* 2017; 4238139.

2 Inflammatory Dermatoses during Pregnancy
Papulosquamous Disease and Eczema

Prashantha GB and Shekhar Neema

2.1 INTRODUCTION

Pregnancy is a life-changing experience characterised by physiological changes that go beyond the womb and influence many different bodily systems, including the skin. There are significant changes in the immune system that results in immune tolerance towards the genetically different fetus. Cell-mediated immunity is impaired, and the immune system is skewed towards T helper type 2 immunity. These changes result in new-onset immune-mediated skin disease in pregnancy or alter the behaviour of immune-mediated skin diseases. We will discuss papulosquamous disorders and eczema in this chapter.

2.2 PAPULOSQUAMOUS DISORDERS

Papulosquamous disorders encompass a diverse array of skin conditions such as psoriasis, lichen planus, pityriasis rosea, and seborrheic dermatitis, each distinguished by their specific clinical presentations and underlying pathogenic mechanisms. These conditions can present both physical and psychological difficulties when they affect pregnant women, which can have an effect on both the mother's health and the pregnancy as a whole. The course and severity of papulosquamous disorders can be influenced by immunological changes that take place during pregnancy.

2.3 PSORIASIS

2.3.1 INTRODUCTION

Psoriasis is a T-cell–mediated disorder of unknown aetiology that results in significant morbidity. The estimated lifetime prevalence of this condition in the population ranges from 1.5% to 2.2% (1), and about three-quarters manifest symptoms before the age of 40 (2). Incidence is similar for both sexes; however, women often have an earlier onset of the disease compared to males (3). The prevalence in pregnant women is uncertain.

2.3.2 THE EFFECTS OF PREGNANCY ON PSORIASIS

Psoriasis is a Th1-mediated disorder, while in pregnancy, the immune system is skewed towards Th2 immunity. The effect of pregnancy on psoriasis is unpredictable; in most cases it has a favourable impact on psoriasis (4). A significant improvement in psoriasis has been documented in around 60–70% of cases(5,6), while worsening is observed in around 10%–20% of pregnancies (5,7). Breastfeeding does not affect psoriasis significantly (5). It may be exacerbated during the postpartum period. The impact of pregnancy on pustular psoriasis appears to be relatively less pronounced when compared to other subtypes (8). The most significant improvement is often observed in the latter part of the first and second trimesters. This has been correlated with elevated levels of progesterone, which downregulates the proliferative response of T cells (9,10).

2.3.3 THE EFFECTS OF PSORIASIS ON PREGNANCY

There is no evidence to suggest that psoriasis has any impact on fertility, pregnancy outcomes, or timing of delivery (11). The treatment used for psoriasis may cause adverse pregnancy outcomes. Methotrexate and acitretin are contraindicated during pregnancy. Other systemic agents should also be used carefully. Generalised pustular psoriasis can result in adverse pregnancy outcome if not treated promptly. An early induction is indicated in patients not responding to treatment (12).

- **Psoriasis variants**: The variants of psoriasis such as chronic plaque psoriasis, guttate psoriasis, erythrodermic psoriasis, pustular psoriasis, scalp psoriasis (Figure 2.1), nail psoriasis, inverse psoriasis, and arthropathic psoriasis can be seen in pregnancy. Generalised pustular psoriasis will be discussed in detail in the following.

2.3.4 PUSTULAR PSORIASIS OF PREGNANCY

Impetigo herpetiformis, also known as generalised pustular psoriasis of pregnancy, is a rare gestational dermatosis that shares clinical and histological features with pustular psoriasis. It is controversial whether it should be classified as a true variety of pustular psoriasis or as a distinct entity (13,14). It is a rare condition with a high risk of severe consequences, necessitating immediate diagnosis and supportive treatment. Associated complications are high risk of stillbirth, perinatal mortality, placental insufficiency, premature rupture of membranes, preterm labour, and fetal abnormalities.

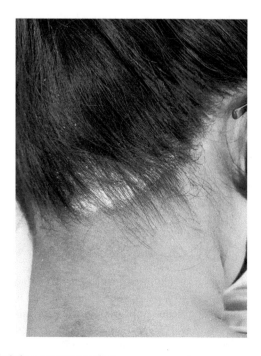

FIGURE 2.1   Scalp psoriasis in a pregnant patient.

The disease is believed to be caused by hormonal changes induced by pregnancy, with pathogenic roles of high progesterone levels and low calcium levels (14). It typically develops during the last trimester of pregnancy and usually resolves after delivery. Recurrences can occur in subsequent pregnancies, sometimes with earlier onset and greater severity or after oral contraceptives. Clinically, impetigo herpetiformis is characterised by erythematous plaques surrounded by micro-pustules and constitutional symptoms including fever, chills, malaise, diarrhoea, nausea, and arthralgia (Figures 2.2 and 2.3). Laboratory examinations may reveal leucocytosis, neutrophilia, elevated erythrocyte sedimentation rate, anaemia, and hypoalbuminemia.

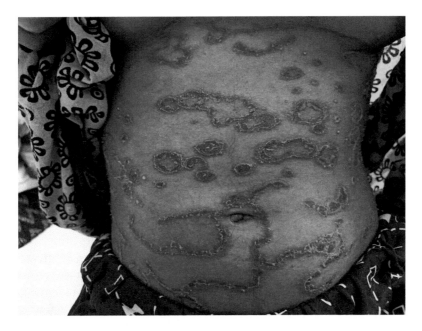

FIGURE 2.2 Generalised pustular psoriasis in an early pregnancy. Patient presented at 14 weeks period of gestation with generalised pustular psoriasis without any prior or family history of psoriasis.

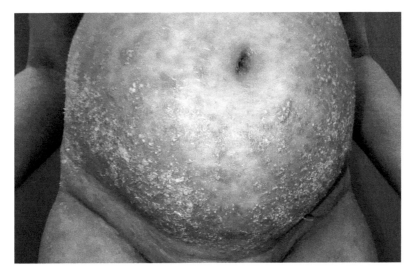

FIGURE 2.3 Generalised pustular psoriasis in late pregnancy. Patient presented with widespread pustules at 26 weeks of period of gestation.

2.4   MANAGEMENT OF PSORIASIS IN PREGNANCY

2.4.1   GENERAL ASPECTS

Psoriasis can improve during pregnancy, making it a reasonable strategy to discontinue the treatment. However, treatment discontinuation may not be possible for those with severe psoriasis. First-line therapy for pregnant patients includes moisturisers, emollients, and topical steroids (15). If moderate-to-severe psoriasis persists or worsens, systemic treatment may be necessary. However, making the appropriate treatment decision can be challenging due to the lack of safety data for many medications during pregnancy. Some medications are known teratogens and mutagens, requiring cautious drug avoidance (16).

2.4.2   TOPICAL THERAPY

Moisturisers and emollients, such as petroleum jelly, should be tried initially, followed by low- to-moderate-potency topical corticosteroids. The safety of topical glucocorticoids varies with the strength of the agent and the specific vehicle employed. Mild/moderate topical corticosteroids are preferred, followed by high-potency topical corticosteroids, if necessary, in the second and third trimesters. High-potency steroids applied on large body surface area can lead to adverse effects due to systemic absorption. It is associated with higher risk of cleft lip in newborns. Pregnancy may alter the bioavailability of topical corticosteroids by modifying skin hydration and blood flow (17,18). The use of anthralin, calcipotriene, coal tar, and topical salicylic acid is not recommended during pregnancy (15).

2.4.3   PHOTOTHERAPY

Second-line treatment for pregnant women involves narrowband UVB (NB-UVB) phototherapy or broadband UVB if NB-UVB is unavailable (15). High cumulative NB-UVB doses can induce folate photodegradation and decrease serum folate levels in psoriasis patients. To minimise low folate levels, some authors advise measuring serum folate levels before and throughout UVB treatment (19,20). Despite theoretical mutagenic and teratogenic effects, PUVA (cat C) treatment does not carry a significant risk for abnormal delivery outcomes (21,22). NB-UVB along with folate supplementation is the preferred treatment for psoriasis in pregnant women.

2.4.4   SYSTEMIC THERAPY

Systemic corticosteroids (FDA Category C): Steroids are not routinely used in common forms of psoriasis but are the treatment of choice for impetigo herpetiformis. The use of systemic steroids during the period of organogenesis (first trimester) has been linked with development of oro-facial clefting in neonates. Fortunately, the onset of disease occurs in the late second trimester when steroids can be safely used.

The effect of corticosteroids on the fetus depends on the transplacental passage, which is influenced by 11β-HSDH activity. Prolonged use of corticosteroids increases the risk of preterm delivery; intrauterine growth restriction; premature membrane rupture; and maternal side effects such as hypertension, pre-eclampsia, eclampsia, gestational diabetes mellitus, and osteoporosis (23,24). It is recommended that prolonged use of prednisone be limited to 7.5 mg/d and avoidance of more than 20 mg/d (25).

- **Cyclosporine (CsA)** is considered a safe oral medication approved for psoriasis during pregnancy (26,27). However, few studies have found an increase in premature delivery and low birth weight but no increase in congenital malformations.
- **Methotrexate** is absolutely contraindicated in pregnancy due to its abortifacient, mutagenic, and teratogenic properties (28).

- **Acitretin** is contraindicated in pregnancy due to teratogenicity, especially in the first trimester. Initially introduced to replace etretinate, is contraindicated in human pregnancy and up to 2 years after the end of therapy, making it an impractical and unsuitable therapy for women in their reproductive years (29,30).

2.4.5 BIOLOGIC THERAPY

The biologics approved for the management of psoriasis are TNF inhibitors (etanercept, infliximab, adalimumab, certolizumab pegol), IL12/23 inhibitors (Ustekinumab), IL17 inhibitors (secukinumab, ixekizumab, brodalumab), IL23p19 inhibitors (Guselkumab, tildrakizumab, Risankizumab), and IL17 A and F inhibitors (Bimekizumab). Monoclonal antibodies are transported through the placenta, reaching high levels in newborn blood after exposure in the late second and third trimester (31). The most experience is with TNF inhibitors, and these drugs are considered relatively safe in pregnancy. When used later in pregnancy, they can lead to neonatal immunosuppression, and live vaccines are contraindicated in infants up to 6 months of age. The drug needs to be stopped earlier to prevent neonatal immunosuppression; the time to stop the drug depends on half-life of the drug (infliximab—16 weeks, adalimumab—28 weeks, etanercept—32 weeks). The transplacental transfer of monoclonal antibodies is mediated by neonatal Fc receptors. Certolizumab Pegol is an Fc-free, pegylated, anti-TNF monoclonal antibody. This drug does not cross the placenta and is safer in pregnant women as compared to other TNF inhibitors (32). There are no published data on other biologics, and the manufacturer recommends stopping the drug prior to conception (33,34). See further Boxes 2.1 and 2.2.

BOX 2.1   KEY POINTS FOR PSORIASIS IN PREGNANCY

- Psoriasis generally improves in pregnancy (60–70%)
- First-line therapy for pregnant patients includes moisturisers, emollients, and topical steroids
- NB-UVB can be used in more extensive disease
- Severe pustular psoriasis may need oral corticosteroids or cyclosporine
- Oral retinoids and methotrexate are contraindicated
- Biological therapies are not currently licensed for use in psoriasis during pregnancy. TNF inhibitors, especially certolizumab pegol, are considered safer as compared to other biologics
- 80% of affected patients will flare postpartum

BOX 2.2   KEY POINTS FOR IMPETIGO HERPETIFORMIS

- Type of generalised pustular psoriasis in pregnancy
- Presents in the third trimester and may recur in subsequent pregnancies (earlier onset and with increased severity)
- Increased risk of stillbirth, neonatal death, and fetal abnormalities due to placental insufficiency
- Maternal constitutional upset—with fever, delirium, tetany, vomiting, and diarrhoea
- Treatment is with oral corticosteroids or cyclosporine
- Infliximab can be used in patients not responding to first-line agents. Early induction and delivery may be indicated in case of non-responsive disease

2.5   PITYRIASIS ROSEA

Pityriasis rosea is a prevalent dermatological condition characterised by the appearance of papulo-squamous skin lesions (35). This condition is often self-limiting and linked to the reactivation of human herpesvirus 6/7 (36). Pityriasis rosea (PR) can manifest spontaneously or as a result of certain medications or vaccinations. While PR is typically regarded as a harmless condition, it may be linked to a higher neonatal risk. There is a correlation between the occurrence of PR during pregnancy and higher incidence of miscarriage, newborn hypotonia, and general delivery problems. Secondary syphilis is a differential diagnosis and should be ruled out. Pruritic urticarial papules and plaques of pregnancy (PUPPP) is another differential diagnosis. It manifests during the third trimester in primigravid pregnancies, while PR can occur at any stage of gestation. PUPPP is a very pruritic condition, while the degree of pruritus in PR varies. The initial lesions in PUPPP typically occur in close proximity to abdominal striae distensae (37). The periumbilical region is commonly unaffected in PR. Peripheral collarette scaling and orientation along the lines of skin cleavage is not observed in PUPPP.

Pruritus can range from being absent to extremely pruritic. Ensuring sufficient symptomatic relief is crucial. Topical emollients are often sufficient for the majority of people diagnosed with pityriasis rosea. If pruritus is severe, sedative antihistaminic may be used (38). Topical and systemic corticosteroids are not very effective in the management and are not advisable (39,40). The data on use of antiviral medicines and macrolides are limited, and they are not advisable in pregnant women (41,42).

2.6   LICHEN PLANUS

Lichen planus, a chronic inflammatory skin condition, can sometimes manifest during pregnancy, raising concerns for both expectant mothers and treating dermatologists. It is characterised by flat-topped, purple papules on the skin or mucous membranes. Lichen planus can manifest in various forms, including cutaneous lichen planus, oral lichen planus, genital lichen planus, and nail lichen planus (Figure 2.4).

It might appear or worsen during pregnancy. Hormonal shifts, shifts in the immune system, and genetic predisposition are all possible contributors, although the exact causes of this phenomenon

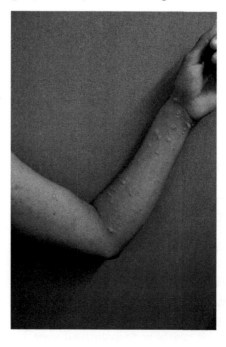

FIGURE 2.4 Eruptive lichen planus in a pregnant patient. The clinical presentation is not different from non-pregnant patient.

remain unclear. The symptoms of lichen planus during pregnancy are similar to those in non-pregnant individuals.

The management of lichen planus during pregnancy can pose challenges, as the available treatment options may be limited due to potential risks to the developing fetus. Management strategies include use of topical steroids in mild to moderate cases, administration of oral antihistamines, and oral corticosteroids are typically used as a last resort in severe cases where symptoms are significantly affecting the quality of life. Cyclosporine can also be used in patients not responding to first line treatment. NB-UVB can also be used safely in pregnant women.

2.7 PITYRIASIS LICHENOIDES ET VARIOLIFORMIS ACUTA

Pityriasis lichenoides (PLC) has diverse range of presentations that affect both the skin and the mucous membranes. Its acute form is known as pityriasis lichenoides et varioliformis acuta (PLEVA). The aetiology of PLEVA remains elusive; however, its sporadic manifestation implies the potential involvement of a viral or bacterial pathogen. Only a few case reports have been published in the literature of PLEVA occurring in pregnant women (43).

PLEVA manifests as an eruption characterised by the appearance of pink, orange, or purpuric papules that develop central vesiculation, may ulcerate, and eventually resolve with the formation of haemorrhagic crusts. Scarring and alterations in pigmentation are often-seen outcomes. The lesions are numerous, mostly concentrated on the trunk and flexural regions of the extremities (44). Lesions affecting the mucous membranes of the vagina and cervix have been implicated with premature labour and/or rupture of membranes (43).

2.7.1 LICHEN SCLEROSUS ET ATROPHICUS

Lichen sclerosus (LS) is an inflammatory condition mostly impacting the anogenital area. The incidence of LS increases with age; however, it has the potential to impact any age group. There is a higher occurrence of LS in females relative to males. It is associated with long-term implications, such as the modification of vulvar architecture, which may potentially affect the mode of delivery (45). Treatment is as same as in non-pregnant women, with potent topical steroids.

One uncommon dermatological condition that can present or worsen during pregnancy is pityriasis rubra pilaris (PRP). There are only a few cases reported in the literature as of now. Treatment options during pregnancy must prioritise the safety of both the mother and the fetus. Topical therapies, such as emollients and moisturisers, are generally considered safe and should be considered first-line therapy. NB-UVB is a safe second-line treatment option in pregnancy. However, systemic treatments, such as retinoids and methotrexate, must be avoided due to potential teratogenicity.

2.8 ECZEMA

The term 'eczema' derives from the Greek word 'ekzein,' meaning 'to boil out.' Eczema periodically flares up, with triggers including skin irritation, infection, stress, and other factors. Eczema encompasses various forms, including atopic, seborrheic, allergic contact, primary irritant, photo-allergic, phototoxic, nummular, asteatotic, stasis, dyshidrotic, and drug-induced eczema. Atopy, a genetic predisposition to allergies, plays a role in atopic eczema.

2.8.1 ATOPIC ERUPTION OF PREGNANCY

2.8.1.1 Introduction

The specific dermatoses of pregnancy represent a group of skin conditions unique to pregnancy; one such entity is atopic eruption of pregnancy (AEP). AEP, also known as atopic eczema of pregnancy, is more common in pregnant individuals with a history of atopy. Approximately 50% of pregnancy-related pruritic rashes are caused by AEP, making it by far the most prevalent pregnant dermatosis (46). The prevalence of this condition appears to be increasing, possibly because of environmental changes (47,48). While AEP affects all three trimesters of pregnancy and appears throughout, it often manifests earlier than the other specific dermatoses of pregnancy (75% onset before the third trimester) (49). It can be further divided into two forms: E-type atopic eruption of pregnancy and P-type atopic eruption of pregnancy.

2.8.2 AETIOLOGY

The hypothesised pathophysiology of AEP is believed to be based on the immunological adaptations of the mother, which are necessary to tolerate her fetus, who has distinct antigens. During the course of pregnancy, there is a downregulation of maternal Th1 cytokine production and cell-mediated activities, accompanied by an increase in Th2 cytokines and humoral response (46). These changes in TH1/TH2 cytokine balance are considered responsible for the remission in predominant TH1-driven autoimmune diseases during pregnancy (50). TH2 shift associated with pregnancy may favour the worsening of atopic dermatitis during pregnancy as well as the appearance of AEP, since atopic dermatitis generally is thought to be a TH2-dominant illness, which accounts particularly for acute lesions (51,52).

2.8.3 CLINICAL AND DIAGNOSTIC FEATURES

A worsening of pre-existing atopic dermatitis with the typical clinical symptoms occurs in 20% of patients. The presence of acute skin lesions, characterised by pruritic, erythematous papules and vesicles or extensive weeping areas with serous exudates, may be observed. Additionally, subacute and chronic manifestations, such as excoriated papules and plaques, scaling, and lichenification, may also be present. However, in 80% of individuals, atopic skin signs appear for the first time ever either during pregnancy or following a protracted remission (i.e., childhood eczema) (Figure 2.5).

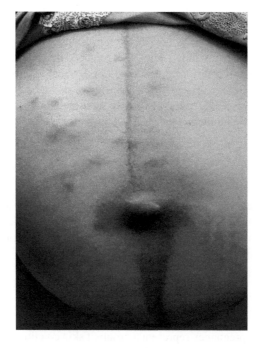

FIGURE 2.5 Atopic eruption of pregnancy presented with pruritic papules. Linea nigra can be also be seen.

E-type atopic eruption of pregnancy refers to individuals with a clear atopic background whose skin lesions first appear during pregnancy and resemble exacerbated atopic dermatitis. P-type atopic eruption of pregnancy also affects those with an atopic background, but it presents with pruritic papules that can lead to excoriation, ulceration, and secondary infection.

Diagnosis relies on clinical findings and the patient's history, with no specific laboratory test for its diagnosis. Histopathology shows non-specific characteristics and varies with clinical presentation. Elevated levels of total serum immunoglobulin (Ig) E are found in 20–70% of patients (53). Complications may include herpes simplex virus (HSV) infection and *Staphylococcus aureus* super-infection. Maternal smoking during pregnancy may increase the risk of atopic eczema in the newborn.

The differential diagnosis mostly includes various specific dermatoses of pregnancy. The presence of spared striae distensae and the earlier onset of symptoms can be used to distinguish between AEP and polymorphic eruption of pregnancy. Normal levels of total serum bile acids differentiate AEP from intrahepatic cholestasis of pregnancy. In addition, it is necessary to consider other dermatoses that occur during pregnancy, including scabies, pityriasis rosea, allergic rashes, and medication eruptions, as well as viral and/or bacterial exanthemata. See further Box 2.3.

BOX 2.3   DIFFERENTIAL DIAGNOSIS

- Polymorphic eruption of pregnancy
- Pemphigoid gestationis
- Intrahepatic cholestasis of pregnancy
- Pityriasis rosea
- Scabies
- Drug eruption
- Contact dermatitis

2.8.4   MANAGEMENT

Management involves liberal use of emollients (moisturisers), avoiding triggers like soap and bubble baths, and moderate to potent topical steroids for mild to moderate eczema. Systemic steroids are rarely indicated but can provide rapid control (54). Topical calcineurin inhibitors and NB-UVB therapy are second-line options. Tacrolimus and pimecrolimus are topical calcineurin inhibitors, with limited systemic absorption (55).

In cases of inadequate control, systemic treatments such as cyclosporine may be considered, with caution and close monitoring during pregnancy.

AEP patients frequently require systemic antibiotics due to secondary bacterial infections, particularly those caused by *Staphylococcus aureus* (56). Pregnancy-safe medications include penicillin, erythromycin, and cephalosporins. For skin infections, penicillinase-resistant penicillins such as ampicillin are advised. See further Box 2.4.

2.9   SEBORRHEIC DERMATITIS

Seborrheic dermatitis is a chronic and recurring skin condition that primarily affects areas rich in sebaceous glands, such as the scalp, face, chest, and back. It is thought to result from a combination of factors, including genetic predisposition, excessive sebum production, and an overgrowth of a yeast called Malassezia (57,58). During pregnancy, the body experiences hormonal changes—particularly elevated levels of oestrogen and progesterone—which can exacerbate seborrheic dermatitis.

BOX 2.4   KEY POINTS FOR ATOPIC ERUPTION OF PREGNANCY

- Approximately 50% of pregnancy-related pruritic rashes are caused by AEP, making it the most prevalent pregnant dermatosis
- AEP affects all three trimesters of pregnancy, with 75% of cases onset before the third trimester
- Pregnancy's TH2 shift may contribute to the development of AEP and the aggravation of atopic dermatitis
- It can be divided into two forms: E-type AEP and P-type AEP
- Two-thirds of patients exhibit patchy eczematous changes (E-type AEP), while one-third show papular lesions (P-type AEP)
- Management includes liberal application of emollients (moisturisers), avoidance of triggers such as soap and bubble baths, and moderate to potent topical steroids

Seborrheic dermatitis is characterised by redness and scaling on the scalp, as well as the para-nasal, submental, post-auricular, sternal, infra-mammary, axillary, umbilical, and inguinal areas. These symptoms can become more pronounced during pregnancy due to hormonal fluctuations and increased blood flow to the skin. Pregnant women may notice flare-ups or worsening of pre-existing seborrheic dermatitis.

The treatment regimen includes the use of topical corticosteroids, ketoconazole shampoo, and selenium sulphide foam. The use of occlusive compounds, such as moisturisers and petrolatum, has the risk of triggering dermatitis.

2.10   NIPPLE ECZEMA

Nipple eczema might provide challenges to breastfeeding. Painful fissures may form and then get infected with pathogens, including *S. aureus*. This issue might be attributed to anatomical characteristics, such as the presence of relatively flat nipples. The treatment for nipple eczema often involves the regular use of moisturisers and the use of a moderate-strength topical corticosteroid, such as hydrocortisone. The use of a topical corticosteroid in conjunction with a topical antibiotic has demonstrated efficacy in the treatment of eczema that has been infected. In certain cases, the use of a systemic antibiotic, such as erythromycin, may become necessary.

2.11   HAND ECZEMA

The recommended treatment approach is preventive, focusing on safeguarding the hands from all skin irritants by rubber gloves. Additionally, the application of topical corticosteroids with moderate potency (class 4 or 5) is necessary. Frequent application of emollients is additionally recommended. The possibility of contact dermatitis should be considered when patients do not exhibit improvement with conventional therapy. However, it is advisable to postpone patch testing until breastfeeding has stopped.

2.12   CONCLUSION

Understanding the impact of various dermatologic disorders on pregnancy is crucial for closely monitoring fetal development and overall pregnancy health. This knowledge enables the anticipation of and preparation for potential issues during pregnancy and childbirth, contributing to more effective management. Conversely, awareness of the typical course of these disorders during pregnancy empowers physicians to proactively identify complications, making necessary adjustments in treatment plans to address potential flares or remissions. Despite these critical implications, there remains a shortage of literature in this field. For instance, studies on the influence of psoriasis on pregnancy outcomes are notably scarce, underscoring the need for more comprehensive research. This chapter sheds light on these literature gaps, highlighting significant opportunities for future investigation.

REFERENCES

1. Gelfand JM, Weinstein R, Porter SB, et al. Prevalence and treatment of psoriasis in the United Kingdom: a population-based study. *Arch Dermatol* 2005;141:1537–1541.
2. Tauscher AE, Fleischer AB Jr, Phelps KC, Feldman SR. Psoriasis and pregnancy. *J Cutan Med Surg* 2002;6:561–570.
3. Barker J. Genetic aspects of psoriasis. *Clin Exp Dermatol* 2001;26:321–325.
4. Dunna SF, Finlay AY. Psoriasis: improvement during and worsening after pregnancy. *Br J Dermatol* 1989;120:584.
5. Mowad CM, Margolis DJ, Halpern AC, et al. Hormonal influences on women with psoriasis. *Cutis* 1998;61:257–260.
6. Boyd AS, Morris LF, Phillips CM, et al. Psoriasis and pregnancy: hormone and immune system interaction. *Int J Dermatol* 1996;35:169.
7. Cecere FA, Persellin RH. The interaction of pregnancy and the rheumatic diseases. *Clin Rheum Dis* 1981;7:748–768.
8. Park BS, Youn JI. Factors influencing psoriasis: an analysis based upon the extent of involvement and clinical type. *J Dermatol* 1998;25:97–102.
9. Pham CT, Koo JY. Plasma levels of 8-methoxypsoralen after topical paint PUVA. *J Am Acad Dermatol* 1993;28:460–466.
10. Ellis CN, Fradin MS, Messana JM, et al. Cyclosporine for plaque-type psoriasis. Results of a multidose, double-blind trial. *N Engl J Med* 1991;324:277–284.
11. Seeger JD, Lanza LL, West WA, et al. Pregnancy and pregnancy outcome among women with inflammatory skin diseases. *Dermatology* 2007;214(1):32–39.
12. Lewden B, Vial T, Elefant E, et al. Low dose methotrexate in the first trimester of pregnancy: results of a French collaborative study. *J Rheumatol* 2004;31:2360–2365.
13. Lotem M, Katzenelson V, Rotem A, et al. Impetigo herpetiformis: a variant of pustular psoriasis or a separate entity? *J Am Acad Dermatol* 1989;20(2 Pt 2):338–341.
14. Roth MM. Pregnancy dermatoses: diagnosis, management, and controversies. *Am J Clin Dermatol* 2011;12(1):25–41.
15. Bae YS, Van Voorhees AS, Hsu S, et al. Review of treatment options for psoriasis in pregnant or lactating women: from the Medical Board of the National Psoriasis Foundation. *J Am Acad Dermatol* 2012;67(3):459–477.
16. Horn EJ, Chambers CD, Menter A, Kimball AB. International Psoriasis Council Pregnancy outcomes in psoriasis: Why do we know so little? *J Am Acad Dermatol* 2009;61(2):e5–e8.
17. Ruiz V, Manubens E, Puig L. Psoriasis in pregnancy: a review (I). *Actas Dermosifiliogr* 2014;105(8):734–743.
18. Chi CC, Mayon-White RT, Wojnarowska FT. Safety of topical corticosteroids in pregnancy: a population-based cohort study. *J Invest Dermatol* 2011;131(4):884–891.
19. El-Saie LT, Rabie AR, Kamel MI, et al. Effect of narrowband ultraviolet B phototherapy on serum folic acid levels in patients with psoriasis. *Lasers Med Sci* 2011;26(4):481–485.
20. Rose RF, Batchelor RJ, Turner D, Goulden V. Narrowband ultraviolet B phototherapy does not influence serum and red cell folate levels in patients with psoriasis. *J Am Acad Dermatol* 2009;61(2):259–262.
21. Stern RS, Lange R. Outcomes of pregnancies among women and partners of men with a history of exposure to methoxsalen-photochemotherapy (PUVA) for the treatment of psoriasis. *Arch Dermatol* 1991;127(3):347–350.
22. Gunnarskog JG, Källén AJ, Lindelöf BG, Sigurgeirsson B. Psoralen photochemotherapy (PUVA) and pregnancy. *Arch Dermatol* 1993;129(3):320–323.
23. Bay Bjørn AM, Ehrenstein V, Hundborg HH, et al. Use of corticosteroids in early pregnancy is not associated with risk of oral clefts and other congenital malformations in offspring. *Am J Ther* 2014;21(2):73–80.
24. Park-Wyllie L, Mazzotta P, Pastuszak A, et al. Birth defects after maternal exposure to corticosteroids: prospective cohort study and meta-analysis of epidemiological studies. *Teratology* 2000;62(6):385–392.

25. Murase JE, Heller MM, Butler DC. Safety of dermatologic medications in pregnancy and lactation: Part I. Pregnancy. *J Am Acad Dermatol* 2014;70(3):401.e1–e14.
26. Paziana K, Del Monaco M, Cardonick E, et al. Ciclosporin use during pregnancy. *Drug Saf* 2013;36(5):279–294.
27. Altomare G, Ayala F, Bardazzi F, et al. Consensus on the use of cyclosporine in dermatological practice. *G Ital Dermatol Venereol* 2014;149(5):607–625.
28. Lam J, Polifka JE, Dohil MA. Safety of dermatologic drugs used in pregnant patients with psoriasis and other inflammatory skin diseases. *J Am Acad Dermatol* 2008;59(2):295–315.
29. Larsen FG, Jakobsen P, Knudsen J, et al. Conversion of acitretin to etretinate in psoriatic patients is influenced by ethanol. *J Invest Dermatol* 1993;100(5):623–627.
30. Vena GA, Cassano N. The effects of alcohol on the metabolism and toxicology of anti-psoriasis drugs. *Expert Opin Drug Metab Toxicol* 2012;8(8):959–972.
31. Kane SV, Acquah LA. Placental transport of immunoglobulins: a clinical review for gastroenterologists who prescribe therapeutic monoclonal antibodies to women during conception and pregnancy. *Am J Gastroenterol* 2009;104(1):228–233.
32. Stensen M, Förger F. How safe are anti-rheumatic drugs during pregnancy? *Curr Opin Pharmacol* 2013;13(3):470–475.
33. Martin PL, Sachs C, Imai N, et al. Development in the cynomolgus macaque following administration of ustekinumab, a human anti-IL-12/23p40 monoclonal antibody, during pregnancy and lactation. *Birth Defects Res B Dev Reprod Toxicol* 2010;89(5):351–363.
34. Chambers CD, Johnson DL. Emerging data on the use of antitumor necrosis factor-alpha medications in pregnancy. *Birth Defects Res A Clin Mol Teratol* 2012;94(8):607–611.
35. Chuh AA, Lee A, Chan PK. Pityriasis rosea in pregnancy-specific diagnostic implications and management considerations. *Aust N Z J Obstet Gynaecol* 2005;45(3):252–253.
36. Chuh A. Narrow band UVB phototherapy and oral acyclovir for pityriasis rosea. *Photodermatol Photoimmunol Photomed* 2004;20(1):64–65.
37. Kroumpouzos G, Cohen LM. Specific dermatoses of pregnancy: an evidence-based systematic review. *Am J Obstet Gynecol* 2003;188(4):1083–1092.
38. Chuh AA, Au TS. Pityriasis rosea—a review of the specific treatments. *Proceed Royal Coll Phys Edinburgh* 2001;31(3):203–207.
39. Tay YK, Goh CL. One-year review of pityriasis rosea at the National Skin Centre, Singapore. *Ann Acad Med Singapore* 1999;28(6):829–831.
40. Parsons JM. Pityriasis rosea update: 1986. *J Am Acad Dermatol* 1986;15(2):159–167.
41. Chuh AA, Chan HH, Zawar V. Is human herpesvirus 7 the causative agent of pityriasis rosea? A critical review. *Int J Dermatol* 2004;43(12):870–875.
42. Sharma PK, Yadav TP, Gautam RK, et al. Erythromycin in pityriasis rosea: a double-blind, placebo-controlled clinical trial. *J Am Acad Dermatol* 2000;42(2):241–244.
43. Fukada Y, Okuda Y, Yasumizu T, Hoshi K. Pityriasis lichenoides et varioliformis acuta in pregnancy: a case report. *J Obstet Gynaecol Res* 1998;24(5):363–366.
44. Khachemoune A, Blyumin ML. Pityriasis lichenoides: pathophysiology, classification, and treatment. *Am J Clin Dermatol* 2007;8:29–36.
45. Kirtschig G. Lichen sclerosus-presentation, diagnosis and management. *Dtsch Arztebl Int* 2016;113:337–343.
46. Ambrose-Rudolph CM. The specific dermatoses of pregnancy revisited and reclassified: results of a retrospective two-center study on 505 pregnant patients. *J Am Acad Dermatol* 2006;54:395–404.
47. Charman C. Atopic eczema. *Br Med J* 1999;318:1600–1604.
48. Williams HC. Is the prevalence of atopic dermatitis increasing? *Clin Exp Dermatol* 1992;17:385–391.
49. Kemmett D, Tidman MJ. The influence of the menstrual cycle and pregnancy on atopic dermatitis. *Br J Dermatol* 1991;125(1):59–61.
50. Elenkov IJ, Chrousos GP. Stress hormones, proinflammatory and antiinflammatory cytokines, and autoimmunity. *Ann New York Acad Sci* 2002;966(1):290–303.
51. Cicek D, Kandi B, Berilgen MS, et al. Does autonomic dysfunction play a role in atopic dermatitis? *Br J Dermatol* 2008;159(4):834–838.
52. Akdis M, Trautmann A, Klunker S, et al. T cells and effector functions in atopic dermatitis. *Allergy Clin Imunol Int* 2002;14(4):161–164.
53. Hanifin JM, Rajka G. Diagnostic features of atopic eczema. *Acta Dermatol Venereol (Stockh.)* 1980; 92:44–47.

54. Yates LM, Thomas SH. Prescribing medicines in pregnancy. *Medicine* 2012;40(7):386–390.
55. Weatherhead S, Robson SC, Reynolds NJ. Eczema in pregnancy. *Br Med J* 2007;335(7611):152–154.
56. Weisshaar E, Diepgen TL, Luger TA, et al. Pruritus in pregnancy and childhood—do we really consider all relevant differential diagnoses? *Eur J Dermatol* 2005;15(5):320–331.
57. Skinner RB, Jr, Noah PW, Zanolli MD, et al. The pathogenic role of microbes in seborrheic dermatitis. *Arch Dermatol* 1986;122:16–17.
58. Heng MC, Henderson CL, Barker DC, et al. Correlation of Pityosporum ovale density with clinical severity of seborrheic dermatitis as assessed by a simplified technique. *J Am Acad Dermatol* 1990;23:82–86.

3 Specific Dermatoses of Pregnancy

Vinitha Varghese Panicker and Radhika Krishna

3.1 INTRODUCTION

Pregnancy is frequently accompanied by disturbances of the skin; these include physiological changes of skin, pre-existing dermatological diseases modified by pregnancy, and specific dermatoses of pregnancy. The specific dermatoses of pregnancy are a diverse set of intensely pruritic inflammatory dermatoses which are associated exclusively with pregnancy and/or the immediate postpartum period. With the exception of immunofluorescence in pemphigoid gestationis (PG), these diseases are uncommon and have several confusing terminologies, variable clinical morphologies, and fewer treatment options, all of which have led to diagnostic dilemmas and challenged their management over the years.[1] Though most of them are benign and resolve post-delivery, a few can endanger fetal life and hence necessitate antenatal surveillance.[2]

3.2 CLASSIFICATION

In 1982, Holmes and Black put forward the first simplified classification of dermatoses of pregnancy, which included Pemphigoid Gestationis (PG), olymorphic eruption of pregnancy (PEP), and prurigo of pregnancy.[1] A further dermatosis, pruritic folliculitis of pregnancy, was later added.[3,4] This classification of Holmes and Black was in use for almost two decades until 1998, when Shornick[5] proposed an advanced adaptation. He suggested that folliculitis of pregnancy belonged to the category of prurigo of pregnancy rather than being an independent entity. Shornick further include Intrahepatic Cholestasis of Pregnancy (ICP) in the specific dermatoses of pregnancy classification. This disease had previously not been added, as there were no primary skin lesions, and it presented with only secondary skin changes. However, it is essential to include it in the classification, as a delay or error in diagnosis is associated with potential fetal risk. Though PG, PEP, and ICP are widely accepted as independent diagnoses, prurigo of pregnancy is considered a questionable independent entity according to both Holmes and Black as well as Shornick.[1]

The most recent classification in use was introduced by Ambros-Rudolph et al.[6] in 2006, based on their retrospective study, which included 505 pregnant patients with dermatologic disorders. This classification had four main categories: PG, PEP, atopic eruption of pregnancy (AEP), and ICP. AEP denoted a new umbrella term to include three distinct entities—eczema in pregnancy, pruritic folliculitis of pregnancy, and prurigo of pregnancy.

3.3 PEMPHIGOID GESTATIONIS (SYN: GESTATIONAL PEMPHIGOID, HERPES GESTATIONIS)

PG is a rare, autoimmune bullous disorder that usually presents toward the last trimester or the immediate postpartum period; however, it can present in any of the three trimesters. Rarely, it may also be seen in association with certain trophoblastic tumours (choriocarcinoma, hydatidiform

DOI: 10.1201/9781003449690-3

TABLE 3.1

Classification of the Specific Dermatoses of Pregnancy

Classification	Synonyms
Pemphigoid gestationis	• Herpes gestationis
Polymorphic eruption of pregnancy	• Pruritic urticarial papules and plaques of pregnancy (PUPPP) • Toxaemic rash of pregnancy • Late onset prurigo of pregnancy • Toxic erythema of pregnancy
Atopic eruption of pregnancy	• Prurigo of pregnancy • Prurigo gestationis • Early onset prurigo of pregnancy • Papular dermatitis of pregnancy • Pruritic folliculitis of pregnancy • Eczema of pregnancy
Intrahepatic cholestasis of pregnancy	• Cholestasis of pregnancy • Prurigo gravidarum • Obstetric cholestasis • Jaundice of pregnancy • Icterus gravidarum

Source: From Ref. 6, with permission.

mole).[1] PG may be associated with higher fetal risks. In a study of 61 cases of gestational pemphigoid, 20 (34%) were complicated by preterm births.[7]

3.3.1 PATHOGENESIS

PG is attributed to circulating complement fixing IgG antibodies belonging to the subclass IgG1 (previously called "herpes gestationis factor") directed against the 180-kDa hemidesmosomal antigen (BP180) or bullous pemphigoid antigen 2 (BPAg2), causing tissue damage and subsequent blister formation.[8] As in bullous pemphigoid, the immune response is even more highly restricted to the NC16A domain. The epidermis and dermis separate as a result of an inflammatory cascade that is triggered by the binding of these autoantibodies to antigens in the basement membrane zone.[9] An observation of association between PG and class II HLA-DR3/HLA-DR4 phenotype supports the hypothesis that there is a genetic predisposition.[10]

3.3.2 CLINICAL FEATURES

PG classically presents in the second or third trimester of pregnancy. Intense pruritus occasionally may precede the onset of skin lesions. The skin lesions, which are erythematous urticarial papules and plaques, initially appear on the abdomen and usually involve the umbilical area but can later become generalised. It can be challenging to distinguish between PG and PEP at this prebullous stage, both clinically and histopathologically. Once there is blister formation, the diagnosis becomes relatively simple. The face and mucus membranes are commonly spared. PG may remit a few weeks after delivery; however, a protracted course, progression to bullous pemphigoid, and recurrence with use of oral contraceptives or menstrual cycles have been described.[11]

3.3.3   DIAGNOSIS

A diagnosis of PG requires the combination of clinical findings, routine histopathological examination of a lesional skin biopsy and a perilesional skin biopsy for direct immunofluorescence (DIF), and measurement of serum anti-BP180 antibody level.[12]

- **Pathology**—The stage and severity of the disease determine the histopathological findings.
  - In the pre-bullous stage, oedema of the upper and middle dermis along with a predominant perivascular inflammatory infiltrate of lymphocytes, histiocytes, and eosinophils are seen.
  - In the bullous stage, there is characteristic subepidermal blistering which is present at the lamina lucida of the dermoepidermal junction.
- **DIF**—DIF of snap-frozen perilesional skin is the gold standard method of diagnosis. On DIF, there is a linear deposition of C3 along the DEJ in 100% of cases and in 30% of cases an additional IgG deposition. The antibasement membrane zone (BMZ) antibodies bind to the roof on the salt split technique.[13]
- **Indirect immunofluorescence (IIF)**—Circulating IgG antibodies can be detected by IIF in 30–100% of cases. On salt-split skin, these antibodies bind to the roof of the artificial cleft.
- **ELISA**—A commercially available ELISA technique (BP180 NC16A ELISA) detects antibodies against the non-collagenous extracellular domain of BP180 (NC16A) in the serum.[12] In a patient with typical clinical symptoms, this test is both sensitive and specific for the diagnosis of PG.[14,15]

3.3.4   TREATMENT

Treatment varies according to the stage and severity of the disease. The aim of treatment is to control pruritus and prevent blister formation. Topical corticosteroids along with oral antihistamines may suffice for mild cases in the pre-bullous stage. Bullous lesions require systemic steroids like prednisolone (usually initiated at a dose of 0.5 mg/kg/day), which are considered safe during pregnancy.[12] The dose of steroids can usually be tapered once the lesions improve but should be increased near the time of delivery to prevent a common flare that occurs at delivery. After delivery, if lesions persist, other immunosuppressive agents may be administered. Azathioprine, high-dose intravenous immunoglobulins (2 g/kg per cycle),[16,17] cyclosporine,[18,19] cyclophosphamide,[20] doxycycline and nicotinamide,[21] rituximab,[22,23] immunoapheresis,[24] and omalizumab[25] are some of the alternative therapies that have been reportedly used successfully in patients with severe, persistent postpartum PG.

3.3.5   PROGNOSIS

- **Fetal prognosis**—The general fetal prognosis is good; however, PG may be associated with fetal risks such as premature birth and small-for-gestational-age babies.[26] About 10% of newborns may develop mild urticaria-like or vesicular skin lesions due to passive transfer of antibodies from the mother to the fetus (neonatal pemphigoid).[27]
- **Maternal prognosis**—Recurrence in subsequent pregnancies is likely; the symptoms may usually be more severe, with earlier onset.[28]

3.4   POLYMORPHIC ERUPTION OF PREGNANCY (SYN: PRURITIC URTICARIAL PAPULES AND PLAQUES OF PREGNANCY, TOXIC ERYTHEMA OF PREGNANCY, TOXAEMIC RASH OF PREGNANCY, LATE-ONSET PRURIGO OF PREGNANCY)

In 1962, Bourne described a pregnancy-related dermatoses named toxaemic rash of pregnancy that often affected small women with excessive weight gain and marked striae and appeared over the abdomen.[29] Pruritic urticarial papules and plaques of pregnancy (PUPPP) were described by Lawley in 1979.[30] The term PEP was later proposed by Holmes and Black[31,3] to incorporate all clinical manifestations, including urticarial papules, plaques, polycyclic erythematous wheals, vesicles, targetoid lesions, and occasionally bullae. The prevalence is about 1 in 160 births, and it is hence the most common specific pregnancy dermatosis.[32] (See Figures 3.1 and 3.2.)

3.4.1 PATHOGENESIS

The pathogenesis of PEP is unclear. Proposed theories include abdominal distension and immunological and hormonal factors.[1] It is believed that damage to connective tissue due to overstretching plays a major factor, as PEP starts within striae distensae at the time of greatest abdominal distension.

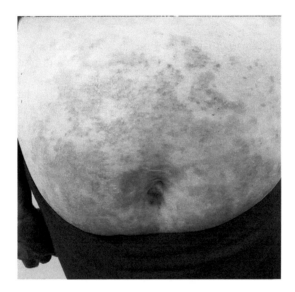

FIGURE 3.1   Polymorphic eruption of pregnancy.

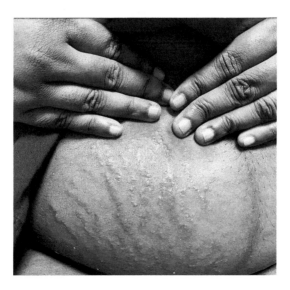

FIGURE 3.2   Polymorphic eruption of pregnancy.

Immunohistochemical (IHC) studies showed an infiltrate composed of predominantly helper T-cells. Activated T-cells (e.g. HLA DR+, CD25+, LFA-1+) are found in the dermis, associated with increased number of CD1a epidermal Langerhans cells and CD1a+, CD54+ dendritic cells. The concept that previously inactive structures acquire antigenic character and hence start the inflammatory process may be confirmed by the rise in CD1a cells in the inflammatory infiltrate. Another factor that may contribute to PUPPP is fetal DNA deposition in skin which contains damaged collagen.[33] The involvement of hormonal and immunological changes, as well as an association with higher birth weight or male sex in the newborn, have not been conclusively demonstrated.[34,35] A study[36] suggests that human keratinocytes serve as progesterone targets, as they express the progesterone receptor (PR). Suprabasal keratinocytes from samples of lesional epidermis of PEP displayed strong PR immunoreactivity, whereas nonlesional epidermis did not.

3.4.2   CLINICAL FEATURES

PEP typically develops in nulliparous women towards the end of the third trimester (average onset 35 weeks) but can occur post-delivery. There are also rare case reports of disease onset in the first and second trimesters.[37,38] The disease onset is typically over the abdomen, within the striae distensae, with urticarial papules and plaques that are severely pruritic, which may later spread to the buttocks and thighs. The lesions can generalise in severe cases. The sparing of the umbilical area is a characteristic feature which helps in differentiation from PG. The morphology of lesions may become more polymorphic as time progresses, and tiny vesicles (1–2 mm in size, never bullae), widespread non-urticarial erythema, and eczematous and targetoid lesions appear in almost 50% of patients. Regardless of delivery, the rash normally subsides in 4–6 weeks.[35] PEP can be classified into three categories:[37]

- *Type 1*: Urticarial papules and plaques
- *Type 2*: Nonurticarial erythema, papules, or vesicles
- *Type 3*: A combination of type I and II

3.4.3   HISTOPATHOLOGY

Histopathology is nonspecific and depends upon the stage of the disease. Early biopsies show a perivascular lymphohistiocytic infiltrate intermingled with eosinophils in the superficial to mid-dermis and prominent dermal oedema, whereas later biopsies frequently show epidermal changes like hyperkeratosis, parakeratosis, and spongiosis.

IHC reveals a predominantly T helper lymphocytic infiltrate with an increase of CD1a+, CD54+ (ICAM-1+) dendritic cells and CD1a+ epidermal Langerhans cells in lesional skin.[12]

Direct and indirect immunofluorescence investigations are negative in PEP, which aid in differentiation from PG.

3.4.4   TREATMENT

The mainstay of treatment is symptomatic, which includes topical corticosteroids along with antihistamines such as loratadine and cetirizine. This is usually sufficient for symptomatic relief. A short course of systemic corticosteroids (prednisolone 40–60 mg/day, in tapering doses, for a few days) may be required in severe generalised cases.[39] Rarely, if ever, is an early delivery necessary for symptomatic relief.[40]

3.4.5   PROGNOSIS

There is no cutaneous involvement in the newborn, and the prognosis for both the mother and fetus is favourable.[37] Lesions are self-resolving and the recurrence is rare, the exception being in multiple pregnancies.[41]

3.5 ATOPIC ERUPTION OF PREGNANCY

AEP, a benign pruritic condition of pregnancy, manifests in individuals with an atopic history as an eczematous or papular eruption (see Figure 3.3).

The term AEP is an umbrella term that includes eczema in pregnancy, prurigo of pregnancy, and pruritic folliculitis of pregnancy, which were all considered separate entities earlier.[6] This classification system was put together based on the existence of common clinical characteristics, along with a possible history suggestive of atopy. However, there is a debate amongst experts as to whether prurigo of pregnancy and pruritic folliculitis of pregnancy are to be classified under the entity of AEP.[42]

AEP is characterised by onset prior to the third trimester (75% of cases), a history of atopy in the patient or family, and recurrence in further pregnancies.[6]

3.5.1 EPIDEMIOLOGY

AEP accounts for about 50% of the pregnancy dermatoses.[6] Its exact incidence is unclear.

3.5.2 PATHOGENESIS

Pregnancy-related immunologic changes are hypothesised to be the cause of AEP. There is significant downregulation of maternal Th1 cytokine production and cell-mediated functions during pregnancy; however, Th2 cytokine production and humoral functions are elevated. An underlying atopic diathesis may unmasked in this context, as it is a Th2-dominant illness, leading to AEP.[6,42] AEP may also be the initial manifestation of atopic skin changes and is often associated with a personal/family history of atopy (atopic dermatitis, seasonal rhinitis, and/or asthma).[6,34]

3.5.3 CLINICAL FEATURES

The classical presentation is during the first or second trimester in most cases. It could either be the first manifestation of atopic skin change or indicate the recurrence of atopic dermatitis after a period

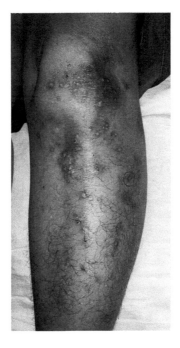

FIGURE 3.3 Atopic eruption of pregnancy.

of remission (20% cases).[5,34] The eruption is commonly seen in primigravids with single gestation and can affect any part of the body, including the face, palms, or soles.

3.5.4 ECZEMA (E-TYPE AEP)

E-type AEP presents in a similar pattern to classic atopic dermatitis, with a widespread eczematous eruption involving the face, neck, and flexural areas; however, it can involve any area of the body.[6] Clinical manifestations include eczematous patches or papules and excoriations, which may be discrete, grouped, or follicular. Skin dryness is almost always associated and may be severe.

3.5.5 PRURIGO OF PREGNANCY (P-TYPE AEP)

Synonyms include prurigo gestationis of Besnier, Spangler's papular dermatitis of pregnancy, linear immunoglobulin M (IgM) disease of pregnancy, and nurse's early-onset prurigo of pregnancy. It presents with erythematous, excoriated papules or nodules over the extensor aspect of the upper and lower limbs as well as trunk.[5,34] Lesions are grouped and may appear eczematous or crusted. Although the eruption usually resolves post-delivery,[34] it may persist for up to 3 months.

3.5.6 PRURITIC FOLLICULITIS OF PREGNANCY

It is a rare presentation of AEP (see Figure 3.4). Multiple follicular papules and pustules present initially on the abdomen and may later spread to the trunk and extremities and subsequently become generalised.[34,43] It resembles steroid-induced acne in appearance and, contrary to its name, is only mildly pruritic.[43] It commonly manifests in the second trimester and affects approximately 1 in 3,000 pregnancies.[44]

The lesions usually clear within 2 weeks postpartum.[4,34] However, one report noted a case with persistent symptoms for 6 weeks after delivery,[45] and another study observed resolution of symptoms in all 14 cases before delivery.[34]

3.5.7 DIAGNOSIS

AEP is a clinical diagnosis, based upon the personal or family history of atopy and characteristic clinical features. Though histopathological features are nonspecific, a biopsy is advisable in case of diagnostic uncertainty or a suspicion of PG. Serum IgE level may be raised in AEP in up to 70% cases.[6]

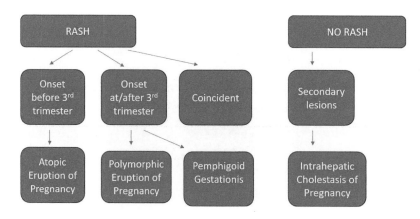

FIGURE 3.4   Approach to pruritus in pregnancy. (See further Ref. 1.)

A pus culture is necessary to rule out bacterial/candidal infection in cases presenting with folliculitis.

Histopathology of AEP:

- In eczematous eruptions, spongiosis and a perivascular mononuclear infiltrate are the common features.[34] Epidermal hyperkeratosis, parakeratosis and acanthosis may be present. Perivascular lymphocytic infiltrate in the dermis without eosinophils may also be seen.
- In prurigo of pregnancy, nonspecific findings may be seen with parakeratosis, acanthosis, and a perivascular lymphohistiocytic infiltrate with or without lymphocytic vasculitis.[46]
- In pruritic folliculitis of pregnancy, a follicle-centred lymphohistiocytic infiltrate containing neutrophils, eosinophils, and plasma cells along with neutrophilic pustules with histopathologic findings of sterile folliculitis may be noted.[4,34,45]
- Both direct as well as indirect immunofluorescence are negative in AEP.

3.5.8 Differential Diagnosis

The differential diagnosis of AEP include early stage of PG and PEP also other conditions with spongiotic dermatitis on histopathology like allergic contact dermatitis, maculopapular drug eruption, and pityriasis rosea. One can differentiate eczema-type AEP from PEP and early PG by its early onset, involvement of skin flexures, and absence of urticarial plaques in abdominal striae. Prurigo-type AEP may be difficult to differentiate clinically from PEP or early PG. Such cases warrant a skin biopsy for the correct diagnosis. Although P-type AEP and PEP share several biopsy features, the findings of lymphocytic vasculitis, oedema, eosinophils in the interstitial dermis, and deposition of mucin in the dermis suggest PEP rather than AEP.[46] Secondary lesions of ICP and conditions not related to pregnancy (e.g., scabies, drug reactions) should be excluded by adequate history and investigations (e.g., bile acids) as necessary.[5]

3.5.9 Treatment

Symptomatic relief is the goal of treatment. Just as in patients with eczema, frequent use of moisturisers should be advised in order to maintain adequate hydration of skin. AEP responds well to low to moderately potent steroids along with first-generation oral antihistamines (e.g. chlorpheniramine) or second-generation antihistamines (e.g. loratadine, cetirizine). Calamine lotion and menthol are considered to be safe in pregnancy and give a soothing effect. Pramoxine and other topical anaesthetics are better avoided in pregnancy, as they may cause topical sensitisation.

Narrow-band UVB is a safe modality for treating AEP and control of pruritus. Though Naltrexone is FDA Category C, there are only limited data on the use in pregnancy-related pruritus.

3.5.10 Prognosis

AEP has not been associated with maternal or fetal morbidity.[34] Recurrence may occur in subsequent pregnancies.[5]

3.6 INTRAHEPATIC CHOLESTASIS OF PREGNANCY (SYN: OBSTETRIC CHOLESTASIS, JAUNDICE OF PREGNANCY, CHOLESTASIS OF PREGNANCY PRURITUS/PRURIGO GRAVIDARUM, ICTERUS GRAVIDARUM)

Svanborg and Thorling first described cholestasis of pregnancy in 1954.[47,48]

It is defined as "generalized pruritus, with or without jaundice and without active hepatitis or hepatotoxic medicines; the presence of biochemical abnormalities; the absence of primary lesions; the spontaneous resolution of symptoms following delivery; and recurrence in subsequent pregnancies."[5]

The onset of intrahepatic cholestasis of pregnancy (ICP) is usually in the second or third trimester of pregnancy, and there is spontaneous remission within 2–3 weeks post-delivery.[49] ICP is the only pregnancy dermatosis that has no primary skin changes.[50] (See Figure 3.5.)

3.6.1 Pathogenesis

The mother experiences acute pruritus due to defective bile salt excretion and increased bile acids in serum. These toxic bile acids reach the fetal circulation and can cause acute placental anoxia as well as cardiac depression, which may prove detrimental to the fetus. It is believed that a number of variables, including genetic, hormonal, and exogenous factors, are responsible for this metabolic abnormality.[51]

Genetic—Familial clustering, higher risk in first-degree relatives and in certain ethnic groups, and a high recurrence rate (60–70%) all point to a genetic predisposition.[52] Mutations of certain genes, such as the ABCB4 (MDR3) gene, encoding for transport proteins necessary for bile excretion have been recognised in some ICP patients.[1,53] If hormone levels are normal, this defect has no clinical significance; it manifests only with high concentrations, for example, with hormonal contraception and/or in late pregnancy.

Hormonal—Oestrogen and progesterone metabolites contribute to cholestasis.[54] ICP typically manifests in the second half of pregnancy when there is a peak in serum concentrations of oestrogen, in twin pregnancies, and in individuals taking oestrogen-progestin contraceptives.

Environmental factors—ICP is more commonly noted during the winter months in countries like Sweden, Chile, and Finland.[55]

Underlying liver disease—Underlying liver disease may contribute to development of ICP.[56] Several liver and biliary diseases such as hepatitis C, non-alcoholic liver cirrhosis gallstones, and cholecystitis have been found to have a significantly higher incidence in patients with ICP.[53]

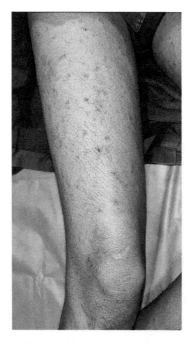

FIGURE 3.5   Intrahepatic cholestasis of pregnancy.

3.6.2 Clinical Manifestations

The classical presentation of ICP is severe, generalised pruritus of abrupt onset, predominantly on the palms and soles, but it quickly progresses to become generalised and may present with excoriations as a result of scratching. There are usually no primary skin lesions associated. Skin lesions secondary to scratching may range from subtle excoriations to severe prurigo nodules due to persistent pruritus. The common sites involved are the extensor surfaces of the extremities; however, other sites such as the buttocks and abdomen may also be involved. Nausea, pain in the right upper quadrant, poor appetite, sleep deprivation, or steatorrhea may be associated.

The most severe and prolonged episodes may be complicated by jaundice, usually after 2–4 weeks, due to concomitant extrahepatic cholestasis, intrahepatic jaundice of pregnancy, or obstetric cholestasis, which occurs in about 10% of patients.[57] There is an increased risk of steatorrhea, cholelithiasis, malabsorption of fat-soluble vitamins (e.g., vitamin K), and potential haemorrhagic complications.[1]

3.6.3 Diagnosis

An increase in serum bile acid levels is the most sensitive indicator for the diagnosis of ICP, while in up to 30%, liver function test including transaminases may be within normal limits.[1] Total serum bile acid levels in healthy pregnancies are slightly higher than in nonpregnant women. Therefore, an upper cutoff of 11.0 μmol/L (normal range: 0–6 μmol/L) is accepted as normal in late gestation.[58,59] The primary bile acids like cholic acid and chenodeoxycholic acid are elevated. The cholic/chenodeoxycholic acid ratio is markedly elevated due to an increase in the serum cholic acid, more than chenodeoxycholic acid.[60]

In case hyperbilirubinemia is noted, which occurs in only 10–20%, it should always lead to close monitoring of prothrombin, along with an ultrasound examination of the liver to exclude cholelithiasis. Serum aminotransferases are increased in 60% of cases,[61] and alkaline phosphatase may also be increased; however, it is not specific for ICP due to expression of the placental isoenzyme. Histopathology is nonspecific and direct and indirect immunofluorescence is negative.

3.6.4 Treatment

Treatment is targeted at symptomatic relief as well as reduction of perinatal morbidity and mortality.

Most obstetricians advise labour induction at 36 weeks of pregnancy (severe cases) and at 38 weeks (mild cases) in order to minimise fetal risk.

Currently, ursodeoxycholic acid (UDCA) is the most effective pharmacologic treatment for ICP for both the mother and fetus. UDCA (450–1200 mg/day or 10–15 mg/kg/day) reduces total bile acids in cord blood, colostrum, and amniotic fluid. It has a multifactorial mechanism of action; it reduces the biliary secretion of endogenous and toxic bile acids and also protects cholangiocytes from cytotoxic bile acids and hepatocytes from apoptosis due to bile acids.[62] On comparison to cholestyramine, UDCA is seen to be safer, has faster onset of action, has a more sustained anti-pruritic effect, and shows better efficacy in improving the liver function abnormalities of ICP.[63] Apart from these, emollients, topical antipruritic agents, rest, and a low-fat diet may also help alleviate the symptoms of ICP.

Other treatment options, such as cholestyramine, S-adenosyl-methionine, rifampicin, phenobarbital, and ultraviolet B light, can be added if the pruritus remains intolerable despite the administration of maximum dose of UDCA.[64]

Repeat measurements of maternal TBA concentrations can be considered as frequently as once per week, which would favour an earlier delivery, considering the greatly increased risk of stillbirth in individuals with TBA ≥ 100 mol/L.[65]

3.6.5 PROGNOSIS

The main fetal complications include increased risk of prematurity (19–60%), intrapartum fetal distress (22–33%), and stillbirths (1–2%), which correlates with increased bile acid levels, particularly if >40 μmol/L. Toxic bile acids may affect fetal cardiomyocytes, causing sudden fetal death, or may enter lungs, causing neonatal respiratory distress syndrome.[65,66]

The maternal prognosis is usually favourable. With the exception of jaundice, which usually subsides within 2 weeks post-delivery, ICP symptoms often resolve within 48 hours postpartum.[51,67] Glantz et al. classified ICP into two types in 2004:

1. *Mild ICP*—total bile acid value up to 40 μmol/mL.
2. *Severe ICP*—total bile acid value > 40 μmol/mL. This reference value lowered the risk of adverse fetal outcomes.[67]

There is spontaneous remission of pruritus within days to weeks post-delivery, along with normalisation of TBA levels and other liver function tests. However, recurrence may occur with subsequent pregnancies in 60–70% of cases and with oral contraception. Therefore, prompt early diagnosis, adequate treatment, obstetric monitoring, and maternal counselling are essential.

3.7 CONCLUSION

Though pruritus and skin changes are often benign and self-limiting in pregnancy, a detailed history, thorough clinical examination, and necessary investigations are of vital importance both in the diagnosis and management of specific dermatoses of pregnancy (see further Figure 3.5). An interdisciplinary approach involving dermatologists, paediatricians, obstetricians, and gastroenterologists is imperative for management and prevention of both maternal as well as fetal complications.

REFERENCES

1. Ambros-Rudolph CM. Dermatoses of pregnancy—clues to diagnosis, fetal risk and therapy. *Ann Dermatol* 2011;23(3):265–275.
2. Sachdeva S. The dermatoses of pregnancy. *Indian J Dermatol* 2008;53(3):103.
3. Holmes RC, Black MM. The specific dermatoses of pregnancy. *J Am Acad Dermatol* 1983;8(3):405–412.
4. Zoberman E, Farmer ER. Pruritic folliculitis of pregnancy. *Arch Dermatol* 1981;117(1):20–22.
5. Shornick JK. Dermatoses of pregnancy. *Semin Cutan Med Surg* 1998;17(3):172–181.
6. Ambros-Rudolph CM, Müllegger RR, Vaughan-Jones SA, et al. The specific dermatoses of pregnancy revisited and reclassified: results of a retrospective two-center study on 505 pregnant patients. *J Am Acad Dermatol* 2006;54(3):395–404.
7. Chi CC, Wang SH, Charles-Holmes R, et al. Pemphigoid gestationis: early onset and blister formation are associated with adverse pregnancy outcomes. *Br J Dermatol* 2009;160(6):1222–1228.
8. Tunzi M, Gray GR. Common skin conditions during pregnancy. *Am Fam Physician* 2007;75(2):211–218.
9. Kasperkiewicz M, Zillikens D, Schmidt E. Pemphigoid diseases: pathogenesis, diagnosis, and treatment. *Autoimmunity* 2012;45(1):55–70.
10. Shornick JK, Jenkins RE, Artlett CM, et al. Class II MHC typing in pemphigoid gestationis. *Clin Exp Dermatol* 1995;20(2):123–126.
11. Kroumpouzos G, Cohen LM. Specific dermatoses of pregnancy: an evidence-based systematic review. *Am J Obstet Gynecol* 2003;188(4):1083–1092.
12. Pomeranz M. Dermatoses of pregnancy. In: *UpToDate*, Post TW (Ed.). Waltham, MA: UpToDate; 2023.
13. Vaughan Jones SA, Bhogal BS, Black MM, et al. A typical case of pemphigoid gestationis with a unique pattern of intercellular immunofluorescence. *Br J Dermatol* 1997;136(2):245–248.
14. Powell AM, Sakuma-Oyama Y, Oyama N, et al. Usefulness of BP180 NC16a enzyme-linked immunosorbent assay in the serodiagnosis of pemphigoid gestationis and in differentiating between pemphigoid gestationis and pruritic urticarial papules and plaques of pregnancy. *Arch Dermatol* 2005;141(6):705–710.

15. Al Saif F, Jouen F, Hebert V, et al. Sensitivity and specificity of BP180 NC16A enzyme-linked immuno-sorbent assay for the diagnosis of pemphigoid gestationis. *J Am Acad Dermatol* 2017;76(3):560–562.
16. Gan DCC, Welsh B, Webster M. Successful treatment of a severe persistent case of pemphigoid gestationis with antepartum and postpartum intravenous immunoglobulin followed by azathioprine. *Australas J Dermatol* 2012;53(1):66–69.
17. Rodrigues CDS, Filipe P, Solana MDM, Soares de Almeida L, Cirne de Castro J, Gomes MM. Persistent herpes gestationis treated with high-dose intravenous immunoglobulin. *Acta Derm Venereol* 2007; 87(2):184–186.
18. Huilaja L, Mäkikallio K, Hannula-Jouppi K, et al. Cyclosporine treatment in severe gestational pemphigoid. *Acta Derm Venereol* 2015;95(5):593–595.
19. Özdemir Ö, Atalay CR, Asgarova V, et al. A resistant case of pemphigus gestationis successfully treated with cyclosporine. *Interv Med Appl Sci* 8(1):20–22.
20. Castle SP, Mather-Mondrey M, Bennion S, et al. Chronic herpes gestationis and antiphospholipid antibody syndrome successfully treated with cyclophosphamide. *J Am Acad Dermatol* 1996;34(2 Pt 2):333–336.
21. Amato L, Coronella G, Berti S, et al. Successful treatment with doxycycline and nicotinamide of two cases of persistent pemphigoid gestationis. *J Dermatolog Treat* 2002;13(3):143–146.
22. Narayanan A, Pangti R, Agarwal S, et al. Pemphigoid gestationis: a rare pregnancy dermatosis treated with a combination of IVIg and rituximab. *BMJ Case Rep* 2021;14(3):e241496.
23. Cianchini G, Masini C, Lupi F, et al. Severe persistent pemphigoid gestationis: long-term remission with rituximab. *Br J Dermatol* 2007;157(2):388–389.
24. Wohrl S, Geusau A, Karlhofer F, et al. Pemphigoid gestationis: treatment with immunoapheresis. [Pemphigoid gestationis: behandlung durch Immunapherese]. *J Deut Dermatol Gesell* 2003;1(2):126–130.
25. Konstantinou MP, Jendoubi F, Fortenfant F, et al. Successful treatment of recalcitrant pemphigoid gestationis with omalizumab: report of two cases. *J Eur Acad Dermatol Venereol* 2022;36(9):e720–e722.
26. Shornick JK, Black MM. Fetal risks in herpes gestationis. *J Am Acad Dermatol* 1992;26(1):63–68.
27. Sävervall C, Sand FL, Thomsen SF. Pemphigoid gestationis: current perspectives. *Clin Cosmet Investig Dermatol* 2017;10:441–449.
28. Huilaja L, Mäkikallio K, Tasanen K. Gestational pemphigoid. *Orphanet J Rare Dis* 2014;9:136.
29. Bourne G. Toxaemic rash of pregnancy. *Proc R Soc Med* 1962;55(6):462–464.
30. Lawley TJ, Hertz KC, Wade TR, et al. Pruritic urticarial papules and plaques of pregnancy. *JAMA* 1979;241(16):1696–1699.
31. Holmes RC, Black MM. The specific dermatoses of pregnancy: a reappraisal with special emphasis on a proposed simplified clinical classification. *Clin Exp Dermatol* 1982;7(1):65–73.
32. Charles-Holmes R. Polymorphic eruption of pregnancy. *Semin Dermatol* 1989;8(1):18–22.
33. Ahmadi S, Powell FC. Pruritic urticarial papules and plaques of pregnancy: current status. *Australas J Dermatol* 2005;46(2):53–58; quiz 59.
34. Vaughan Jones SA, Hern S, Nelson-Piercy C, et al. A prospective study of 200 women with dermatoses of pregnancy correlating clinical findings with hormonal and immunopathological profiles. *Br J Dermatol* 1999;141(1):71–81.
35. Rudolph CM, Al-Fares S, Vaughan-Jones SA, et al. Polymorphic eruption of pregnancy: clinicopathology and potential trigger factors in 181 patients. *Br J Dermatol* 2006;154(1):54–60.
36. Im S, Lee ES, Kim W, et al. Expression of progesterone receptor in human keratinocytes. *J Korean Med Sci* 2000;15(6):647–654.
37. Aronson IK, Bond S, Fiedler VC, et al. Pruritic urticarial papules and plaques of pregnancy: clinical and immunopathologic observations in 57 patients. *J Am Acad Dermatol* 1998;39(6):933–939.
38. Yancey KB, Hall RP, Lawley TJ. Pruritic urticarial papules and plaques of pregnancy. Clinical experience in twenty-five patients. *J Am Acad Dermatol* 1984;10(3):473–480.
39. Taylor D, Pappo E, Aronson IK. Polymorphic eruption of pregnancy. *Clin Dermatol* 2016;34(3):383–391.
40. Beltrani VP, Beltrani VS. Pruritic urticarial papules and plaques of pregnancy: a severe case requiring early delivery for relief of symptoms. *J Am Acad Dermatol* 1992;26(2 Pt 1):266–267.
41. Chouk C, Litaiem N. Pruritic urticarial papules and plaques of pregnancy [Internet]. In: *StatPearls*. Treasure Island (FL): StatPearls Publishing; 2023. Available from: www.ncbi.nlm.nih.gov/books/NBK539700/
42. Wilder RL. Hormones, pregnancy, and autoimmune diseases. *Ann N Y Acad Sci* 1998;840:45–50.
43. Roth MM, Cristodor P, Kroumpouzos G. Prurigo, pruritic folliculitis, and atopic eruption of pregnancy: facts and controversies. *Clin Dermatol* 2016;34(3):392–400.
44. Delorenze LM, Branco LG, Cerqueira LF, et al. Pruritic folliculitis of pregnancy. *An Bras Dermatol* 2016;91(5 Suppl 1):66–68.

45. Kroumpouzos G, Cohen LM. Pruritic folliculitis of pregnancy. *J Am Acad Dermatol* 2000;43(1 Pt 1):132–134.
46. Massone C, Cerroni L, Heidrun N, et al. Histopathological diagnosis of atopic eruption of pregnancy and polymorphic eruption of pregnancy: a study on 41 cases. *Am J Dermatopathol* 2014;36(10):812–821.
47. Svanborg A. A study of recurrent jaundice in pregnancy. *Acta Obstet Gynecol Scand* 1954;33(4):434–444.
48. Thorling L. Jaundice in pregnancy; a clinical study. *Acta Med Scand Suppl* 1955;302:1–123.
49. Pusl T, Beuers U. Intrahepatic cholestasis of pregnancy. *Orphanet J Rare Dis* 2007;2:26.
50. Hillman SC, Stokes-Lampard H, Kilby MD. Intrahepatic cholestasis of pregnancy. *BMJ* 2016;353:i1236.
51. Lammert F, Marschall HU, Matern S. Intrahepatic cholestasis of pregnancy. *Curr Treat Options Gastro* 2003;6(2):123–132.
52. Pataia V, Dixon PH, Williamson C. Pregnancy and bile acid disorders. *Am J Physiol Gastrointest Liver Physiol* 2017;313(1):G1–G6.
53. Ropponen A, Sund R, Riikonen S, et al. Intrahepatic cholestasis of pregnancy as an indicator of liver and biliary diseases: a population-based study. *Hepatology* 2006;43(4):723–728.
54. Reyes H, Sjövall J. Bile acids and progesterone metabolites in intrahepatic cholestasis of pregnancy. *Ann Med* 2000;32(2):94–106.
55. Geenes V, Williamson C. Intrahepatic cholestasis of pregnancy. *WJG* 2009;15(17):2049.
56. Marschall HU, Wikström Shemer E, Ludvigsson JF, et al. Intrahepatic cholestasis of pregnancy and associated hepatobiliary disease: a population-based cohort study. *Hepatology* 2013;58(4):1385–1391.
57. Rioseco AJ, Ivankovic MB, Manzur A, et al. Intrahepatic cholestasis of pregnancy: a retrospective case-control study of perinatal outcome. *Am J Obstet Gynecol* 1994;170(3):890–895.
58. Brites D, Rodrigues CM, Oliveira N, et al. Correction of maternal serum bile acid profile during ursodeoxycholic acid therapy in cholestasis of pregnancy. *J Hepatol* 1998;28(1):91–98.
59. Carter J. Serum bile acids in normal pregnancy. *Br J Obstet Gynaecol* 1991;98(6):540–543.
60. Kondrackiene J, Kupcinskas L. Intrahepatic cholestasis of pregnancy—current achievements and unsolved problems. *WJG* 2008;14(38):5781.
61. Bacq Y, Sapey T, Bréchot MC, et al. Intrahepatic cholestasis of pregnancy: a French prospective study. *Hepatology* 1997;26(2):358–364.
62. Joshi D, James A, Quaglia A, et al. Liver disease in pregnancy. *Lancet* 2010;375(9714):594–605.
63. Kroumpouzos G. Intrahepatic cholestasis of pregnancy: what's new. *J Eur Acad Dermatol Venereol* 2002;16(4):316–318.
64. Lindor K, Lee R. Intrahepatic cholestasis of pregnancy. In: *UpToDate*, Post TW (Ed.). Waltham, MA: UpToDate; 2023.
65. Ovadia C, Seed PT, Sklavounos A, et al. Association of adverse perinatal outcomes of intrahepatic cholestasis of pregnancy with biochemical markers: results of aggregate and individual patient data meta-analyses. *Lancet* 2019;393(10174):899–909.
66. Zecca E, De Luca D, Baroni S, et al. Bile acid-induced lung injury in newborn infants: a bronchoalveolar lavage fluid study. *Pediatrics* 2008;121(1):e146–e149.
67. Glantz A, Marschall HU, Mattsson LA. Intrahepatic cholestasis of pregnancy: relationships between bile acid levels and fetal complication rates. *Hepatology* 2004;40(2):467–474.

4 Vesiculobullous Diseases and Pregnancy

Renata Heck, Hossein Akbarialiabad and Dedee F Murrell

4.1 INTRODUCTION

In the study of autoimmune blistering diseases (AIBDs), certain conditions exhibit pronounced relevance during pregnancy, significantly impacting both maternal and fetal health. This chapter focuses on three pivotal AIBD conditions: pemphigoid gestationis, pemphigus vulgaris, and pemphigus foliaceus. These diseases were specifically chosen due to their prevalence and distinct clinical implications in pregnant patients, contrasting sharply with other types of AIBD that are rarely encountered during pregnancy. By examining these conditions, the chapter aims to illuminate the unique challenges and considerations necessary for managing AIBD in a pregnancy context, providing a comprehensive overview that supports clinical decision-making and enhances understanding of pregnancy-associated dermatological autoimmunity.

4.2 PEMPHIGOID GESTATIONIS

4.2.1 INTRODUCTION

Pemphigoid gestationis (PG), gestational pemphigoid, or herpes gestationis is a rare autoimmune skin disorder that exclusively affects pregnant women in the second or third trimester. As an illness influenced by hormonal and immunological changes during pregnancy, PG presents specific challenges in diagnosis and management. Understanding its aetiology, associated genetic markers, and the immune response that leads to skin lesions is crucial for timely and effective treatment.

4.2.2 EPIDEMIOLOGY

The annual incidence of the disease ranges between 0.5 and 2.0 cases per 1 million people, with no difference in racial distribution [1–4].

It is more commonly seen in multiparous females and usually recurs in subsequent pregnancies with early onset and increased severity. It presents most often in the second or third trimester of pregnancy and has also been reported in association with trophoblastic tumours [5].

4.2.3 ETIOPATHOLOGY

The pathogenesis of PG is not fully understood [6]. There is a genetic predisposition associated with MHC class II antigens DR3 and DR4 in the mothers, and HLA-DR2 was found in 50% of the husbands of patients with PG [7]. The HLA mismatch between the mother and fetus leads to the loss of fetal-placental immune privilege. This leads to the presentation of foreign paternally derived placental antigens from the fetus to the maternal immune system and the production IgG class antibodies (predominantly IgG1 and IgG3) directed to collagen XVII/BP180, a transmembrane hemidesmosomal glycoprotein expressed in the basement membrane zone of the placenta—the chorionic and amniotic epithelial BMZ. Paternal MHC class II on the chorionic villi are thought to induce maternal antibodies which cross-react with the skin in the mother and rarely the newborn [7].

DOI: 10.1201/9781003449690-4

Most commonly, the antibodies are directed against the epitopes found in NC16A, the largest domain of BP180, but antibodies against intracellular domains and other extracellular domains of BP180 have also been observed [8].

Th2 cells, found in the skin lesions of PG patients, may be implicated in the very early stages of the autoimmune response and influence blister formation [9,10].

4.2.4 CLINICAL FEATURES

Intense pruritus usually precedes the onset of skin lesions, which typically begin on the trunk around the umbilicus as papules, urticarial plaques, or annular target lesions (erythema multiforme-like), followed by vesicles or tense blisters after a few weeks (Figure 4.1) [1]. It can affect the entire skin surface, but the face and the mucous membranes are usually not affected [11].

PG may remit prior to delivery but typically resolves within weeks to months postpartum [5]. The remitting, relapsing course of the disease can be associated with progestin levels [12]. More than half of PG patients have a flare postpartum, and at least a quarter of them subsequently have a flare with the use of oral contraceptive pills or during menses [13].

PG is related to an increased risk of fetal growth restriction and preterm birth [14,15]. Adverse pregnancy outcomes are assumed to be due to mild placental dysfunction secondary to impaired BP180 as a result of an immune attack of the placental BMZ [14,16,17]. Premature delivery is more likely to occur with the early onset of PG in the first or second trimester or when the disease is blistering [18]. With the advent of egg donor pregnancies, in which all the fetal DNA is foreign to the pregnant mother, not surprisingly, there has been a rise in PG cases among patients receiving such fertility treatments [19].

A systematic review showed that more than 80% of newborns and mothers with PG do not have skin disease [20]. The minority who are born with skin lesions due to the transplacental passage of maternal IgG autoantibodies has a mild course and resolves within weeks without treatment [21]. The antibody titers, in patients with PG, do not correlate with the magnitude of adverse fetal outcomes [14].

4.2.5 DIAGNOSIS

The diagnosis of pemphigoid gestationis is based on clinical findings, lesional skin histopathology, perilesional skin direct immunofluorescence, and serology. The clinical picture of the disease may

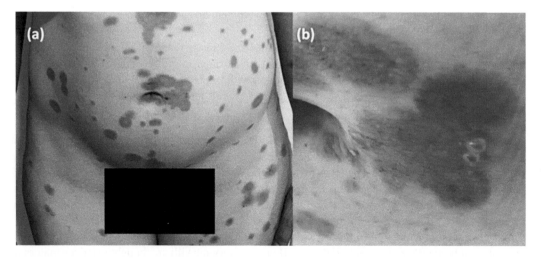

FIGURE 4.1 Annular urticarial plaques predominantly in the trunk (a). In detail, the presence of blisters (b).

not be conclusive, being particularly difficult to differentiate from the polymorphic eruption of pregnancy, often with similar clinical presentation.

Histopathological findings include subepidermal vesicles with lymphocytes and eosinophils in a perivascular distribution within the dermis. Eosinophils can be found at the dermo-epidermal junction and in the blister cavity (Figure 4.1a). Papillary dermal oedema with eosinophilic spongiosis can be found in urticarial lesions [1].

Direct immunofluorescence examination reveals linear deposition of complement C3 in the basement membrane zone at the interface of the epidermis and dermis in 100% of cases. Immunoglobulin G (IgG) deposits can also be present in a smaller number of patients (25–50% of the cases) [5,14] (Figure 4.1b). These linear deposits of C3 and IgG bind to the epidermal side of salt-split skin. Other deposits (IgM, IgA, C1, C4, C5) are very rare. If no sample has been obtained for DIF, C4 staining, immunohistochemistry (IHC) can be done on the paraffin-embedded tissue [12].

Serum-circulating antibodies against BP180 (particularly against the NC16A domain) can be found in ELISA and immunoblotting tests [12,22,23]. Where these tests are not available, another technique of indirect IF with complement fixation may be employed. After 24-hour incubation of normal human skin in NaCl 1M to split the lamina lucida, the cut slices are incubated with the patient serum, then with fresh complement (serum of a healthy person), and lastly with fluorescein-labelled human C3. This leads to the detection of auto-Ab ("HG factor") in 75–100% of patients.

4.2.6 TREATMENT

Pregnancy and breastfeeding impose limitations on the therapeutic management of PG. The treatment aims to suppress excessive itching, heal the blisters and erosions, and prevent the formation of new blisters. Early diagnosis and management of the disease are important for a favourable pregnancy outcome.

High-potency class A topical corticosteroids, such as betamethasone, are used as the first option for patients with localised disease and antihistamines can be used to control pruritus. The use of

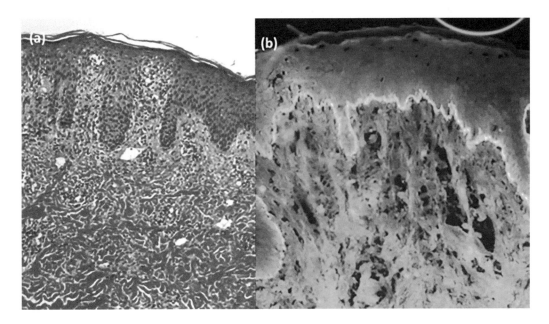

FIGURE 4.2 Histopathology of lesional skin showing spongiotic dermatitis with eosinophils; Hematoxylin and eosin, 20× (a). Linear deposition of C3 at the dermo-epidermal junction in direct immunofluorescence of perilesional skin, 20× (b).

topical corticosteroids appears to be safe concerning the risk of congenital abnormality, preterm delivery, or stillbirth. However, limited data suggest an association between potent topical corticosteroids and low birth weight [24–26].

More severe patients require the use of systemic corticosteroids, starting with prednisolone or prednisone at a dosage of 0.5–1 mg/kg per day [14,24]. Other safe treatment interventions during pregnancy include intravenous immunoglobulin, immunoadsorption, and plasmapheresis [27–30]. The corticotherapy is generally safe during pregnancy, but long-term use of corticosteroids may lead to severe long-term consequences. A study of 61 women with pemphigoid gestationis found an increased risk of low birth weight for women treated with ≥60 mg prednisone per day after adjusting for maternal age and comorbidities (odds ratio 16.65, 95% CI 1.15–241.46). However, because of the small sample size and wide confidence interval, the magnitude of the risk remains uncertain. Postpartum PG may need higher systemic CS up to 2 mg/kg/d until disease control is achieved, then a slow taper.

Intravenous immunoglobulin (IVIG) is another safe option during pregnancy and the postpartum period [24,31,32]. There are reports of safety with the use of azathioprine and dapsone during pregnancy for the treatment of other diseases, being drug options in refractory cases or in the unavailability of IVIG [20,31,33–36].

There are reports of the use of several drugs, such as rituximab, tetracyclines, cyclosporine, and omalizumab, in resistant cases in the postpartum period, but these drugs do not have a fetal safety profile during pregnancy [24,36–40].

There are reports of safety with the use of azathioprine and dapsone during pregnancy for the treatment of other diseases, being drug options in refractory cases or in the unavailability of IVIG [20,31,33,34].

FcRN inhibitors rapidly reduce IgG from recirculation. Nipocalimab has been successfully used in an open-label phase 2 trial to prevent haemolytic disease of the newborn by reducing IgG. In the proof-of-concept trial, 92% of pregnancies treated with nipocalimab resulted in a live birth, of which 54% achieved the primary endpoint of a live birth at or after 32 weeks of gestation without intrauterine transfusions (IUTs) [41].

As these drugs rapidly reduce IgG levels in the blood, and one of these (efgartigimod) has shown good activity in a phase 2 clinical trial in bullous pemphigoid, it is likely that these drugs may be used off-label in the future. A phase 3 trial of efgartigimod in BP is currently recruiting worldwide, and another phase 2/3 RCT of nipocalimab is registered with clinicaltrials.gov.

4.2.7 CONCLUSION

Timely and accurate diagnosis of pemphigoid gestationis is critical, as it allows for the initiation of treatments that can mitigate the disease's impact on both the mother and fetus. Effective management strategies, primarily involving corticosteroids and immunosuppressants, must be balanced against potential risks to the fetus, underscoring the need for multidisciplinary care involving dermatologists and obstetricians.

4.3 PEMPHIGUS VULGARIS

Pemphigus vulgaris is known for its potentially life-threatening mucocutaneous blistering, which may intensify during pregnancy due to hormonal influences on the immune system. The disease's propensity to worsen in this period necessitates a deep understanding of its pathophysiology and the careful selection of treatments that are safe for pregnant patients. Clinicians must be vigilant to differentiate PV from other pregnancy-associated dermatoses to ensure appropriate management. (Figures 4.3, 4.4 and 4.5).

Pemphigus can be exacerbated during pregnancy, but generally to a mild degree [42]. The disease tends to improve after the third trimester, probably due to the rising endogenous corticosteroid

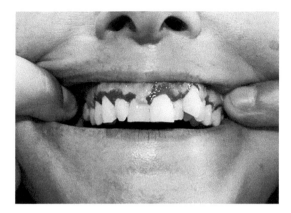

FIGURE 4.3 Mucosal involvement in pemphigus vulgaris appearing like desquamative gingivitis.

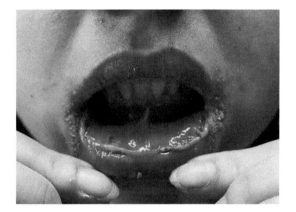

FIGURE 4.4 Mucosal involvement in pemphigus vulgaris.

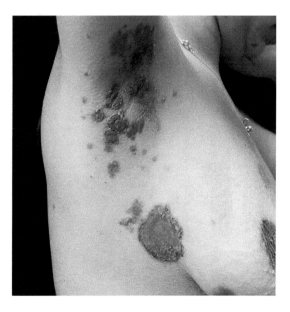

FIGURE 4.5 Cutaneous lesions in pemphigus vulgaris in a seborrheic distribution.

TABLE 4.1

Summary of Key Aspects of Pemphigoid Gestationis, Pemphigus Vulgaris, and Pemphigus Foliaceus

Disease	Epidemiology	Key Clinical Features	Diagnosis	Treatment
Pemphigoid Gestationis (PG)	Annual incidence of 0.5 to 2.0 cases per 1 million people. More commonly seen in multiparous females and can recur in subsequent pregnancies.	Intense itching, blisters begin around the umbilicus; affects skin but not mucous membranes. Recurs in subsequent pregnancies with possible early onset and severity.	Clinical findings, histopathology, direct immunofluorescence showing C3 and IgG deposits; ELISA for BP180 antibodies.	Primarily corticosteroids and immunosuppressants, balanced to mitigate fetal risks. Topical for localized cases, systemic for severe cases. Safe use of IVIG and plasmapheresis.
Pemphigus Vulgaris (PV)	Not specific to pregnancy; affects a broader population. May see changes in disease activity due to hormonal influences during pregnancy.	Painful blisters and erosions on skin and mucosa. May worsen or improve during pregnancy due to immune system changes.	Clinical assessment, histopathology, direct immunofluorescence showing intercellular IgG and C3 deposits.	Corticosteroids are first-line; azathioprine and mycophenolate mofetil are options, depending on trimester. Rituximab is not recommended during pregnancy.
Pemphigus Foliaceus (PF)	Similar to PV in terms of population but less aggressive and not typically affecting mucous membranes. Course can vary significantly during pregnancy.	Superficial skin lesions, less aggressive than PV, variable course during pregnancy.	Similar to PV with focus on antibodies against desmoglein 1.	Treatment mirrors PV; focuses on corticosteroids and immunosuppressive agents as needed.

production by the chorion and consequent immunosuppression, but also tends to reactivate in the postpartum period [42–45].

Neonatal pemphigus can occur caused by the passive transplacental transfer of IgG pemphigus autoantibodies, and no correlation was established between maternal antibody levels and severity of neonatal disease [46]. The absence or presence of clinical disease in the mother is not a predictor of whether the infant will have neonatal pemphigus [43]. It is a self-limiting condition that responds to topical therapy and usually resolves within 1 to 4 weeks [43,47]. The rate of stillbirth is estimated to be around 10% [43].

Corticosteroids are considered the treatment of choice. Azathioprine, IVIG, or plasmapheresis are therapeutic options in refractory disease [47,48].

Rituximab, the drug that is highly successful in achieving disease remission of PV, is not contra-indicated during pregnancy. It crosses the placenta, depleting fetal B cells and increasing the risk of newborn infections [48,49]. It is recommended to avoid pregnancy for 1 year after infusing the drug [50]. There is insufficient evidence to consider breastfeeding safe while using rituximab; however, the concentrations found in breast milk appear to be very low [51,52].

In conclusion, management of pemphigus vulgaris, as a life-threatening blistering disease, during pregnancy requires careful consideration of the therapeutic options that can control disease activity without posing undue risk to the fetus. Corticosteroids remain the mainstay of treatment, but newer biologics and other immunosuppressive therapies offer potential, albeit with limited evidence in pregnancy. Continued research and case studies are vital to enhance our understanding and treatment of PV in pregnant patients.

4.4 PEMPHIGUS FOLIACEUS

Pemphigus foliaceus (PF) is a less aggressive form of pemphigus that does not typically affect mucous membranes and presents with superficial skin lesions. Its course during pregnancy can vary significantly, requiring dermatologists to adapt treatment strategies based on the severity of symptoms and the overall health of the patient [44].

Fetal involvement is extremely rare. The coexpression of desmoglein 3 in the superficial epidermis in neonates protects their skin from blistering caused by passively transferred maternal antibodies against desmoglein 1 [53].

The variable nature of pemphigus foliaceus during pregnancy necessitates a flexible approach to management, prioritising treatments that are efficacious yet safe for the developing fetus. The primary goals are to maintain disease control, prevent new blister formation, and manage symptoms without compromising fetal safety. Collaboration between dermatologists and obstetricians is crucial to achieve these outcomes effectively. The treatment is the same as that recommended for pemphigus vulgaris.

See further Table 4.1.

REFERENCES

1. Huilaja L, Mäkikallio K, Tasanen K. Gestational pemphigoid. *Orphanet J Rare Dis* 2014; 9:136.
2. Nanda A, Dvorak R, Al-Saeed K, et al. Spectrum of autoimmune bullous diseases in Kuwait. *Int J Dermatol* 2004; 43(12):876–881.
3. Bernard P, Vaillant L, Labeille B, et al. Incidence and distribution of subepidermal autoimmune bullous skin diseases in three French regions. Bullous Diseases French Study Group. *Arch Dermatol* 1995; 131(1):48–52.
4. Bertram F, Brocker E, Zillikens D, et al. Prospective analysis of the incidence of autoimmune bullous disorders in Lower Franconia. *J Dtsch Dermatol Ges* 2009; 7(5):434–439.
5. Intong LRA, Murrell DF. Pemphigoid gestationis: pathogenesis and clinical features. *Dermatol Clin* 2011; 29(3):447–452.
6. Sadik CD, Lima AL, Zillikens D. Pemphigoid gestationis: toward a better understanding of the etiopathogenesis. *Clin Dermatol* 2016; 34(3):378–382.

7. Shornick JK, Stastny P, Gilliam JN. Paternal histocompatibility (HLA) antigens and maternal anti-HLA antibodies in herpes gestationis. *J Invest Dermatol* 1983; 81:407–409.

8. Di Zenzo G, Calabresi V, Grosso F, et al. The intracellular and extracellular domains of BP180 antigen comprise novel epitopes targeted by pemphigoid gestationis autoantibodies. *J Invest Dermatol* 2007; 127(4):864–873.

9. Fabbri P, Caproni M, Berti S, et al. The role of T lymphocytes and cytokines in the pathogenesis of pemphigoid gestationis. *Br J Dermatol* 2003; 148(6):1141–1148.

10. Lu PD, Ralston J, Kamino H, et al. Pemphigoid gestationis. *Dermatol Online J* 2010; 16(11):10.

11. Castro LA, Lundell RB, Krause PK, et al. Clinical experience in pemphigoid gestationis: report of 10 cases. *J Am Acad Dermatol* 2006; 55(5):823–828.

12. Semkova K, Black M. Pemphigoid gestationis: current insights into pathogenesis and treatment. *Eur J Obstet Gynecol Reprod Biol* 2009; 145(2):138–144.

13. Jenkins RE. Clinical features and management of 87 patients with pemphigoid gestationis. *Clin Exp Dermatol* 1999; 24(4):255–259.

14. Abdelhafez MMA, Ahmed KAM, Daud MNBM, et al. Pemphigoid gestationis and adverse pregnancy outcomes: a literature review. *J Gynecol Obstet Hum Reprod* 2022; 51(5):102370.

15. Holmes RC, Black MM. The fetal prognosis in pemphigoid gestationis (herpes gestationis). *Br J Dermatol* 1984; 110(1):67–72.

16. Huilaja L, Meakikallio K, Sormunen R, et al. Gestational pemphigoid: placental morphology and function. *Acta Derm Venereol* 2013; 93(1):33–38.

17. Shimanovich I, Brocker EB, Zillikens D. Pemphigoid gestationis: new insights into the pathogenesis lead to novel diagnostic tools. *BJOG* 2002; 109(9):970–976.

18. Chi CC, Wang SH, Charles-Holmes R, et al. Pemphigoid gestationis: early onset and blister formation are associated with adverse pregnancy outcomes. *Br J Dermatol* 2009; 160(6):1222–1228.

19. Cowan TL, Makhija M, Murrell DF. Pemphigoid gestationis and preeclampsia in a donor-egg IVF pregnancy. *Int J Womens Dermatol* 2022; 8(3):e026.

20. Genovese G, Derlino F, Cerri A, et al. A systematic review of treatment options and clinical outcomes in pemphigoid gestationis. *Front Med* 2020; 7:1–10.

21. Aoyama Y, Asai K, Hioki K, et al. Herpes gestationis in a mother and newborn: immunoclinical perspectives based on a weekly follow-up of the enzyme-linked immunosorbent assay index of a bullous pemphigoid antigen noncollagenous domain. *Arch Dermatol* 2007; 143:1168.

22. Al Saif F, Jouen F, Hebert V, et al. Sensitivity and specificity of BP180 NC16A enzyme-linked immunosorbent assay for the diagnosis of pemphigoid gestationis. *J Am Acad Dermatol* 2017; 76:560.

23. Sitaru C, Dähnrich C, Probst C, et al. Enzyme-linked immunosorbent assay using multimers of the 16th non-collagenous domain of the BP180 antigen for sensitive and specific detection of pemphigoid autoantibodies. *Exp Dermatol* 2007; 16:770.

24. Intong LRA, Murrell DF. Pemphigoid gestationis: current management. *Dermatol Clin* 2011; 29(4):621–628.

25. Chi CC, Mayon-White RT, Wojnarowska FT. Safety of topical corticosteroids in pregnancy: a population-based cohort study. *J Invest Dermatol* 2011; 131:884–891.

26. Chi CC, Wang SH, Kirtschig G, et al. Systematic review of the safety of topical corticosteroids in pregnancy. *J Am Acad Dermatol* 2010; 62:694–705.

27. Kreuter A, Harati A, Breuckmann F, et al. Intravenous immune globulin in the treatment of persistent pemphigoid gestationis. *J Am Acad Dermatol* 2004; 51(6):1027–1028.

28. Westermann L, Hügel R, Meier M, et al. Glucocorticosteroid-resistant pemphigoid gestationis: successful treatment with adjuvant immunoadsorption. *J Dermatol* 2012; 39(2):168–171.

29. Patsatsi A, Vavilis D, Tsikeloudi M, et al. Refractory pemphigoid gestationis postpartum. *Acta Obstet Gynecol Scand* 2012; 91(5):636–637.

30. Doiron P, Pratt M. Antepartum intravenous immunoglobulin therapy in refractory pemphigoid gestationis: case report and literature review. *J Cutan Med Surg* 2010; 14:189–192.

31. Natekar A, Pupco A, Bozzo P, et al. Safety of azathioprine use during pregnancy. *Can Fam Physician* 2011; 57:1401–1402.

32. Yang A, Uhlenhake E, Murrell DF. Pemphigoid gestationis and intravenous immunoglobulin therapy. *Int J Womens Dermatol* 2018; 4(3):166–169.

33. Alstead EM, Ritchie JK, Lennard-Jones JE, et al. Safety of azathioprine in pregnancy in inflammatory bowel disease. *Gastroenterology* 1990; 99:443–446.

34. Brabin BJ, Eggelte TA, Parise M, et al. Dapsone therapy for malaria during pregnancy: maternal and fetal outcomes. *Drug Saf* 2004; 27(9):633–648.

35. Ozturk Z, Tatliparmak A. Leprosy treatment during pregnancy and breastfeeding: a case report and brief review of literature. *Dermatol Ther* 2017; 30:12414.
36. Butler DC, Heller MM, Murase JE. Safety of dermatologic medications in pregnancy and lactation Part II. Lactation. *J Am Acad Dermatol* 2014; 70(3):417.e1–417.e10.
37. Huilaja L, Mäkikallio K, Hannula-Jouppi K, et al. Cyclosporine treatment in severe gestational pemphigoid. *Acta Derm Venereol* 2015; 95:593.
38. Amato L, Coronella G, Berti S, et al. Successful treatment with doxycycline and nicotinamide of two cases of persistent pemphigoid gestationis. *J Dermatolog Treat* 2002; 13:143.
39. Cianchini G, Masini C, Lupi F, et al. Severe persistent pemphigoid gestationis: long-term remission with rituximab. *Br J Dermatol* 2007; 157:388.
40. Konstantinou MP, Jendoubi F, Fortenfant F, et al. Successful treatment of recalcitrant pemphigoid gestationis with omalizumab: report of two cases. *J Eur Acad Dermatol Venereol* 2022; 36:e720.
41. *New Phase 2 Data Demonstrate Potential Benefit of Nipocalimab for Pregnant Individuals at High Risk of Early-Onset Severe Hemolytic Disease of the Fetus and Newborn (HDFN)*. Janssen. Press release. Published June 2023; available at: www.janssen.com/us/sites/www_janssen_com_usa/files/new_phase_2_data_demonstrate_potential_benefit_of_nipocalimab_for_pregnant_individuals_at_high_risk_of_early-onset_severe_hemolytic_disease_of_the_fetus_and_newborn_hdfn.pdf
42. Daneshpazhooh M, Chams-Davatchi C, Valikhani M, et al. Pemphigus and pregnancy: a 23-year experience. *Indian J Dermatol Venereol Leprol* 2011; 77(4):534.
43. Kardos M, Levine D, Gurcan HM, et al. Pemphigus vulgaris in pregnancy: analysis of current data on the management and outcomes. *Obstet Gynecol Surv* 2009; 64:739–749.
44. Fagundes PPS, Santi CG, Maruta CW, et al. Autoimmune bullous diseases in pregnancy: clinical and epidemiological characteristics and therapeutic approach. *An Bras Dermatol* 2021; 96:581–590.
45. Ruach M, Ohel G, Rahav D, et al. Pemphigus vulgaris and pregnancy. *Obstet Gynecol Surv* 1995; 50:755–760.
46. Bonifazi E, Milioto M, Trashlieva V, et al. Neonatal pemphigus vulgaris passively transmitted from a clinically asymptomatic mother. *J Am Acad Dermatol* 2006; 5(5):S113–S114.
47. Kianfar N, Dasdar S, Mahmoudi H, et al. Burden of pemphigus vulgaris with a particular focus on women: a review. *Int J Womens Dermatol* 2022; 8(3):e056.
48. Kushner CJ, Concha JSS, Werth VP. Treatment of autoimmune bullous disorders in pregnancy. *Am J Clin Dermatol* 2018; 19:391–403.
49. Chakravarty EF, Murray ER, Kelman A, et al. Pregnancy outcomes after maternal exposure to rituximab. *Blood* 2011; 117(5):1499–1506.
50. Braunstein I, Werth V. Treatment of dermatologic connective tissue disease and autoimmune blistering disorders in pregnancy. *Dermatol Ther* 2013; 26(4):354–363.
51. Skorpen CG, Hoeltzenbein M, Tincani A, et al. The EULAR points to consider for use of antirheumatic drugs before pregnancy, and during pregnancy and lactation. *Ann Rheum Dis* 2016; 75(5):795–810.
52. Bragnes Y, Boshuizen R, de Vries A, et al. Low level of Rituximab in human breast milk in a patient treated during lactation. *Rheumatology* 2017; 56(6):1047–1048.
53. Wu H, Wang ZH, Yan A, Lyle S, et al. Protection against pemphigus foliaceus by desmoglein 3 in neonates. *N Engl J Med* 2000; 343:31–35.

5 Pigmentary Disorders in Pregnancy

Rashmi Sakar and Vidya Yadav

5.1 INTRODUCTION

During pregnancy, skin and skin appendages both undergo a plethora of changes. These changes include both physiological as well as pathological entities. The course of pre-existing dermatoses during pregnancy is variable; it may worsen, improve or remain the same. Vice versa, the impact of pre-existing dermatoses on pregnancy is also variable. Many skin disorders are pregnancy specific, which may have adverse effects on the fetus and require regular fetal monitoring; hence it is very important to recognise them and intervene in a timely way. This list of pigmentary disorders of skin in pregnancy is usually similar to the pigmentary disorders in non-pregnant females of the reproductive age group. Elevated levels of oestrogen and progesterone increase melanogenesis, which leads to hyperpigmentation.[1] Increased amounts of circulating hormones also lead to vascular alterations and affect hair growth cycles.[1] Melasma is the most common pathological pigmentary disorder of skin in pregnancy. This chapter shall provide insights on the various types of pigmentary disorders in skin, their impact on pregnancy and vice versa.

5.2 MECHANISM OF MELANOGENESIS

Melanin, haemoglobin and to a lesser extent carotenoids are the main chromophores that contribute to normal skin colour. Racial and ethnic differences in skin colour are attributed to the number, size, shape, distribution and degradation of melanin-laden organelles called melanosomes. These are produced by melanocytes and are transferred to the surrounding epidermal keratinocytes.

Two types of melanin pigment production occur in humans, constitutive (genetically determined) and facultative (inducible), which result from sun exposure. Increased pigmentation can also be due to endocrine (estragon, progesterone), paracrine and autocrine factors. UV radiation and melanocyte-stimulating hormones are known to stimulate both melanogenesis and transfer of melanin to keratinocytes via melanosomes.

Based on the increasing amount of melanin pigment in skin, it is categorised into six types, known as Fitzpatrick skin typing.

5.3 CLASSIFICATION OF PIGMENTARY DISORDERS

There is lack of standard classification of disorders of pigmentation in the normal population as well as in pregnant females. The causes of pigmentary disorders in pregnancy are the same as in the normal population. In Table 5.1, the causes of pigmentary disorders are categorised. Up to 90% of pregnant women experience pigmentary changes. Freckles, nevi, hyperpigmentation of the areolae and nipples and linea nigra are most commonly observed. Melasma is also a common cause of pigmentation, seen in approximately 70% of pregnant women, which often regresses after delivery.[2]

DOI: 10.1201/9781003449690-5

TABLE 5.1

List of Causes of Hyperpigmentation during Pregnancy

Class	Entity	Examples
	Disorders of Hyperpigmentation	
1	Physiological hyperpigmentation	Increased pigmentation on nipple areola and genitalia, linea nigra, changes in melanocytic naevi, stria gravidarum, longitudinal melanonychia of nails
2	Pathological hyperpigmentation	Localised, generalised
A. Localised disorders of hyperpigmentation based on aetiology and site	1. Post-inflammatory hyperpigmentation (PIH)	Secondary to infections, inflammatory dermatoses (acne, rosacea, hidradenitis suppurativa, lichen planus, psoriasis-impetigo herpetiformis, atopic dermatitis), pregnancy-specific dermatoses, tumours (pyogenic granuloma)
	2. Facial melanosis	Melasma, periorbital hyperpigmentation, EDP, PCD, LPP, EFFC, *Acanthoses nigricans*
B. Localised disorders of hyperpigmentation based on depth of pigmentation	1. Epidermal	CALM, ephelids, lentiginoses
	2. Dermal	Nevus of ota, nevus of ito
	3. Mixed	Melasma
C. Generalised disorders of hyperpigmentation	1. Systemic illness	Endocrine and metabolic disorders, nutritional disorders, drug-induced, autoimmune disorders (pemphigoid gestationis), connective tissue disorders (SLE, DM, SS, MCTD), malignancy (melanoma)
	2. Linear	PDL
	3. Miscellaneous	Pregnancy and pre-existing congenital/early age onset pigmentation (no change in pregnancy)
	Disorders of Hypopigmentation	
A. Localised disorders of hypopigmentation	Post-inflammatory hypopigmentation	Secondary to infection (Leprosy, PKDL). trauma, inflammatory disorder (seborrheic dermatitis, atopic dermatitis, PLC, lichen striatus) Autoimmune: lichen sclerosis, morphea, vitiligo
B. Generalised disorders of hypopigmentation	Autoimmune	Vitiligo
	Tumour	Mycoses fungoides
	Miscellaneous	Pregnancy and pre-existing congenital/early age onset hypopigmentation (no change in pregnancy)

5.4 PHYSIOLOGICAL HYPERPIGMENTATION

Significant hormonal, circulatory, metabolic, mechanical and immunological changes occur throughout pregnancy which may predispose pregnant women to different physiological and pathological alterations in their skin, hair, nails, connective tissue and vascular system.[3] Increased pigmentation of nipple areola, genitalia, linea nigra and striae gravidarum are determined to be the most prevalent physiological alterations developed during pregnancy (Figure 5.1). These pigmentary changes develop more frequently in women of darker complexion. Linea nigra is a linear

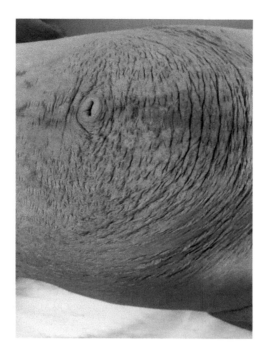

FIGURE 5.1 Physiological alterations are shown here, which developed during pregnancy such as increased pigmentation, linea nigra, striae gravidarum, and laxity of skin after delivery of a multiparous female.

hyperpigmentation that runs vertically from the pubis to the umbilicus to the top of the abdomen along the midline, with a width of 0.4 inches or 1 centimetre.

In a north Indian study done on 100 pregnant females, linea nigra was found in 82%, secondary areola in 62%, and pigmentation of flexures in 16%, and darkening of nevi was observed in 8% participants. Striae gravidarum and melasma were seen in 68% and 40% cases, respectively.[3]

In a study from Brazil on 157 postpartum females, photographic recording of supra- and infra-umbilical linea nigra was done on day 1 or 2 and analysed according to three directions (left, centre and right of the umbilical scar). The formations of nine distinct patterns were found. The "anticlockwise spiralization of the linea nigra" was the most frequent pattern seen in primiparous (72.2%) and multiparous women (50.0%).[4]

This increase in pigmentation during pregnancy is presumed to be caused by oestrogen and progesterone's melanocyte-stimulating impact.[5] An increased level of melanocyte-stimulating hormone stimulates melanogenesis and melanin transfer to keratinocytes. The majority of the alterations are temporary and regress after delivery, although others may persist in a less noticeable form.[3]

The rate of nail growth is faster during pregnancy. Nails may become dystrophic, brittle and soft. Transverse ridging, longitudinal melanonychia and leukonychia can also be found in the nails of pregnant females.[3] Melanonychia striata are uniformly homogenous dark brown streaks, with a distinct margin and width of 2–5 mm, that develop in nails during the 12th week of pregnancy without any evidence of Hutchinson sign in the affected nails.[6] Hormonal change during pregnancy prolongs the anagen phase, leading to increased thickness of hairs. After delivery, a large proportion of hairs enter the telogen stage, leading to telogen effluvium at the postpartum stage.[1]

Most of these physiological skin changes of pregnancy are self-limiting and need to be distinguished from pathological causes to avoid needless medication and tests and to improve patient care and counselling.

5.5 PATHOLOGICAL CAUSES OF HYPERPIGMENTATION

5.5.1 LOCALISED DISORDERS OF HYPERPIGMENTATION

Post-inflammatory hyperpigmentation (PIH) and facial melanosis shall be discussed in this section.

5.5.1.1 PIH

1. **Infections**: Most infections in pregnancy have the same prognosis as in non-pregnant females, but some infections, such as rubella, cmv and syphilis, have adverse maternal and fetal outcomes post-pregnancy. These infections require screening during the antenatal period. Common cutaneous infections during pregnancy include folliculitis, furunculosis, dermatophyte infection, herpes simplex viral infection, varicella zoster virus infection, scabies, cellulitis and secondary bacterial infections, which heal with PIH. It is a common notion that pregnancy is a state of immunosuppression; hence there is increased risk of infection, but recent advices show that there is immune modulation in pregnancy which responds differentially to microorganisms and will provide adequate protection to mother and fetus.[8]

2. **Disorders of pilosebaceous units—Acne, rosacea and hidradenitis suppurativa (HS)**: Acne in pregnancy shows many similarities with adult-onset acne and can heal with PIH. It has been found that acne vulgaris often improves in early pregnancy but worsens in the third trimester because of raised maternal androgen levels.[9] Acne in pregnancy is managed with topical antibiotics, systemic antibiotics (macrolides) and benzoyl peroxide depending upon its severity. Retinoids and doxycycline are absolutely contraindicated during pregnancy (Figure 5.2).
   - **Rosacea** usually worsens during **pregnancy**. It is managed with topical azelaic acid and metronidazole, but sometimes it may be severe enough to require systemic treatment during pregnancy, called rosacea fulminans.[9]

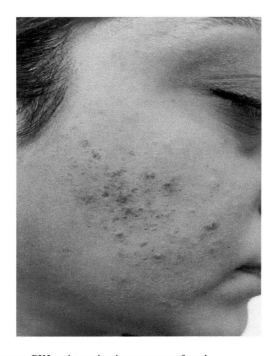

FIGURE 5.2   Acne, post-acne PIH and scarring in a pregnant female.

- **HS** is a chronic debilitating inflammatory skin disease. Although a small percentage of people (20%) report experiencing symptom remission during pregnancy, the great majority (72%) do not, and only a small percentage (8%) experience clinical worsening. Postpartum disease flare-ups have also been seen. There is currently no established pathophysiological explanation for pregnancy-related changes in clinical state. Topical antibiotics, such as clindamycin (1%), metronidazole (0.75%), and erythromycin (2%), can be used twice a day to active HS lesions until they resolve. These drugs fall under Pregnancy Category B.[10]

3. **Papulosquamous disorders—lichen planus, psoriasis**: Data about the course of lichen planus in pregnancy are limited, but it heals, leaving behind PIH. Lichen planus pigmentosus is a variant of lichen planus in which dark brown to grey macular pigmentation develops on sun-exposed areas of the face, neck and flexures, commonly found in dark-skinned patients. Due to a shift in immunity from a predominantly T helper 1 lymphocyte profile to a T helper 2 profile, diseases driven by T helper 1 lymphocyte such as psoriasis tend to improve in 80% of cases during pregnancy but may worsen in 20% of pregnant females with psoriasis.[9] Topical corticosteroids and calcipotriol for localised disease can be used to treat psoriasis during pregnancy. There has been no evidence of prenatal harm in trials. Emollients and topical corticosteroids are the primary treatments for mild psoriasis.[9]
   - Severe psoriasis can be adequately treated in secondary care with prednisolone and phototherapy with narrowband ultraviolet B radiation. Psoralen mixed with ultraviolet A light should be avoided during pregnancy, and systemic medications such as methotrexate, hydroxyurea and acetretin should be avoided, as they are all teratogenic.
   - Impetigo herpetiformis is a severe form of pustular psoriasis and occurs mostly during the third trimester, improving after delivery. It causes adverse pregnancy and fetal outcomes; hence, it is managed with systemic corticosteroids (first-line treatment) or cyclosporine (second-line treatment).

4. **Atopic dermatitis**: Due to shift in immunity from a predominantly T helper 1 lymphocyte profile to a T helper 2 profile, diseases driven by T helper 2 lymphocytes such as atopic dermatitis tend to worsen during pregnancy.[9] While 80% of women have atopic skin changes for the first time during pregnancy, 20% of women experience an aggravation of pre-existing eczema for the first time or following a long-lasting remission.[3] One-third of these have papular lesions (P-type atopic eruption of pregnancy), and about two-thirds have widespread eczematous changes (so-called E-type atopic eruption of pregnancy), frequently affecting typical atopic sites like the face, neck and flexural surfaces of the arms and legs. Maternal and fetal prognosis is good, but there is increased risk of atopy to the newborn baby and in subsequent pregnancy.[9]

5. **Tumours (pyogenic granuloma)**: There is increased prevalence of pyogenic granuloma in the oral cavity, especially during pregnancy. It is also called granuloma gravidarum, pregnancy tumour and pregnancy granuloma. It may cause bleeding and significant morbidity. Although excisional surgery is the preferred treatment for it, numerous other treatment procedures have been offered, including the use of Nd:Yag lasers, flash lamp pulsed dye lasers, cryosurgery, intralesional injections of ethanol or corticosteroid and sodium tetradecyl sulphate sclerotherapy.[11]

6. **Pregnancy-specific dermatoses**: Certain dermatoses are peculiar to pregnancy and may heal with pigmentation. These disorders cause severe itching and secondary excoriation, which may heal with PIH. These disorders include atopic eruption of pregnancy, polymorphic eruption of pregnancy, pemphigoid gestationis and intrahepatic cholestasis of pregnancy. Among these pregnancy-specific dermatoses, pemphigoid gestationis may also be associated with poor fetal outcome, leading to prematurity and small for date babies, although intrahepatic cholestasis of pregnancy imposes the risk of fetal distress, prematurity and stillbirth.[9] Itching is frequently nocturnal in intrahepatic cholestasis and affects

the palms and soles. It is critical to exclude pregnancy-related intrahepatic cholestasis in patients with pruritus and an absence of skin abnormalities other than excoriations. It is important to assess signs of liver disease, performing liver function tests and tests for bile acid and carrying out regular fetal monitoring. These disorders are treated with antihistamines (chlorpheniramine is safe in first trimester), emollients and mild to moderate topical corticosteroids, and in resistant or severe cases, systemic steroids may be required.

5.5.1.2 Facial Melanosis

The common causes of facial melanoses include melasma, PIH, Riehls melanosis, poikiloderma of Civatte/erythromelanosis interfollicularis colli, lichen planopilaris, erythema dyschromicum perstans (EDP), periorbital melanosis, exogenous ochronosis, Addisonian pigmentation, acanthosis nigricans and peribuccal pigmentation of Brocq. The prevalence of this entity is increasing, the reason being easily visible pigmentation on the face causes low self-esteem and significant psychological comorbidity, leading to more patients presenting to a dermatologist seeking consultation.

Besides the complex interplay of genetic, racial and environmental factors, increased oestrogen and progesterone levels during pregnancy lead to increased frequency of melasma, acanthosis nigricans, darkening of pre-existing naevi and periocular pigmentation. Other causes of facial melanosis are also common in pregnant women, as in nonpregnant women. In an Indian study on pregnant females, melasma in was documented in 40% of the pregnant females and pigmentation on flexures in 16%, and pre-existing naevi were found in 8% of study subjects, with a centrofacial pattern of pigmentation the most common (Figures 5.3, 5.4, 5.5).[3] Melasma during pregnancy is known as chloasma or mask of pregnancy, and its frequency varies between 50% and 70%. Melasma is an acquired pigmentary disorder characterised by bilateral symmetric, light to dark brown or brown-grey patches with an irregular outline, occurring on the face. The aggravating factors for this entity include sun exposure, pregnancy, thyroid disorders and certain drugs such oral contraceptive pills and hormone replacement therapy. Based on the site of pigmentation, it has three classic patterns:

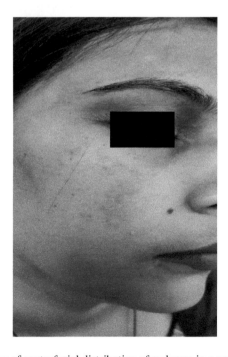

FIGURE 5.3   Left lateral view of centrofacial distribution of melasma in a pregnant female.

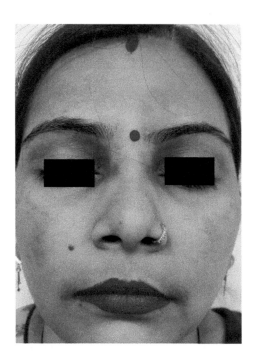

FIGURE 5.4   Left front view of centrofacial distribution of melasma in a pregnant female.

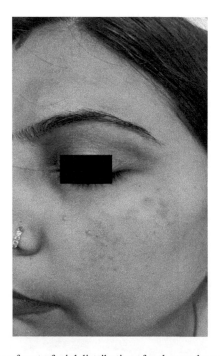

FIGURE 5.5   Right lateral view of centrofacial distribution of melasma along with milia in a pregnant female.

centrofacial (forehead, cheeks, nose, upper lip, sparing the philtrum and nasolabial folds), malar (cheeks and nose) and mandibular (along jawline).[12] Centrofacial is the most common pattern among all three. Based on depth of pigmentation in skin, it has been subdivided into four types: epidermal dermal, mixed and indeterminate.[12]

Riehl's melanosis is caused by a phototoxic reaction that occurs following skin contact with photoactive substances. such as tar compounds, cosmetics and scents which should be avoided during pregnancy. It is more common in middle-aged women. Brownish-grey pigmentation appears promptly throughout the majority of the face but is more pronounced on the forehead and temples.[12]

Poikiloderma of Civatte presents clinically with atrophy, telangiectasia and dyschromic pigmentation (hyper- and hypo-pigmentation). It develops after years of persistent UV exposure and occurs on the sides of the face and neck, as well as the upper anterior chest. Light exposure and photodynamic chemicals in cosmetics are influencing factors.

Although the specific cause of lichen plano pigmentosus (LPP) is unknown, cosmetics such as fragrances, hair dyes and mustard oil have been implicated. LPP is distinguished by a largely asymptomatic and diffuse (most frequent) reticular, blotchy and perifollicular pattern of hyperpigmented dark-brown to slate-grey macules that appear predominantly in overexposed areas and flexures (Figures 5.6 and 5.7).[12] The lesions do not have the erythematous border of EDP. EDP is considered a variant of LPP. The literature about LPP in pregnancy is limited.

Increased frequency of acanthosis nigricans and acrochordons is commonly seen in pregnant females with gestational diabetes, but there are a few reports of these lesions present in pregnant females without gestational diabetes (Figure 5.8).[13]

Periorbital pigmentation can be because of physiological periorbital darkening, shadowing from lax skin or PIH secondary to atopic or allergic contact dermatitis.

Exogenous ochronosis develops after prolonged use of hydroquinone. Its use is not recommended during pregnancy.

5.5.2 LOCALISED DISORDERS OF HYPERPIGMENTATION BASED ON DEPTH OF PIGMENTATION

Increased pigmentation of ephelids has been reported in pregnant females. Increased numbers of neurofibromatosis 1 associated lentigines and CALM have been reported in pregnancy.[14]

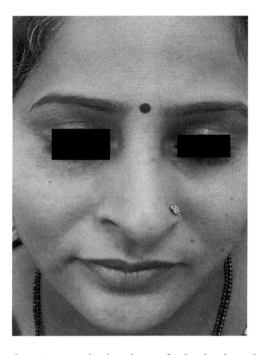

FIGURE 5.6 Lichen plano pigmentosus predominantly over forehead and temple area in a pregnant female.

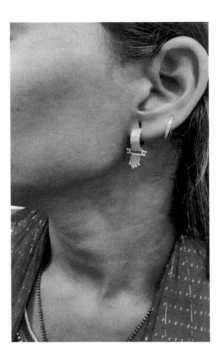

FIGURE 5.7   Distribution of lichen plano pigmentosus over cheek and neck in a pregnant female.

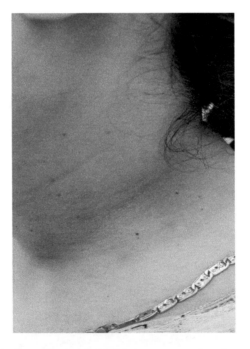

FIGURE 5.8   Acanthosis nigricans along with skin tag in a pregnant female.

Nevus of Ota is caused by the arrest of embryonic migration of melanocytes from the neural crest to the epidermis. It is characterised by unilateral speckled or mottled blue-grey pigmentation along the areas supplied by the ophthalmic and maxillary divisions of the trigeminal nerve. It may involve the oral mucosa and the eye (conjunctiva, sclera, retrobulbar fat, cornea and retina) as well

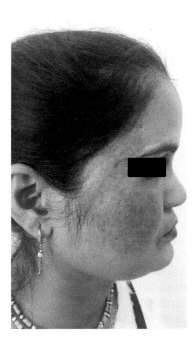

FIGURE 5.9   Blue-grey pigmentation over left cheek, temple area in a primigavida female suggestive of nevus of Ota.

(Figure 5.9).[12] Nevus of Ito is an entity similar to nevus of Ota, with different sites of distribution (along the posterior supraclavicular and cutaneous brachii lateralis nerve). Both nevus of Ota and Ito usually appear at birth but may appear during puberty and pregnancy due to hormonal changes. In a study from Singapore done on females of reproductive age with Hori nevus (acquired, bilateral naevus of Ota-like macules), the two most common individual triggering factors reported were sun exposure (27.3%) and pregnancy (19.3%).[15]

5.6   MANAGEMENT OF LOCALISED HYPERPIGMENTATION IN PREGNANCY

Management of hyperpigmentation during pregnancy is usually conservative, and it is advised to avoid medications which may have adverse pregnancy outcomes. Counselling the pregnant female about the pros and cons of available treatment options and their impact on pregnancy outcome is an essential step for managing hyperpigmentation disorders in pregnancy. Due to ethical concerns, clinical trials and systematic reviews on the safety profile of topical treatments in pregnancy are quite restricted. Although the majority of the treatments are only suggested after birth, there are some alternative approaches for preventing and treating hyperpigmentory disorders during pregnancy.

Physical/mineral sunscreens and emollients go hand in hand a long way to slow down the disease process.

Azelaic acid (US FDA Pregnancy Category B)—it has antioxidant, anti-inflammatory and comedolytic and melanogenesis properties; hence it can be used for mild to moderate acne, PIH and melasma during pregnancy. Use of 10–20% azelaic acid twice a day is considered safe during pregnancy and lactation.[16]

Topical corticosteroids (Pregnancy Category C)—The current best data favour the use of mild-to-moderate TCS in pregnancy over potent/super-potent alternatives due to the risk of fetal growth limitation with the latter. When mild-to-moderate TCs are used in pregnancy, there is no statistically increased risk of orofacial clefts, premature birth, growth retardation or fetal mortality. However, it should be highlighted that potent or super-potent TCs should only be administered as second-line therapy for as brief a time as feasible. When high-potency corticosteroids are administered, attentive obstetric care is required since they increase the probability of a baby being born with a low birth weight.[16]

Kojic acid—Kojic acid (KA) is a fungal derivative that inhibits tyrosinase by chelating copper in the enzyme's active site. It is used in concentrations ranging from 1% to 4%.[17] A USFDA rating is not available for this product. Because kojic acid was found to be non-toxic in acute, chronic, reproductive and genotoxicity examinations, the Cosmetic Ingredient Review (CIR) Expert Panel determined that these findings created no safety concerns. The panel did highlight, however, that some animal studies suggest tumour promotion and low carcinogenicity. Kojic acid does not reach a significant systemic level where these effects were observed. The known human sensitisation studies indicate the safety of kojic acid in leave-on cosmetics at a concentration of 2%, implying that a 2% limit may be reasonable.[18]

Niacinamide—It is the active amide of vitamin B3 that decreases pigmentation by inhibiting the transfer of melanosomes to keratinocytes.[17] A US FDA pregnancy category has not been assigned, and although this is an essential micronutrient, data about its use in pregnancy are limited.

Tranexamic acid (US FDA Pregnancy Category B) (trans-4-aminomethylcyclohexane-carboxylic acid)—This is a synthetic lysine derivative. It binds reversibly to plasminogen lysine binding sites, inhibiting plasminogen activator (PA) and hence the conversion of plasminogen to plasmin. Plasminogen can also be found in basal epidermal cells and keratinocytes, and UV radiation induces melanogenesis through the formation of prostaglandins and leukotrienes. TA reduces UV-induced plasmin activity in keratinocytes by preventing plasminogen binding, consequently lowering melanogenesis through decreased prostaglandin synthesis.[17]

Hydroquinone (Pregnancy Category C)—Also demands vigilance during pregnancy. Although systemic exposure from this medication's topical use is unknown, it does not appear to pose a major risk to the fetus. There was an elevated risk of structural malformations in the fetus in one of two animal species studied during pregnancy at levels that were likewise toxic to the mother. As a result, the risk of fetal abnormalities during pregnancy from topical usage is considered modest.

Vitamin C (US FDA Pregnancy Category A if dose < RDA and Category C if dose is > RDA)—Vitamin C inhibits melanogenesis by acting as a reducing agent at various oxidative steps in melanin synthesis and can be used in pregnancy.

5.7   CHEMICAL PEELS

Topical beta hydroxy (salicylic) and alpha hydroxy (glycolic) acids are anti-acne and anti-pigmentation agents that are available in a variety of over-the-counter medications. Because of their minimal systemic absorption, they are regarded as safe during all trimesters of pregnancy and lactation, despite the lack of FDA pregnancy safety ratings. To avoid enhanced systemic absorption, pregnant patients should avoid applying topical salicylic acid to broad areas for extended periods of time or beneath occlusive dressings. Because of their minimal skin penetration, lactic and glycolic acid peels are considered safe during pregnancy and lactation.[16]

Trichloroacetic acid (US FDA Pregnancy Category C)—While trichloroacetic acid can be beneficial as a chemical peel, it is also associated with an increased risk of pigmentary alterations or very superficial scarring.

Procedures safe in pregnancy—Any procedure must take maternal and fetal health concerns into account. With the growing popularity of aesthetic procedures, dermatologic surgeons will be confronted with situations requiring knowledge of the safety of such procedures during pregnancy. During pregnancy, definitive advice on the safety of procedures including chemical peels, injectables, fillers and most laser therapies cannot be given. Lidocaine can be used as topical aesthesia in pregnancy because it is relatively safe in pregnancy. According to the FDA established drug risk category of pregnancy, lidocaine has been kept in Category B (safe in animal studies, but no controlled study has been conducted in human beings).

The data about safety of the Nd:Yag laser in pregnancy are limited. Its use for condylomas during pregnancy implies that it is safe to use for dermatologic disorders. Pulsed dye laser has been used to treat pyogenic granulomas and warts during pregnancy. This laser may be effective for striae treatment as well; however, it is advised to wait until childbirth as data about the safety of these lasers in pregnancy are sparse.[19]

5.7.1 Generalised Disorders of Hyperpigmentation

1. **Systemic Illness**—Generalised hyperpigmentation secondary to endocrine (Addisonian pigmentation) metabolic disorders (metabolic syndrome, acanthosis nigricans), nutritional disorders (vitamin B12 deficiency), drug induced (minocycline, tetracycline), autoimmune disorders (pemphigoid gestationis), connective tissue disorders (systemic lupus erythematosus, dermatomysitis) and malignancy (melanoma) can be seen during pregnancy.

During pregnancy or puerperium, around 60% of women with pre-existing systemic lupus erythematosus (SLE) have a flare, compared to 40% of non-pregnant women.[20] Corticosteroids are the preferred treatment. Anti-Ro antibodies are present in around 30% of women with systemic lupus erythematosus. They are more common in people with Sjögren's syndrome and subacute lupus erythematosus.[20] Congenital heart block (2–3% risk) is commonly discovered in gestation between the ages of 18 and 20 weeks.[20]

Autoimmune bullous disorders such as Pemphigus vulgaris can manifest or worsen during pregnancy, and it can also be passed on to the fetus. The prognosis of the fetus is diverse, and there is no direct link between the severity of the mother's condition and the level of neonatal involvement.[20] Both hypopigmentation and hyperpigmentation are seen in systemic sclerosis patients. Salt-and-pepper, diffuse, vitiligo-like and Addisonian pigmentation are seen in systemic sclerosis (Figures 5.10 and 5.11).

2. **Pigmentary Demarcation Lines (PDLs)**—PDLs are borders of abrupt transition between more deeply pigmented skin and that of lighter pigmentation. The five types of defined PDLs are (see also Figures 5.12 and 5.13):

1. Upper anterior arms across pectoral area
2. Lower posteromedial limbs
3. Pre- and parasternal area
4. Posteromedial area of spine
5. Bilateral chest marking from mid-third of clavicle to peri-areolar skin

Many case reports show the appearance of type 2 PDL symmetrically on the bilateral medial aspect of the thigh during the last trimester of pregnancy.[21]

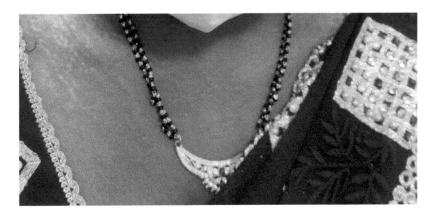

FIGURE 5.10 Salt and pepper pigmentation over neck in a pregnant female with systemic sclerosis.

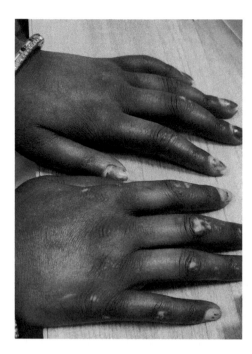

FIGURE 5.11   Acral distribution of hyperpigmentation and vitiligo like depigmentation in a pregnant female with systemic sclerosis.

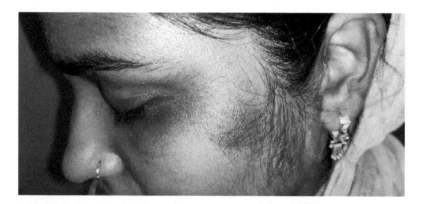

FIGURE 5.12   Distribution of V-shaped F-type facial pigmentary demarcation line over lateral aspect of temple and malar area in a pregnant female.

5.8   MANAGEMENT OF LOCALISED HYPERPIGMENTATION IN PREGNANCY

For systemic illness, obstetricians and dermatologists must work closely together to prevent mother and newborn mortality. If immunosuppressants are required, then oral corticosteroids are the first-line and cyclosporine is the second-line treatment for management of autoimmune bullous disorder, and hydroxychroloquine and systemic corticosteroids are used for SLE. Treating the cause may reduce hyperpigmentation spontaneously. No intervention is done for pigmentary demarcation lines during pregnancy, but counselling is a key step to reduce anxiety and cosmetic concerns.

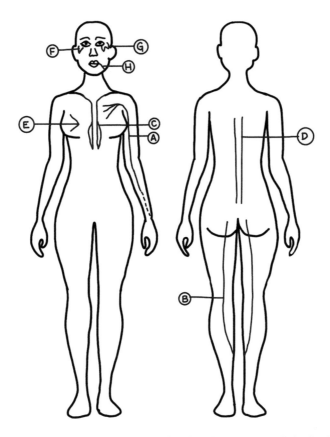

FIGURE 5.13   Various types of pigmentary demarcation lines based on site of distribution.

5.9   DISORDERS OF HYPOPIGMENTATION

5.9.1   LOCALISED DISORDERS OF HYPOPIGMENTATION

Postinflammatory hypopigmentation secondary to infection (leprosy, PKDL), trauma, inflammatory disorder (seborrheic dermatitis, atopic dermatitis, pityriasis rosea, lichen striatus) and autoimmune disorders (lichen sclerosis, morphea, vitiligo) may develop.

5.9.1.1   Management of Localised Disorders of Hypopigmentation in Pregnancy

For treatment of leprosy, a complete course of MB-MDT id given. For PKDL, amphotericin (Pregnancy Category B) is a safer treatment option during pregnancy. For inflammatory disorders, symptomatic treatment can be done, and for autoimmune disorders, mild to moderate topical corticosteroids can be used.

5.9.2   GENERALISED DISORDERS OF HYPOPIGMENTATION

A common cause of generalised hypopigmentation is autoimmune-mediated vitiligo, whereas rarely it may be because of a hypopigmented variant of mycoses fungoides. In a study done on pregnant females with vitiligo, a majority of patients reported steady or improved vitiligo vulgaris activity during pregnancy (Figure 5.14). These findings could be explained by pregnancy-related immunological, hormonal or other physiological changes, pregnancy having a protective effect against the extension of vitiligo vulgaris.[22]

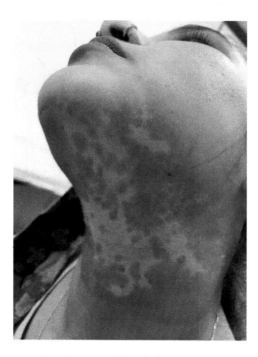

FIGURE 5.14   Repigmentation and erythema in vitiligo lesions of a pregnant female.

5.10   MANAGEMENT OF LOCALISED HYPOPIGMENTATION IN PREGNANCY

Treatment of a cause such as a tumour or any systemic illness is advised. For the time being, there are just a few therapeutic options for vitiligo in pregnancy. Topical corticosteroids and phototherapies may be among them. Folic acid supplementation is especially recommended for women who are undergoing phototherapy. The combination of steroids and ultraviolet light has the most evidence for vitiligo treatment, particularly during pregnancy.[23]

We must emphasise that the majority of systemically used drugs for the treatment of vitiligo are classified as Category C pregnancy drugs, and their continued use during pregnancy is only subject to the drugs' disparaging risk–benefit ratio: oral corticosteroids, calcineurin inhibitors and vitamin D analogues such as calcipotriol and tacalcitol. Psoralens, Minocycline, Cyclophosphamide and Azathioprine are all Category D pregnancy medicines that should be avoided during pregnancy and breastfeeding. The pregnancy category status of other peptides generated from basic fibroblast growth factor (bFGF) is unknown, while there is no contraindication to administering intravenous immunoglobulin (IVIG) and zinc during preganacy.[23] Due to limited data availability about biologics and new immunomodulates, it is better to avoid these medications during pregnancy

5.11   CONCLUSION

Many disorders of pigmentation may have an altered impact on pregnancy and vice versa. The exact aetiology, pathogenesis and behaviour of these disorders during pregnancy is a subject which needs to be explored more by researchers. Due to ethical considerations, there is a lack of randomised controlled trials about aetiopathogenesis and treatment modalities of these disorders in pregnancy. It is better to avoid non-essential medications during pregnancy, and they should be given only after assessing the risk–benefit ratio. Adequate counselling of the mother about the self-limiting nature of the disorder reduces disease-related anxiety. Since few of these disorders may alter the course of pregnancy, they may necessitate multi-specialty consultation including obstetricians, dermatologists, paediatricians and the physician. Therefore, the mother should be educated about regular follow-up.

REFERENCES

1. Errickson CV, Matus NR. Skin disorders of pregnancy. *Am Fam Physician*. 1994;49(3):605–610.
2. Scoggins RB. Skin changes and diseases in pregnancy. In: Fitzpatrick TB, Eisen A, Wolff K, eds. *Dermatology in General Medicine*. New York, McGraw-Hill; 1979, p. 1363.
3. Sharma A, Jharaik H, Sharma R, et al. Clinical study of pregnancy associated cutaneous changes. *Int J Clin Obstet Gynaecol*. 2019;3(4):71–75.
4. Klotzel D, Zamuner M, Machado AM, et al. The anti-clockwise spiralization of the linea nigra sign. *Einstein (São Paulo)*. 2020;18:eAO5432.
5. Tyler KH. Physiological skin changes during pregnancy. *Clin Obstet Gynecol*. 2015;58:119–124.
6. Plachouri KM, Kolonitsiou F, Georgiou S. Melanonychia striata: Nail alterations during pregnancy. *Skinmed*. 2019;17(6):413–414.
7. James WD, Meltzer MS, Guill MA, et al. Pigmentary demarcation lines associated with pregnancy. *J Am Acad Dermatol*. 1984;11(3):438–440.
8. Mor G, Cardenas I. The immune system in pregnancy: A unique complexity. *Am J Reprod Immunol*. 2010;63(6):425–433.
9. Jones SV, Ambros-Rudolph C, Nelson-Piercy C. Skin disease in pregnancy. *BMJ* 2014;348–349.
10. Perng P, Zampella JG, Okoye GA. Management of hidradenitis suppurativa in pregnancy. *J Am Acad Dermatol*. 2017;76(5):979–989.
11. Jafarzadeh H, Sanatkhani M, Mohtasham N. Oral pyogenic granuloma: A review. *J Oral Sci*. 2006;48(4):167–175.
12. Dharman BK, Sridhar S. Diffuse facial melanosis—an overview of etiology and dermoscopic findings. *J Skin Sex Transmitted Dis*. 2020;2(2):86–93.
13. Kroumpouzos G, Avgerinou G, Granter SR. Acanthosis nigricans without diabetes during pregnancy. *Br J Dermatol*. 2002;146(5):925–928.
14. Sifakis S, Kalmantis K, Karagiannopoulos A. Neurofibromatosis type-1 and pregnancy: A review. *Obstet Gynecol Imaging*. 2021;1(1):26–30.
15. Ee HL, Wong HC, Goh CL, Ang P. Characteristics of Hori naevus: A prospective analysis. *Br J Dermatol*. 2002;154(1):50–53.
16. Ly S, Kamal K, Manjaly P, et al. Treatment of acne vulgaris during pregnancy and lactation: A narrative review. *Dermatol Ther*. 2023;13(1):115–130.
17. Das A, Panda S. Use of topical corticosteroids in dermatology: An evidence-based approach. *Indian J Dermatol*. 2017;62(3):237–250.
18. Burnett CL, Bergfeld WF, Belsito DV, et al. Final report of the safety assessment of kojic acid as used in cosmetics. *Int J Toxicol*. 2010;29(6 Suppl):244S–273S.
19. Lee KC, Korgavkar K, Dufresne Jr RG, Higgins HW. Safety of cosmetic dermatologic procedures during pregnancy. *Dermatol Surg*. 2013;39(11):1573–1586.
20. Vaughan S, Ambros-Rudolph C, Nelson-Piercy C. Skin disease in pregnancy. *BMJ*. 2014;348(9):10–12.
21. Bonci A, Patrizi A. Pigmentary demarcation lines in pregnancy. *Arch Dermatol*. 2002;138(1):127–128.
22. Webb KC, Lyon S, Nardone B, et al. Influence of pregnancy on vitiligo activity. *J Clin Aesthet Dermatol*. 2016;9(12):21.
23. Rodrigues M, Ezzedine K, Hamzavi I, Pandya AG, Harris JE, Vitiligo Working Group. Current and emerging treatments for vitiligo. *J Am Acad Dermatol*. 2017;77(1):17–29.

6 Disorders of Hair in Pregnancy and Postpartum

Soumya Jagadeesan and Prateek Nayak

6.1 INTRODUCTION

Pregnant women are susceptible to cutaneous and appendageal changes, both physiological and pathological, due to the substantial immunologic, metabolic, endocrine, and vascular alterations that accompany pregnancy. Pregnancy-associated cutaneous changes are discussed at length in all available publications, but hair disorders are rarely touched upon. In this chapter, we have tried to focus on hair disorders and their management during pregnancy and postpartum.

As far as hair is considered, pregnant females have universally improved hair growth and increased hair volume due to anagen retention, which can manifest as hypertrichosis and/or hirsutism.[1,2] The subsequent return to normal immunologic and endocrine state postpartum propels hair into the telogen phase, which may manifest as telogen gravidarum in some females. Androgenetic alopecia, alopecia areata, scalp infections and infestations, and other hair-related issues are commonly encountered during motherhood and are discussed subsequently. In addition, we have tried to address the question of the safety of hair treatments and products during pregnancy and/or lactation.

6.2 PHYSIOLOGICAL CHANGES IN HAIR CYCLE DURING PREGNANCY

A human hair follicle's life cycle comprises three distinct phases: the anagen (growing phase), catagen (involuting phase), and telogen (resting phase). The anagen phase of scalp hair follicles lasts for about 2–6 years, and the duration of the anagen phase is a major determinant of maximum hair length. Under physiological conditions, around 85% of scalp hair is in the anagen phase, and only about 10% to 15% of the scalp's terminal follicles are in the telogen phase. The telogen follicles are dispersed at random over the scalp, and the phase lasts for about 2–3 months before the hair is shed. These cyclic transformations are influenced by precisely timed alterations in the local signalling environment, which are based on changes in the expression of cytokines, hormones, neurotransmitters, and their receptors as well as transcription factors and enzymes that operate through endocrine, paracrine, or autocrine pathways.[3]

Hair changes during pregnancy have been only occasionally researched. A small analytical study by Lynfield[4] in the 1960s showed that during pregnancy, the anagen phase is prolonged and transition of hair from anagen to telogen is slowed down, a phenomenon initially addressed as delayed anagen release.[5] The study further documented that the average number of scalp anagen hairs increases from the usual 85% to close to 95% during the second and early third trimester, while the percentage of anagen follicles drops to 76% shortly after birth, possibly due to accelerated conversion from anagen hair to telogen hair. Though the Lynfield study had a very small sample size, it set in place the basic conceptual physiological phenomenon which translates into observable excessive hair growth during pregnancy and subsequent hair shedding postpartum.

The apparent increase in the number of anagen hairs and the associated increased diameter of scalp hair[6] is attributed to high levels of oestrogens.[7] The major steroid receptors expressed in human skin, β-type oestrogen receptors, are present in large numbers in hair follicles and mostly localised to nuclei of the outer root sheath, epithelial matrix, and dermal papilla cells. It is possible that increased oestrogen binding to these receptors promotes and prolongs the anagen phase. The hypothesis is further

DOI: 10.1201/9781003449690-6

supported by trichogram evidence of prolonged anagen phase after the use of topical oestrogens in the treatment of female pattern hair loss and also by apparent scalp hair thinning associated with aromatase inhibitors, which prevent synthesis of oestrogens.[8] However, the state of pregnancy is also characterised by dramatic alteration in thyroid hormone, secondary androgens, and prolactin, and it can be hard to differentiate between the effects of other hormones and the effects of oestrogen on scalp hair.[2,7]

The exuberant hair growth during pregnancy is usually followed by excessive shedding of hair within 1–5 months after childbirth and may also be associated with altered hair colour, texture, and curliness. Several factors contribute to postpartum hair loss, including the stress of labour and delivery (fever, surgical stress, mental stress, and blood loss) and changes in endocrine balance. However, an oestrogen-deficient state immediately after postpartum is postulated to be a major driving force behind accelerated and synchronised conversation of anagen hair to telogen hair and subsequent molt-like shedding of the hair.

6.3 DISORDERS OF HAIR DURING PREGNANCY AND POSTPARTUM

6.3.1 HIRSUTISM AND HYPERTRICHOSIS

Hirsutism is defined as the increased growth of terminal hairs in a female in an androgen-dependent fashion (or male pattern distribution), while hypertrichosis is the excessive growth and thickness of hair on any part of the body.[9,10]

Hirsutism is the result of primary or secondary hyperandrogenism or an increased end-organ androgen sensitivity and is often a cause of cosmetic concern amongst young females. Conventionally, the modified Ferriman–Gallwey's (mFG) scoring system is used to assess the severity, and an mFG score ≥ 8 is considered hirsutism, but various studies have shown that this cut-off value may vary for different races.

In pregnancy, hirsutism is more of a physiological phenomenon, and a majority of pregnant women experience it to some extent, generally in the first trimester. Pregnancy-related hirsutism is most prominent among women with thick dark hair and noticeable mainly on the upper lip, chin, and cheeks (Figure 6.1); however, quite generalised hair growth is not infrequent and hypertrichosis is frequently observed over the mid-suprapubic region.[2,11] Fine lanugo hairs fade after 6 months postpartum, but coarse terminal hairs typically persist and can be a cause of cosmetic concern eventually. Moreover, recurrence with subsequent pregnancies is also frequent.[2]

A minor degree of hirsutism and hypertrichosis is common during pregnancy but when associated with signs of overt hyperandrogenism like significant hirsutism, severe acne, male pattern hair

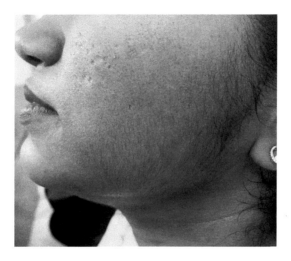

FIGURE 6.1   Hirsutism in a 12-week antenatal woman.

loss, deepening of the voice, and clitoromegaly, further evaluation and the possibility of virilising tumours should be considered. Pre-existing polycystic ovarian disease, benign neoplasms like pregnancy luteoma, or malignant ovarian tumours can present with overt hyperandrogenism secondary to excess androgen and may also lead to masculinised female fetuses.[2,12–14]

6.3.1.1 Treatment

In non-pregnant females, hirsutism is managed with combination of hair removal methods and pharmacotherapy. Hair removal methods include both cosmetic non-permanent measures like depilation, shaving, plucking, chemical depilation, and hair bleaching and permanent hair removal methods like epilation, electrolysis/electroepilation, and photoepilation (Table 6.1).

TABLE 6.1
Hair Removal Methods

Hair Removal Methods	
Cosmetic Measures	
Depilation	Depilation is the removal of the hair shaft from the skin surface.
Shaving	Easiest and patient-administered method.
	Hair is removed down to just below the surface of the skin. It yields a blunt tip of the uncut hair, giving the illusion of thicker hair.
Plucking	Various methods of plucking hairs include the use of tweezers, waxing, sugaring, and threading. Relatively long lasting compared to shaving.
	Associated with tolerable discomfort during the procedure. Localised complications like scarring, folliculitis, and hyperpigmentation can occur.
Chemical depilation	Use of chemicals (2–4% calcium thioglycolate) to dissolve the hair.
Bleaching	It helps to disguise unwanted dark hair by using 6–12% hydrogen peroxide or a 20% ammonia solution.
	Side effects include irritation, pruritus, and possible skin discoloration.
Direct Hair Removal Methods	
Electroepilation/electrolysis	A fine needle is inserted into individual follicles, which are then destroyed using galvanic electrolysis, thermolysis, or a combination of the two.
	Preferred for lightly pigmented hair.
	Regrowth rate of hair with this technique is approximately 40%.
	Major adverse effects of this technique include potential scarring, follicular hyperpigmentation, and pain.
Photoepilation	Removes hair quickly through photo-thermolysis by selectively damaging the pigmented part of the hair follicle while minimising non-selective injury to the surrounding tissues.
	Laser treatments are less painful, are much quicker, and offer better results than electrolysis.
	The ideal patient for photoepilation is one with lighter skin (phototypes I–III) and dark brown to black hair.
	Over the years, many laser systems, including ruby (694 nm), alexandrite (755 nm), diode (800–810 nm), and Nd:YAG (1064 nm) lasers, in addition to a variety of IPL systems with different cut-off filters, have been utilised for photoepilation.
	No system is inherently superior for photoepilation.
	Lighter skin phototypes (I–III) respond better to 755 nm alexandrite or the 800-nm diode laser, while darker skin phototypes (IV–VI) respond better to treatment with the 1064-nm Nd:YAG laser.

Unsatisfactory treatment response due to constant hormonal stimulation during pregnancy, an increased theoretical risk of electrolysis via amniotic fluid during electroepilation, and, in the overall absence of safety data, electrolysis and laser treatment are generally not advised during pregnancy. Topical eflornithine (13.9% cream) used twice daily appears to shorten the anagen phase of hair growth to some extent, and considering the poor systemic absorption, limited use can be permitted in pregnancy. Other systemic therapies such as oral contraceptive pills (OCPs) or antiandrogens were previously classified as Category X drugs and are contraindicated in pregnancy.

Pregnant patients are instead advised to use waxing, shaving, and depilatory lotions to manage excessive hair growth.[11,15] If unwanted hair persists beyond 6 months postpartum, laser hair removal can be considered.[16]

6.3.2 Telogen Effluvium

Telogen effluvium (TE) is a self-limited, diffuse hair loss that typically occurs approximately 2 to 3 months after a triggering event like febrile states, stress, major surgery, altered androgen and oestrogen hormonal profile, and others.[17] Along with diffuse alopecia, patients may have complaints such as tenderness, pain, burning, itching, and stinging. Physical exam findings in TE include shorter regrowing frontal and or bitemporal hair, diffuse hair thinning, and a positive hair pull test. Histopathology reveals an increase in telogen hair follicles but a normal ratio of telogen to vellus follicles and a normal number of hair follicles overall.

Postpartum hair loss is the most common and significant hair complaint which concerns a lactating mother. It is a type of delayed anagen release TE, wherein the elevated levels of oestrogen in circulation during pregnancy promote the lengthening of the anagen phase of the hair cycle and increase the thickness of the hair shaft. After delivery, due to sudden withdrawal of these hormones, numerous hair follicles enter the telogen phase, leading to diffuse hair loss, telogen gravidarum.[2] The recent attempts to reclassify telogen effluvium are based upon an altered teloptosis phase. In adult humans, hairs follow an individual cycle, and hair growth occurs randomly and asynchronously.[4] However, in certain situations hair cycles are synchronised, and collective teloptosis occurs, leading to molt-like shedding.[18]

Gestational diabetes, postnatal decreased levels of thyroxine, iron deficiency due to blood loss during labour, poor nutritional status, and mental/emotional stress during or after delivery can potentially contribute to telogen gravidarum.[19] It is usually seen 1–5 months after childbirth and is most severe during the second and third postpartum months.[16,19,20]

Telogen gravidarum does not have a specific treatment or management protocol; however, nutritional deficiency and subclinical thyroid conditions should be ruled out. The prognosis for hair regrowth is excellent, and most women will return to their usual hair growth cycle and pre-pregnancy thickness within 12 months of birth. Generally, hair loss is a worrisome experience for females and may cause psychosocial anxiety; thus reassurance and appropriate counselling about postpartum alopecia being a common physiological response are the most important therapeutic modalities. Improving nutritional supplementation using ferrous sulphate, L-cysteine, CYP complex, vitamin B12, and vitamin D and ensuring a protein-rich good calorific diet may further help patient alleviate their symptoms and anxiety.[2,16,21]

Telogen gravidarum which is persisting beyond >12 months may be due to common underlying conditions like seborrheic dermatitis, iron deficiency, or hypothyroidism. Persistent hyperprolactinemia (Chiari–Frommel syndrome) and postpartum hypopituitarism (Sheehan syndrome) are other rare conditions which may prolong postpartum TE. Haematological investigations, such as complete blood count (CBC), erythrocyte sedimentation rate (ESR), iron profile, thyroid function tests, and vitamin B12 and D3 levels can be done. Occasionally, persistent telogen gravidarum may unmask underlying hair growth disorders like female androgenetic alopecia and alopecia areata incognito. Scalp biopsy may help differentiate between underlying non-scarring alopecia. Appropriate nutritional supplementation, use of combination of various hair growth peptides, 2% topical minoxidil, PRP therapy, and/or low-level laser therapy can be tried for persistent telogen gravidarum.[21]

6.3.3   FEMALE PATTERN HAIR LOSS

Female pattern hair loss (FPHL) is the most common form of alopecia, usually encountered in middle-aged females, presenting as patterned nonscarring diffuse alopecia, especially involving the central, frontal, and parietal scalp regions. FPHL can present in three different patterns: diffuse thinning of the upper biparietal and vertex regions and preservation of the anterior hair implantation line, thinning of the upper bitemporal region and vertex with frontal accentuation that appears as a triangular or Christmas tree form, and the uncommon pattern of deep recession of the frontal-temporal hairline and true vertex balding; it lacks clinical signs of inflammation, scarring, scaling, or active hair shedding (hair pull test negative) and requires long-term topical, systemic, and adjuvant treatment.[22]

During motherhood, it is often only apparent after the excessive hair shedding in the postpartum period, and the patient may undergo both a telogen gravidarum and then an accelerated process of female pattern hair loss. Rarely, a female in pregnancy may present with male pattern hair loss secondary to virilising tumours.

6.3.3.1   Pathogenesis

Human hair follicles are majorly regulated under the influence of multiple hormones, but in general androgens are considered the main regulator of hair growth. Androgen surge during puberty promotes transformation of vellus to terminal hair over the beard, axillary, trunk, and pubic regions. On the other hand, androgens have a paradoxical effect on hair on the frontal and parietal scalp by decreasing the duration of anagen hair follicles and replacing terminal hair with vellus hair and thus are the main drivers of male pattern hair loss. The role of androgens in FPHL is less clear, and patterned hair loss in females is polygenic and multifactorial.

6.3.3.2   Diagnosis

Hair diameter diversity due to miniaturisation of hair follicles, perifollicular pigmentation/peripilar signs, and yellow dots are common trichoscopic findings. Persistent telogen gradvidarum, diffused alopecia areata, and patterned cicatricial alopecia are common differentials for FPHL, in case history and clinical presentation are inconclusive. An increased number of miniaturised hair follicles and decreased anagen to telogen ratio on histopathology are suggestive of FPHL.

6.3.3.3   Treatment

A plethora of pharmaceutical and non-pharmaceutical treatment options are available for non-pregnant females with FPHL. The most commonly used agent is topical minoxidil (2%, 5%) preparation: 1 mL of minoxidil is applied over the area of hair loss at 12-hour intervals with peak effect seen at a 1-year interval. Antiandrogens (finasteride, dutasteride, and spironolactone) and oral minoxidil, though not FDA approved for females, are frequently used in non-pregnant women for FPHL with good results. The newer modalities of treatment are also used as adjuvants despite no conclusive evidence of direct benefit yet. These include topical use of caffeine, melatonin, proanthocyanidins, saw palmetto, oral biotin, L-cysteine and L-arginine supplementation, platelet rich plasma therapy, microneedling, and low-level laser therapy.[23]

In women who are planning pregnancy, the conventional topical minoxidil can be continued until they get pregnant but should be stopped once they conceive, while all other systemic anti-androgens should be stopped a month prior before planning for conception. All pregnant patients should be counselled against the use of all conventional pharmacotherapeutic options for female pattern hair loss. The newer topical medical modalities like caffeine and melatonin are poorly absorbed from skin and can be used during pregnancy. Platelet rich plasma (PRP) therapy falls into the category of "minimally manipulated tissue" and is therefore exempt from the FDA's mandated animal studies and clinical trials. Adjuvant therapy with microneedling and PRP can be tried during the second and early third trimester but is best deferred to postpartum considering the added risk of potential sepsis.

In lactating mothers with FPHL postpartum, 2% topical minoxidil is safe to prescribe. Oral spironolactone appears to be acceptable to use during breastfeeding.[24]

6.4 OTHERS

6.4.1 Alopecia Areata

Alopecia areata (AA) is an autoimmune condition that targets the hair follicles and results in non-scarring hair loss involving any hair-bearing area with no inflammatory signs. The severity varies from small patches of hair loss to complete alopecia. Anagen-stage hair follicles (HFs) exhibit relative "immune privilege" (IP) status from the bulge level to the bulb. This IP status is dependent on absent or minimal expression of intra-follicular MHC class I and II molecules and prominent expression of safe or immunoinhibitory signals like CD200. In AA, interferon-gamma (IFN-γ) cytokine upregulates local expression of MHC class-1 protein and makes hair follicles prone to attack by CD8+ T cells and other immune cells. Alopecia areata is frequently associated with other common autoimmune conditions, further suggesting a role of autoimmunity. Pregnancy-associated hormonal changes and overall psychosocial stress associated with pregnancy can occasionally trigger the onset of AA (Figure 6.2), suggesting a capacity to alter susceptibility to disease onset.[25] The apparent effect of altered hormonal state in pregnancy on alopecia areata is not well documented; however, both luxuriant hair regrowth in chronic AA totalis and apparent onset of AA during pregnancy have been infrequently reported.[10] The improved hair growth in pre-existing AA is transient and relapses postpartum.

6.4.1.1 Clinical Features

AA usually presents as single- or multiple-circumscribed, smooth patches of hair loss involving any hair-bearing area of the body. Multiple patches may coalesce later to form large areas of hair loss, which may evolve in certain specific patterns or progress to involve the whole scalp (alopecia totalis) or loss of hair on the whole body (alopecia universalis). Another severe acute variant, alopecia areata incognita, is more commonly seen in women and presents as severe hair loss and diffuse scalp hair thinning, mimicking telogen effluvium. The hair on the alopecia patch, being weak, tends to kink when forced inwards around 5–10 mm above the scalp surface, and this has been described as "coudability sign". The periphery of the affected scalp may reveal exclamatory mark hair and a positive hair pull test. Dermoscopy of the patch often shows prominent yellow dots, black dots, broken hair, vellus hairs, and exclamation mark hairs.

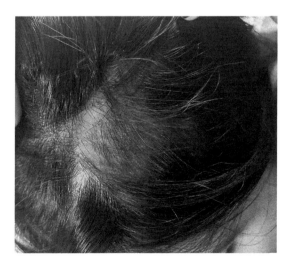

FIGURE 6.2 New-onset alopecia areata patch in a 20-week antenatal woman.

Histopathology of alopecia areata shows dense intrafollicular and perifollicular infiltration resembling a "swarm of bees". This inflammatory infiltration mostly consists of activated T cells mixed with Langerhans cells, macrophages, and cells expressing natural killer cell markers.

6.4.1.2 Treatment

Spontaneous recovery is seen in up to half of patients with single or limited patch disease. Waiting and watching for such patients during pregnancy is an ideal choice.

Topical steroids are commonly prescribed for limited patch disease. Mid-potent or potent topical steroids can be safely used in pregnancy, but lower-potency preparations should be preferred.[26,27] These agents are often used along with irritants like anthralin and keratolytic agents like benzoic acid and salicylic acids (<3%). All these agents are relatively safe and can be used during pregnancy and/or lactation considering their poor systemic absorption.[28,29] Salicylic acid–based products should preferably be used less than 20 g per day and without occlusion.[30]

Intralesional corticosteroids (triamcinolone acetonide 2.5–10 mg/mL) are also commonly used in adults with patchy AA. They are injected in the deep dermis/upper subcutaneous tissue plane, 0.1 mL at multiple sites, 1 cm apart, and repeated after 4–6 weeks. First-trimester exposure to triamcinolone is associated with an increased frequency of congenital anomalies in animal studies, while the initial human data on corticosteroids during early pregnancy show they have been inconsistently associated with orofacial clefts in the offspring and should be avoided, especially during embryogenesis.[31]

Given their potential teratogenic effects and the fact that their potential for systemic absorption is yet unknown, topical sensitisers shouldn't be used during pregnancy.[32]

Systemic therapy is mainly used for multifocal AA, patterned AA, alopecia totalis, and alopecia universalis. Systemic corticosteroids can be used as daily, weekly, or monthly pulses but carry a modest increase in the risk of cleft lip with or without palate, especially during the first trimester.[33] Jak-Stat inhibitors, tofacitinib (off label), baricitinib (FDA approved 2022), and Ritlecitinib (FDA approved 2023) have shown good results and are now being employed for the treatment of severe alopecia areata. However, due to a lack of safety data, Jak stat inhibitors are best avoided during pregnancy and the lactation period.

Phototherapy is another alternative which can be tried for multifocal alopecia areata in pregnant females. Narrow-band UV-B therapy and a 308-nm excimer laser are safer options that can be explored in pregnant females who warrant but are not willing to use systemic therapy.[34,35]

6.4.2 PEDICULOSIS CAPITIS

Pediculosis capitis, or head louse infestation, caused by *Pediculus humanus* var. *capitis*, is one of the most common ectoparasitic infestations and can cause significant distress and discomfort in pregnant females or nursing mothers. Patients with head lice infestations are often asymptomatic but can have itching, mild allergic reactions, irritability, and secondary bacterial infections. A thorough search along with vigorous combing for lice and nits can help in diagnosis.

6.4.2.1 Treatment

Permethrin (Category B) 1% lotion is the recommended treatment for both pregnant and lactating women with pediculosis.[36] After washing the hair with a non-conditioning shampoo and towel drying, permethrin is applied to damp hair until fully saturated, left on for 10–20 minutes, and rinsed off, and then the nits and eggs are combed out with a fine-toothed comb. Permethrin leaves a residue on the hair which is fatal for nymphs emerging from nits not killed after the first application; thus shampooing of hair should be avoided for 24 to 48 hours. A repeat application is recommended between days 9 and 10 after initial treatment. In order to reduce extensive systemic absorption, permethrin should be rinsed off from the hair over a sink instead of a shower or bath.[37] All household members and close contacts should be screened and treated.

Topical ivermectin 1% lotion may be used if permethrin is not effective. A topical suspension of spinosad 0.9% (Category B drug) can also be used. Oral ivermectin is not recommended for use by pregnant women but can be safely used by lactating mothers.[38]

6.4.3 Tinea Capitis

Tinea capitis is infection of the scalp hair follicles and surrounding skin caused by the *Microsporum* and *Trichophyton genera* of dermatophyte species. The most commonly implicated agents are *Trichophyton violaceum* and *T. tonsurans*. Tinea capitis can be inflammatory and noninflammatory. Kerion, favus, abscess, and pustular (agminate folliculitis) are types of inflammatory tinea capitis. Noninflammatory types are grey patch, black dot, seborrheic dermatitis kie, and smooth patch of baldness types.

6.4.3.1 Treatment

Ideally, tinea capitis should be treated with systemic antifungals; however, in pregnancy, systemic antifungals should be deferred until after delivery/lactation, and topical therapy alone should be used. If absolutely required, terbinafine (Category B) is the agent of choice in pregnancy and can be used at 250 mg per day for 2–4 weeks.

6.5 SAFETY OF HAIR PRODUCTS AND PROCEDURES DURING PREGNANCY AND LACTATION

6.5.1 Prescription Medications

1. **Minoxidil**
   - Topical minoxidil (2% solution and 5% foam) is the most commonly prescribed FDA-approved therapeutic option for female pattern hair loss. The anti-hypertensive opens potassium channels, leading to an increased cutaneous blood flow, enhanced levels of vascular endothelial growth factor, and hair growth promoters in the dermal papilla.
   - Minoxidil is a Category C (non-PLR format) drug; however, multiple case reports and series have described fetal minoxidil syndrome. It is characterised by a constellation of symptoms and congenital malformations following accidental maternal exposure to oral or topical minoxidil. Reversible hypertrichosis and neurodevelopmental, gastrointestinal, renal cardiac, and limb malformations have been reported.[39–41,4]
   - Though the use of minoxidil is not advised for pregnant females, the American Academy of Paediatrics considers topical minoxidil relatively safe during lactation, and thus it may be used postpartum.[42]

2. **Antiandrogen Therapies**
   5-Alpha-Reductase Inhibitors

   Finasteride
   - Finasteride is a type 2 5-alpha-reductase inhibitor that decreases the conversion of testosterone to dihydrotestosterone (DHT) and prevents the miniaturisation of hair in males. Though several case series and trials have shown some success with both oral and topical finasteride in FPHL, its mechanism of action is not fully understood, and it is presently used as an off-label indication.[43]
   - Considering the potent teratogenic effect of finasteride on the genitalia of male fetuses, women who are already expecting or could possibly get pregnant should not be prescribed oral or topical finasteride. In contrast, finasteride levels in semen are incredibly low and do not endanger a male fetus in a pregnant sexual partner and thus can be safely used by male partners.[44]

Dutasteride

- Dutasteride blocks the activity of both type 1 and type 2 5-alpha-reductase isoenzymes and reduces DHT serum levels more potently. Few studies have shown better efficacy than finasteride in FPHL, but its use is largely limited to male patients with patterned baldness. Dutasteride has a longer half-life in comparison to finasteride and thus needs to be more cautiously prescribed in women in the reproductive age group. It carries the same teratogenic risk to male fetuses and shouldn't be prescribed to expecting mothers or those planning pregnancies.[39,45]

Androgen Receptor Antagonists
Spironolactone

- Spironolactone is a potassium-sparing diuretic that blocks androgen receptors in peripheral target tissues, thereby reducing testosterone levels. It has been used to treat FPHL (off-label) for many years and provides significant results with tolerable adverse effect profiles.[39,45,46]
- Just like other antiandrogen therapies, spironolactone affects sex differentiation in male fetuses during embryogenesis. Additionally, spironolactone can lead to uncontrolled hypertension in pregnant females and carry an increased risk of cardiac failure and liver cirrhosis in both mother and fetus.

3. **Corticosteroids**
   - Systemic corticosteroids have an immunosuppressive and anti-inflammatory role to play in both scarring alopecia and alopecia areata. The FDA classified systemic corticosteroids as former Pregnancy Category C; however, use of oral corticosteroids during first trimester of pregnancy has been causally associated with cleft lip with or without cleft palate.
   - If systemic corticosteroid treatment cannot be avoided, non-halogenated corticosteroids which are enzymatically inactivated in the placenta are preferred. Prednisone, prednisolone, and cortisol are thus inactivated by placental 11beta-hydroxysteroid dehydrogenase type 2, resulting in suitable maternal-fetal exposure of approximately 10:1. Small doses (≤20 mg/day prednisolone) given for a short-course period is generally safe.
   - In lactating mothers, systemic corticosteroids are considered safe, and patients should be advised to avoid breastfeeding for 4 hours after dosage.
   - Intralesional steroid injections (triamcinolone acetonide) are a frontline treatment option for limited alopecia areata and provide good results with acceptable local adverse effects. First-trimester exposure to triamcinolone is associated with increased frequency of congenital anomalies in animal studies and inconclusive risk in humans and should be avoided, especially during embryogenesis.
   - Use of topical corticosteroids during pregnancy has shown no casual association of maternal exposure and pregnancy outcome, irrespective of the potency of the agent.[47]

4. **Platelet-Rich Plasma Therapy**
   - Platelet rich plasma is often used as an adjuvant for management of androgenetic alopecia and persistent telogen gravidarum. It involves extracting and concentrating platelets from whole blood and then injecting them into the scalp. It is usually offered postpartum and is not indicated in pregnancy considering the added risk of potential sepsis.

5. **Scalp Biopsy**
   - Skin or scalp biopsy with lidocaine for local anaesthesia can be done safely any time during pregnancy and doesn't require any special modification. A small quantity of epinephrine used during local anaesthesia for biopsies is also considered safe.

6.5.2 Non-Prescription Products and Procedures

1. **Hair Dyes**
   - The current literature doesn't provide concrete evidence regarding the safety of hair dyes and other hair care products during pregnancy.
   - Permanent hair colour products usually contain phenylenediamine, aminophenol, resorcinol, toluene-2,5-diaminesulphate, sodium sulphite, oleic acid, sodium hydroxide, ammonium hydroxide, propylene glycol, and isopropyl alcohol. In animal studies, some of these chemicals have shown an increased risk of teratogenicity when used in high doses. In humans, systemic absorption of these chemicals as part of hair dye is very limited unless the scalp has bare exposed skin, and thus they are unlikely to reach the placenta in substantial amounts. A Brazilian case-control survey-based study found some association between first-trimester maternal exposure to hair dyes and hair-straightening cosmetics and the development of early myeloid or lymphocytic leukaemia in their children.[48] Another study conducted in China showed that prolonged and constant pre-pregnancy hair dye exposure was associated with increased incidence of low birth weight, while a Black women's health study on use of hair relaxers revealed no significant association with preterm birth.[49,50]
   - Though hair dyes are minimally absorbed and limited inadvertent use doesn't carry serious teratogenic risk, the general recommendation is to avoid chemical-based products during the first trimester and to use relatively safe alternatives like vegetable based pure henna (*Lawsonia alba*) for hair colouring.[51–53] Female hairdressers who are constantly exposed to these products should ideally work for less than 35 hours per week in a well-ventilated work place with strict use of gloves and possible avoidance of prolonged standing and awkward positions.[53–55]

2. **Hair-Straightening Products**
   - Keratin treatment, hair rebonding, and hair smoothing are a few options available for smoothing and straightening curly hair. These procedures use a variety of powerful chemicals like methylene glycol, methanediol, methanal, and others to break the hydrogen and disulphide bonds of keratin molecules and seal the new molecular crosslinks in a pin-straight alignment using high heat. The entire process lasts a few hours and invariably leads to the production of formaldehyde, a potent toxic and teratogenic gas. Formaldehyde exposure is casually but not conclusively associated with increased risk of spontaneous abortion, perinatal complications, and congenital malformations.[56,57] All these procedures should ideally be avoided during pregnancy.
   - Pregnant hairdressers who work with such products regularly are advised to use non-latex synthetic-based impervious material gloves and a filter cartridge mask or a full mask with a face shield to avoid exposure.[57]

3. **Leave-On Hair Products**
   - Leave-on hair products often contain phthalates, which are well known for their endocrine-disrupting potential. Phthalates have not been associated with congenital defects in humans, but animal studies have shown these substances interfere with male sexual development, so caution is warranted. Overall exposure to phthalate-containing products should be reduced proactively.
   - Use of hair dyes, hair-straightening, and leave-on hair products is generally considered safe during lactation as long as there is no direct exposure to infants.

4. **Shampoos and Conditioners**
   - The regular over-the-counter sulphate-based shampoos used for a minimal contact period and over a limited surface area do not seem to increase any maternal or fetal risk.

- Ketoconazole-based shampoos and lotions, owing to their poor systemic absorption, are safe to use during pregnancy, although systemic ketoconazole is associated with feminisation of male fetuses. Coal tar is one of the major constituents of permanent and semi-permanent hair dyes and is also used in anti-dandruff shampoos. Human studies are limited, and use of coal tar-based products should be avoided during the first trimester.

6.6   CONCLUSION

The state of pregnancy is marked by gross physiological and morphological changes.

Hypertrichosis, hirsutism, postpartum hair loss, and patterned hair loss can potentially be a cause of anxiety and add to the overwhelming experience of motherhood. Pre-existing hair disorders become secondary concerns in the overall care and management of pregnancy, but switching to safe prescription drugs prior to and during pregnancy is crucial for the safety of both the mother and the child. In-depth counselling, guidance about the safety of non-prescription products/procedures, and empowering patients with safe therapeutic options are key to the holistic management of hair disorders during pregnancy. The unsaid dictum is to perform any dermatological procedure preferably in the postpartum period or during the relatively safe second trimester (weeks 13–24). The first trimester is crucial for organogenesis and may increase the risk of spontaneous abortion, while any inadvertent incident during third trimester carries an increased risk of preterm labour.[58]

REFERENCES

1. Motosko CC, Bieber AK, Pomeranz MK, et al. Physiologic changes of pregnancy: A review of the literature. *Int J Women's Dermatol* 2017;3(4):219–224.
2. Ingber A. Hair and nails. In: *Obstetric Dermatology: A Practical Guide*. Berlin, Heidelberg: Springer; 2009, pp. 19–24.
3. Vogt A, McElwee KJ, Blume-Peytavi U. Biology of the hair follicle. In: Whitting DA, Blume-Peytavi U, Tosti A, Trüeb RM, eds. *Hair Growth and Disorders*. Berlin, Heidelberg: Springer; 2008, pp. 1–22.
4. Lynfield YL. Effect of pregnancy on the human hair cycle. *J Invest Dermatol* 1960;35:323–327.
5. Headington JT. Telogen effluvium: New concepts and review. *Arch Dermatol* 1993;129(3):356–363.
6. Trüeb RM. Diagnosis and treatment. In: Trüeb RM, ed. *Female Alopecia: Guide to Successful Management*. Berlin, Heidelberg: Springer; 2013, pp. 59–151.
7. Gizlenti S, Ekmekci TR. The changes in the hair cycle during gestation and the postpartum period. *J Eur Acad Dermatol Venereol* 2014;28(7):878–881.
8. Thornton MJ. Oestrogen functions in skin and skin appendages. *Expert Opin Ther Targets* 2005;9(3):617–629.
9. Messenger AG, Sinclair RD, Farrant P, de Berker DAR. Acquired disorders of hair. In: *Rook's Textbook of Dermatology*, 9th ed. United Kingdom: Wiley; 2016, pp. 1–88.
10. Camacho-Martínez FM. Hypertrichosis. In: Whitting DA, Blume-Peytavi U, Tosti A, Trüeb RM, eds. *Hair Growth and Disorders*. Berlin, Heidelberg: Springer; 2008, pp. 333–356.
11. Nussbaum R, Benedetto AV. Cosmetic aspects of pregnancy. *Clin Dermatol* 2006;24(2):133–141.
12. Mvunta DH, Amiji F, Suleiman M, et al. Hirsutism caused by pregnancy luteoma in a low-resource setting: A case report and literature review. *Case Rep Obstet Gynecol* 2021;2021:e6695117.
13. Papantoniou N, Belitsos P, Hatzipapas I, et al. Excessive hirsutism in pregnancy because of Krukenberg tumor. *J Maternal-Fetal Neonatal Med* 2012;25(6):869–871.
14. Millikan L. Hirsutism, postpartum telogen effluvium, and male pattern alopecia. *J Cosmet Dermatol* 2006;5(1):81–86.
15. Trivedi MK, Kroumpouzos G, Murase JE. A review of the safety of cosmetic procedures during pregnancy and lactation. *Int J Women's Dermatol* 2017;3(1):6–10.
16. Bechtel MA. Physiologic skin changes in pregnancy. In: Tyler KH, ed. *Cutaneous Disorders of Pregnancy*. Cham: Springer; 2020, pp. 3–12.
17. Malkud S. Telogen effluvium: A review. *J Clin Diagn Res* 2015;9(9):WE01–WE03.

18. Rebora A. Proposing a simpler classification of telogen effluvium. *Skin Appendage Disord* 2016;2(1–2): 35–38.
19. Ebrahimzadeh-Ardakani M, Ansari K, Pourgholamali H, Sadri Z. Investigating the prevalence of postpartum hair loss and its associated risk factors: A cross-sectional study. *Iran J Dermatol* 2021; 24(4):295–299.
20. Bergfeld CB, Wilma F. Telogen effluvium. In: McMichael A, Hordinsky M, eds. *Hair and Scalp Disorders*, 2nd ed. London: CRC Press; 2018.
21. Raj Kirit EP, Kumar AS. Chronic telogen effluvium. In: *IADVL Textbook of Trichology*. India: Jaypee Brothers; 2018.
22. Fabbrocini G, Cantelli M, Masarà A, et al. Female pattern hair loss: A clinical, pathophysiologic, and therapeutic review. *Int J Women's Dermatol* 2018;4(4):203–211.
23. Nirmal B. Recent advances in medical management. In: *IADVL Textbook of Trichology*. India: Jaypee Brothers Medical Publishers; 2018.
24. Spironolactone. In: *Drugs and Lactation Database (LactMed®)*. Bethesda, MD: National Institute of Child Health and Human Development; 2006.
25. Freyschmidt-Paul P, Hoffmann R, McElwee KJ. Alopecia areata. In: Whitting DA, Blume-Peytavi U, Tosti A, Trüeb RM, eds. *Hair Growth and Disorders*. Berlin, Heidelberg: Springer; 2008, pp. 311–332.
26. Andersson NW, Skov L, Andersen JT. Evaluation of topical corticosteroid use in pregnancy and risk of newborns being small for gestational age and having low birth weight. *JAMA Dermatol* 2021;157(7):788–795.
27. Alabdulrazzaq F, Koren G. Topical corticosteroid use during pregnancy. *Can Fam Physician* 2012;58(6):643–644.
28. Bozzo P, Chua-Gocheco A, Einarson A. Safety of skin care products during pregnancy. *Can Fam Physician* 2011;57(6):665–667.
29. Little B. Use of dermatologics during pregnancy. In: *Drugs and Pregnancy*. London: CRC Press; 2006.
30. Ferreira C, Azevedo A, Nogueira M, Torres T. Management of psoriasis in pregnancy—a review of the evidence to date. *Drugs Context* 2020;9:2019–11–6.
31. Little BB. *Drugs and Pregnancy: A Handbook*, 2nd ed. Boca Raton: CRC Press; 2022.
32. Vincenzi C, Marisaldi B, Tosti A. Topical Immunotherapy: Step by Step [Internet]. In: Tosti A, Asz-Sigall D, Pirmez R, eds. *Hair and Scalp Treatments: A Practical Guide*. Cham: Springer; 2020, pp. 25–33.
33. Bandoli G, Palmsten K, Forbess Smith CJ, Chambers CD. A review of systemic corticosteroid use in pregnancy and the risk of select pregnancy and birth outcomes. *Rheum Dis Clin North Am* 2017;43(3):489–502.
34. Zakaria W, Passeron T, Ostovari N, et al. 308-nm excimer laser therapy in alopecia areata. *J Am Acad Dermatol* 2004;51(5):837–838.
35. Welsh O. Phototherapy for alopecia areata. *Clin Dermatol* 2016;34(5):628–632.
36. Patel VM, Lambert WC, Schwartz RA. Safety of topical medications for scabies and lice in pregnancy. *Indian J Dermatol* 2016;61(6):583–587.
37. Madke B, Khopkar U. Pediculosis capitis: An update. *IJDVL* 2012;78:429.
38. Harrison CV. Management of dermatological conditions in pregnancy [Internet]. In: Mattison D, Halbert LA, eds. *Clinical Pharmacology during Pregnancy*, 2nd ed. Boston: Academic Press; 2022, pp. 357–375.
39. Kelly Y, Tosti A. Androgenetic alopecia: Clinical treatment [Internet]. In: Tosti A, Asz-Sigall D, Pirmez R, eds. *Hair and Scalp Treatments: A Practical Guide*. Cham: Springer; 2020, pp. 91–108.
40. Smorlesi C, Caldarella A, Caramelli L, et al. Topically applied minoxidil may cause fetal malformation: A case report. *Birth Defects Res A Clin Mol Teratol* 2003;67(12):997–1001.
41. Rampon G, Henkin C, Souza PRM de, Almeida Jr HL de. Infantile generalized hypertrichosis caused by topical minoxidil. *An Bras Dermatol* 2016;91:87–88.
42. American Academy of Pediatrics Committee on Drugs. Transfer of drugs and other chemicals into human milk. *Pediatrics* 2001;108(3):776–789.
43. Iamsumang W, Leerunyakul K, Suchonwanit P. Finasteride and its potential for the treatment of female pattern hair loss: Evidence to date. *Drug Des Devel Ther* 2020;14:951–959.
44. McMichael A, Hordinsky Maria K, eds. *Hair and Scalp Disorders: Medical, Surgical, and Cosmetic Treatments*, 2nd ed. London: CRC Press; 2018.
45. Brough KR, Torgerson RR. Hormonal therapy in female pattern hair loss. *Int J Womens Dermatol* 2017;3(1):53–57.
46. Burns LJ, Souza BD, Flynn E, et al. Spironolactone for treatment of female pattern hair loss. *J Am Acad Dermatol* 2020;83(1):276–278.
47. Chi C, Wang S, Wojnarowska F, et al. Safety of topical corticosteroids in pregnancy. *Cochrane Database Syst Rev* 2015;2015(10):CD007346.

48. Couto AC, Ferreira JD, Rosa ACS, et al. Pregnancy, maternal exposure to hair dyes and hair straightening cosmetics, and early age leukemia. *Chem Biol Interact* 2013;205(1):46–52.
49. Jiang C, Hou Q, Huang Y, et al. The effect of pre-pregnancy hair dye exposure on infant birth weight: A nested case-control study. *BMC Pregnancy Childb* 2018;18(1):144.
50. Rosenberg L, Wise LA, Palmer JR. Hair-relaxer use and risk of preterm birth among African-American women. *Ethn Dis* 2005;15(4):768–772.
51. American College of Obstetricians and Gynecologists. *Is It Safe to Dye My Hair during Pregnancy?* [Internet]. Available from: www.acog.org/en/womens-health/experts-and-stories/ask-acog/is-it-safe-to-dye-my-hair-during-pregnancy
52. Johns Hopkins All Children's Hospital. *Using Hair Dyes and Color During Pregnancy* [Internet]. Available from: www.hopkinsallchildrens.org/Patients-Families/Health-Library/HealthDocNew/Using-Hair-Dyes-and-Color-During-Pregnancy
53. Chua-Gocheco A, Bozzo P, Einarson A. Safety of hair products during pregnancy. *Can Fam Physician* 2008;54(10):1386–1388.
54. Halliday-Bell JA, Gissler M, Jaakkola JJK. Work as a hairdresser and cosmetologist and adverse pregnancy outcomes. *Occup Med* 2009;59(3):180–184.
55. Peters C, Harling M, Dulon M, et al. Fertility disorders and pregnancy complications in hairdressers—a systematic review. *J Occupational Med Toxicol* 2010;5(1):24.
56. Haffner MJ, Oakes P, Demerdash A, et al. Formaldehyde exposure and its effects during pregnancy: Recommendations for laboratory attendance based on available data. *Clin Anat* 2015;28(8):972–979.
57. Barreto T, Weffort F, Frattini S, et al. Straight to the point: What do we know so far on hair straightening? *Skin Appendage Disord* 2021;7(4):265–271.
58. Villasenor-Park J. Dermatologic surgery in pregnancy. In: Tyler KH, ed. *Cutaneous Disorders of Pregnancy*. Cham: Springer; 2020, pp. 113–121.

7 Acne and Rosacea during Pregnancy

Valencia Long and Nisha Suyien Chandran

7.1 ACNE

7.1.1 INTRODUCTION

Acne vulgaris is a condition affecting the pilosebaceous unit with a peak incidence in adolescence. It can also affect individuals during pregnancy and lactation. Acne shows a predominance for females through all decades of adolescent and adult life (1).

The pathogenesis of acne is multifactorial. Updated literature on acne pathogenesis suggests that it is a result of an interplay of various endogenous and exogenous factors, yet very precise mechanisms remain elusive. Historically, four main mechanisms have been described: abnormal follicular hyperkeratinisation, excess sebum production influenced by androgen release, over-colonisation of pilosebaceous units by *Cutibacterium acnes* (*C. acnes*, previously known as *Propionibacterium acnes*; *P. acnes*), and inflammation (2). Interactions between genetic, hormonal, and environmental factors play a crucial role in pathogenesis (3). More recent studies have also suggested the role of skin dysbiosis, where there is an imbalance of skin microbiota, as the skin microbiomes of individuals with acne had been shown to differ significantly when compared to healthy controls (4,5). Resultant proliferation of *C. acnes* leads to the inflammatory cascade, activating innate immunity through expression of protease activated receptors (PARs) and toll-like receptors (TLRs) and the production of inflammatory interleukins, tumour necrosis factor, and matrix metalloproteinases (MMPs) by keratinocytes which in turn causes hyperkeratinisation of the pilosebaceous unit (6).

7.1.2 DISEASE PROGRESSION OF ACNE THROUGH PREGNANCY

Studies reflect that up to 43% of people experience acne during pregnancy (7–9). In a study by Dréno et al. involving 378 pregnant patients, the majority (86.6%) had had acne previously, with relapse during pregnancy of previously cured acne occurring in a third of cases. Half (51.5%) of the cases had unabating acne since adolescence. Pregnancy was noted to be a period of worsening (59.7%), improvement (9.1%), or no change (31.2%) in acne severity (9).

Several studies cited that young pregnant women, especially those ≤25 years of age, had more frequent truncal acne and tended to have severe to very severe acne (9,10). As the pregnancy progresses, there are mixed observations on whether acne improves or worsens. Different subgroups may behave differently. For instance, in a Turkish study of 295 pregnant individuals (10), there was more frequent occurrence of acne during the first and second trimester, compared to a Taiwanese study (8) which revealed more acne in the second and third trimester.

During the first 9 weeks of pregnancy, the corpus luteum and, to a lesser extent, the maternal ovary and the adrenal cortex, contribute to circulating concentrations of maternal oestradiol, estrone, and progesterone (11,12). After this period, the placenta becomes the predominant source of maternal steroid hormones (12). In normal pregnancies, existing literature confirms the substantial increase in maternal serum concentrations of oestradiol, estrone, and progesterone throughout pregnancy. Comparatively, longitudinal studies establish that there is a weaker and more gradual increase in

DOI: 10.1201/9781003449690-7

testosterone concentration across gestation (11). Prolactin, which is produced by the pituitary gland, increases throughout pregnancy. Studies reflect that prolactin levels increase, likely from the stimulatory effect of oestradiol, and to a lesser extent progesterone, on the pituitary gland (13).

In the first trimester, when a significant surge of beta-human chronic gonadotropin takes place, androgen production is stimulated and can induce acne (14). In the second and third trimesters, the levels of oestrogen and progesterone rise even higher than the premenstrual elevation, while the circulating testosterone continues to increase slightly (15). Although oestrogens antagonise the effects of androgens, a parallel surge of progesterone levels can aggravate acne by stimulation of sebum secretion and keratinocyte proliferation. High levels of prolactin in the third trimester also lead to increased secretion of sebum in the skin, directly or indirectly, through partly androgen-dependent pathways that contribute to worsening acne (16–18).

The effect of fetal genders on the maternal plasma level of testosterone is controversial. Although there are reports of an association between female gender of the fetus and higher acne severity, Kuijper et al. demonstrated in a systematic review that maternal serum testosterone concentrations showed no fetal gender-related differences (20) This suggests that factors other than fetal genders cause maternal hormonal changes.

Several risk factors have been suggested to be associated with severe acne in pregnancy. These include young age (≤25 years old), primigravida state, previous irregular menstruation, presence of polycystic ovary syndrome, high maternal weight, female gender of the fetus, and low birth weight for gestational age of the fetus (8,9).

The exact distribution of facial acne during pregnancy varies in different studies. In Yang et al.'s study, cheeks (62%) were most commonly involved, followed by the perioral and mandibular area (37.1%) (8). In contrast, a French study (9) demonstrated that the mandibular region (69.1%) was most commonly affected. In a Turkish study (10), the cheeks and perioral areas were among the most commonly affected areas in the face.

7.1.3 Pathophysiological Targets for Acne Management

Treatment algorithms for acne management may be based upon the recommendations from the Global Alliance to Improve Outcomes in Acne workgroup (21). and the European Evidence-based S3 acne guidelines (22). Updated acne pathogenesis implicates these major factors: androgen-dependent sebogenesis, hyperkeratinisation of the pilosebaceous unit, skin dysbiosis and the proliferation of *C. acnes*, and inflammation (23). Androgens drive sebogenesis, whilst oestrogen decreases serum production. Studies have shown that high local expression and hyperresponsiveness of the androgens in the skin can influence the formation of acne lesions (24). Acne is also known to be focused around the pilosebaceous unit. When hyperkeratinisation occurs in the follicular infundibulum, keratohyaline granules increase in numbers and size, resulting in increased numbers of sticky laminated corneocytes (25). In terms of microbial colonisation of the follicular unit, *C. acnes* has been implicated as a key player in acne pathogenesis, triggering inflammatory responses through innate immunity, and maintains inflammation by acquired cell-mediated responses through Th1 cells (24). *C. acnes* causes the release of extracellular enzymes, reactive oxygen, sebum production, keratin, filaggrin, and IGF, in turn resulting in inflammation and hyperkeratosis (26).

Based on these implicated factors, the armamentarium for acne treatment has included antimicrobials (topical and oral), retinoids and retinoid derivatives (topical and oral), and benzoyl peroxide. In the following section, all available agents for women and men are discussed, with separate considerations for pregnant and lactating individuals addressed subsequently.

7.1.3.1 Targets for Sebogenesis

In recent years, the topical anti-androgen agent clascoterone has attained FDA approval for topical treatment in patients 12 years of age and older. By competing with androgens for binding to androgen receptors, clascoterone blocks androgen receptor signalling cascades—which in turn leads to reduced sebaceous gland proliferation, sebum production, and inflammation (27). Traditional medications to reduce sebogenesis otherwise included isotretinoin (which inhibits sebum production and inhibit the size of the sebaceous glands), combined oral contraceptives (COCs), and spironolactone. The main antiandrogenic effect of COCs is through oestrogen's ability to increase sex hormone-binding globulins, leading to a decrease in free testosterone available for receptors (28). Progestins in birth control may also exert anti-androgenic effects through antagonistic mechanisms (28). Last, spironolactone may be used off-label for the treatment of acne and reduces testosterone levels by a direct inhibition of the 17α-hydroxylase enzyme required in testosterone biosynthesis (29).

7.1.3.2 Targets for Hyperkeratinisation

Retinoids can regulate abnormal keratinisation in the infundibulum of acne lesions. Since 2019, fourth-generation topical retinoid (trifarotene), which specifically targets retinoid acid receptor gamma, had also attained FDA approval for the topical treatment of acne vulgaris in patients 9 years and older (30). BPO is able to exert comedolytic effects, and a combination of adapalene and BPO has been shown to decrease the expression of TLR2 ex vivo (31). Oral isotretinoin also inhibits hyperkeratosis in the infundibulum and blocks TLRs (32).

7.1.3.3 Targets for Microbial Colonisation and Inflammation

Agents that target microbial colonisation include benzoyl peroxide (BPO) and antimicrobials. BPO acts on the bacterial cell wall, ribosomes, and DNA gyrase to inhibit bacterial growth and inflammation in acne. BPO is also comedolytic and can inhibit the production of *C. acnes* biofilms (33). Antimicrobials may have bactericidal or bacteriostatic effects on *C. acnes*. Of these, antibiotics like tetracyclines may also inhibit bacterial DNA gyrase/bacterial protein synthesis, and exert inhibitory effects on inflammatory cytokines such as IL-6/8.

7.1.4 PRINCIPLES OF THERAPEUTIC SELECTION FOR PREGNANT AND LACTATING INDIVIDUALS

First Trimester (Weeks 0 to 13)

During the first 2 weeks of gestation, drugs tend to affect all cells equally, resulting in spontaneous abortion rather than a congenital anomaly. Organogenesis occurs in the 2nd to 8th week of gestation—and is a period where teratogenic drugs should be avoided. Historically, these drugs were labelled FDA Category X or D.

Second Trimester (Weeks 14–26)

During this period of fetal growth, drugs administered have the potential to affect the maturation of fetal organs. This is pertinent for instance, during the selection of antimicrobials and anti-androgenic agents (tetracyclines, which are commonly used in the general population, are contraindicated after 15 weeks of gestation due to deposition in fetal teeth and bones with subsequent malformations, and spironolactone leading to feminisation of the male fetus).

Third Trimester (Weeks 27–40)

In late pregnancy, tetratogenicity is less of a concern, as organogenesis has now been completed. Drugs administered in this period may directly affect the newborn. For example, dapsone may increase the risk of neonatal hyperbilirubinemia and kernicterus if administered in the last month of gestation (34).

7.1.4.1 Previous Pregnancy-Risk Categories

Historically, systems that rated the teratogenicity of medications were derived by the Food and Drug Administration (FDA), Briggs Drugs in Pregnancy and Lactation, and other international health agencies. In use from 1979 to 2015 were categories A (no risk in human studies), B (no risk in animal studies), C (risk cannot be ruled out), D (evidence of risk), and X (contraindicated).

In 2015, the FDA revised traditional labelling with the Pregnancy and Lactation Labeling Rule (PLLR) to provide more detailed safety data specific to pregnant and lactating patients in clinical trials, the new rule also seeking to avoid misinformation by mandating that prescription drug labels remain updated. This has led to a revision of pregnancy risk categories to encompass the subcategories of pregnancy (including labour and delivery), lactation, females and males of reproductive potential.

Under the PLLR, the pregnancy subsection advises any potential risks of medication use to the mother and the developing fetus. The lactation subsection provides advice on the timing of breastfeeding, excretion of drugs in breast milk, and risks to the infant. Finally, the females and males of reproductive potential subsection provide recommendations about fertility, miscarriage, contraception, and pregnancy testing. In this chapter, focus will be placed on considerations in pregnancy and lactation (35).

Despite the PLLR labelling system being more encompassing, prescribing acne medications for pregnant and lactating individuals often requires extensive risk–benefit analysis. Clinical decisions are often obtained via shared decision making, and are tailored to personalised health needs of the expectant individual.

7.1.4.2 Specific Considerations in Pregnancy (Maternal Outcomes)

Apart from the recommendations from the American Board of Family Medicine (ABFM) for treatment of acne during pregnancy, there is a paucity of studies which analyse real-life data of acne management in pregnant patients. As pregnant and lactating patients are also often excluded in clinical trials, data on the safety and efficacy of most acne medications during pregnancy and lactation have mostly been derived from observational case studies and series.

In general, mild-to-moderate acne is best treated with topical agents during pregnancy. When oral antibiotic medications are indicated/desired, particularly for indications of moderate-severe acne, beta-lactams are generally considered first-line agents. Penicillins (such as amoxicillin) and cephalosporins are compatible with pregnancy and show efficacy in the treatment of acne. There is generally no increased risk to the expectant mother with the use of these antibiotics. For individuals with severe acne (nodulocystic acne, acne conglobata, acne fulminans), short courses of low dose oral corticosteroids may be sometimes considered—however, this is not routine unless the benefits clearly outweigh risks.

7.1.4.3 Specific Considerations in Pregnancy (Fetal Outcomes)

Specific maternal and fetal considerations for each class of acne drug are listed in Table 7.2.

TABLE 7.1

Therapeutics for Acne during Pregnancy and Lactation

Agent	Pregnancy (Maternal and Fetal Considerations)	Lactation
	TOPICAL	
Azelaic acid	• Indication: mild-moderate acne • Also effective for treating post-inflammatory hyperpigmentation (61) • Historic labelling 'B' • ☑First trimester ☑second trimester ☑third trimester (62) • Azelaic acid may be preferred in patients who cannot tolerate benzoyl peroxide or are experiencing post-inflammatory hyperpigmentation, particularly patients with skin of colour • Can be used as monotherapy or in combination with BPO (63) *Fetal considerations* None significant *Maternal considerations* Adverse events were transient, mild-to-moderate intensity, with burning, stinging, or irritation most commonly reported	• Minimal systemic absorption after topical application • Moreover, azelaic acid is found in natural foods, and bloodstream and breast milk normally; hence azelaic acid is considered a low risk to the nursing infant (64) • Considered safe in breastfeeding. Extra precautions to avoid application of azelaic acid to the breast or nipple and ensure that the infant's skin does not come into direct contact with the areas of skin that have been treated
Benzoyl peroxide	• Indication: mild-moderate acne • Historic labelling 'C' • ☑First trimester ☑second trimester ☑third trimester • May be used as monotherapy or in combination with antibiotics to prevent antibiotic resistance (37) *Fetal considerations* None significant *Maternal considerations* None significant	• Safe in lactating individuals • A thin layer should be applied, avoiding contact of site of application to baby • Avoid application on breast/nipple • Only 5% absorbed following topical application—considered a low risk to nursing infant

(Continued)

TABLE 7.1 (*Continued*)

Therapeutics for Acne during Pregnancy and Lactation

Agent	Pregnancy (Maternal and Fetal Considerations)	Lactation
	TOPICAL (Contd)	
Clindamycin	• Indication: mild-moderate acne • Historic labelling 'B' • ☑First trimester ☑second trimester ☑third trimester • Clindamycin is a first-line topical antibiotic for acne and when considered can be used in combination with BPO *Fetal considerations* Approximately 50% of maternal serum levels of clindamycin crosses the placenta, but no teratogenic effects have been reported (37) *Maternal considerations* While clindamycin is associated with risk of pseudomembranous colitis in the general population, the risk does not increase during pregnancy (65) These risks are further attenuated with topical application	• Overall regarded as safe in lactating individuals • Clindamycin is present in breast milk in small amounts and can potentially cause adverse effects on the breastfed infant's gastrointestinal flora • If oral or intravenous clindamycin is required by a breastfeeding woman, it is not a reason to discontinue breastfeeding, but an alternative drug may be preferred • Breastfeeding women can be advised to monitor the infant for diarrhoea and bloody stools • These risks are further attenuated with topical application
Dapsone	• Indication: mild-moderate acne • Historic labelling 'C' • ☑First trimester ☑second trimester • Considered a second-line topical agent for acne *Fetal considerations* Existing recommendations for topical dapsone to be discontinued before the last month of pregnancy to minimise the theoretical risk of neonatal hyperbilirubinemia (34) *Maternal considerations* No specific harms to pregnant individual Risk of maternal anaemia is considered low (prescription of oral dapsone in patients with glucose6-phosphate dehydrogenase (G6PD) deficiency leads to haemolytic anaemia; however, this risk is low in topical forms) (62)	• Topical dapsone is excreted in breast milk and is not recommended during lactation (37)

(*Continued*)

TABLE 7.1 (Continued)

Therapeutics for Acne during Pregnancy and Lactation

Agent	Pregnancy (Maternal and Fetal Considerations)	Lactation
Macrolides, such as erythromycin	• Indication: oral—moderate-severe acne • Historic labelling 'B' • Topical: ☑First trimester ☑second trimester ☑third trimester • Although suitable for use during pregnancy, topical erythromycin use and efficacy have generally decreased because of high rates of antibiotic resistance in the community, and other topical antibiotics may be preferred (66) • Oral: ☑second trimester ☑third trimester • Oral erythromycins (only the erythromycin base and ethylsuccinate forms) are safe during the second and third trimester *Fetal considerations* • Usage of oral erythromycin during the first trimester has been associated with increased risks of fetal cardiovascular malformations and pyloric stenosis, but recent studies found no significant relationships (67) *Maternal considerations* • Oral erythromycin in its estolate form is contraindicated during all trimesters because of risk of maternal hepatotoxicity (37)	• Overall regarded safe for lactating individuals *Infant considerations* • Despite some studies suggesting oral erythromycin be avoided during the first 2 weeks of lactation due to concerns of infantile pyloric stenosis, this finding was not replicated in multiple subsequent studies and meta-analyses (68). The AAP classifies erythromycins in its ethylsuccinate, base form (except estolate form) compatible with breastfeeding (69,70)
Metronidazole	• Indication: mild-moderate acne • Historic labelling 'B' • ☑First trimester ☑second trimester ☑third trimester • Metronidazole is a second-line topical antibiotic for acne and when considered can be used in combination with BPO *Fetal considerations* Animal studies with topical formulations have not been reported. Animal studies with the oral formulation have failed to reveal evidence of impaired fertility, teratogenicity, or fetal harm at higher doses; however, some intrauterine deaths were observed in mice when the drug was administered intraperitoneally (71) *Maternal considerations* Adverse events were mild, consisting of pruritus, skin irritation, and dry skin	• Overall safe for lactation • Few cases of diarrhoea, Candida infections, and lactose intolerance in breastfed infants have been reported in mothers taking oral metronidazole (72) • For topical use in breastfeeding individuals, systemic absorption is negligible, and no adverse fetal effects have been reported (37)

(Continued)

TABLE 7.1 (Continued)

Therapeutics for Acne during Pregnancy and Lactation

Agent	Pregnancy (Maternal and Fetal Considerations)	Lactation
	TOPICAL (Contd)	
Beta hydroxy (e.g., salicylic acids and alpha hydroxy (e.g., glycolic acids, lactic acids)	• Indication: mild-moderate acne • No historic FDA labelling • ☑First trimester ☑second trimester ☑third trimester • Prescribed as topical (whilst oral forms exist, not used for acne treatment) • Oral form of salicylic acid (aspirin) is contraindicated *Fetal considerations* • In human studies, a possible association between oral aspirin use during the first trimester and fetal gastroschisis was reported (73,74) • Studies also reported association of application in early and mid-pregnancy with cryptorchidism (75) *Maternal considerations* • In pregnancy-associated diseases, low dose oral aspirin has been employed as an effective prophylaxis and treatment medication	• Glycolic and lactic acid peels are considered safe during lactation because of limited dermal penetration (76)
Sodium sulfacetamide ± sulphur	• Indication: mild-moderate acne • Historic labelling 'C' • ☑First trimester ☑second trimester ☑third trimester • Has bacteriostatic properties and acts via inhibition of bacterial folic acid synthesis • Commonly combined with sulphur for added antimicrobial and keratolytic effects against acne (37) *Fetal considerations* • No fetal anomalies reported *Maternal considerations* • Sulfacetamide is a sulphonamide. As a drug within this class, there is a theoretical risk of severe drug eruptions such as Stevens-Johnson syndrome (SJS) and toxic epidermolytic necrosis (TEN) and risk of agranulocytosis and other blood dyscrasias (77). Sodium sulfacetamide contains sodium metabisulphite (as excipient) that may cause allergic type reactions including anaphylaxis • The overall prevalence of sulphite sensitivity in the general population is unknown and considered low. (Sulphite sensitivity is seen more frequently in asthmatic than in non-asthmatic people) (78)	• Considered safe during lactation except when breastfeeding infants with glucose-6-phosphate dehydrogenase (G6PD) deficiency or hyperbilirubinemia given the risk of infantile jaundice and kernicterus (79)

(Continued)

TABLE 7.1 (*Continued*)

Therapeutics for Acne during Pregnancy and Lactation

Agent	Pregnancy (Maternal and Fetal Considerations)	Lactation
Topical retinoids	• Indication: moderate-severe acne • Tretinoin: Historic labelling 'C' • Adapalene: Historic labelling 'D' • Tazarotene: Historic labelling 'X' • Trifarotene: no historic labelling • Conflicting data on the safety of topical retinoids in pregnant patients, with most safety ratings based on systemic isotretinoin, which is highly teratogenic and strictly contraindicated during pregnancy • Topical retinoids are minimally absorbed, and some studies suggest application to limited areas is unlikely to increase fetal risk • Despite early case reports (80) describing fetal cerebral and ocular malformations associated with topical retinoid use, subsequent studies (81) did not find an increased risk of major fetal malformations for topical tretinoin or adapalene during any trimester of pregnancy • Tazarotene is associated with retinoid-like malformations from high doses in animal studies (82) • Clinical trials for topical trifarotene, the newest FDA-approved topical retinoid, did not identify any maternal or fetal risks among pregnant (37) *Overall recommendation* Experts' advice to avoid all retinoids if possible	• Topical retinoids are considered safe during lactation (34) • Trace amounts are excreted into breast milk • Application of topical retinoids should be avoided on the breasts and other areas that make direct contact with the infant's skin • Topical tazarotene is metabolised into a less lipophilic form than other retinoids, further reducing its risk of transfer to breast milk—hence considered safe during lactation based on existing recommendations (83)
Clascoterone	• Indication: moderate-severe acne • No historic labelling • Conflicting data on safety of clascoterone on pregnancy • Some studies suggest that there is minimal systemic absorption and rapid metabolism to cortexolone (84) *Overall recommendation* Avoid if possible due to uncertainty of risks	• Avoid due to uncertainty of risks

(*Continued*)

TABLE 7.1 (Continued)
Therapeutics for Acne during Pregnancy and Lactation

Agent	Pregnancy (Maternal and Fetal Considerations)	Lactation
	ORAL	
Beta-lactams	• Indication: moderate-severe acne • Penicillins/cephalexin/amoxicillin: historic labelling 'B' • Penicillin and cephalexin: ☑First trimester ☑second trimester ☑third trimester • Amoxicillin: ☑second trimester ☑third trimester *Fetal considerations* • Amoxicillin usage in the first trimester has been associated with risk of cleft lip and palate. Advised for use in second and third trimesters only (85) *Maternal considerations* • No significant maternal considerations	• Safe during lactation • Less than 1% of the concentration of penicillins and cephalosporins is transferred to breast milk (83)
Tetracyclines	• Indication: moderate-severe acne • Historic labelling 'D' • If utilised, ☑first trimester • First-trimester use not associated with increased risk of congenital malformations *Fetal considerations* • However, after the 15th week of gestation, there is risk of permanent fetal teeth discoloration and bone growth inhibition • Tetracyclines may also be associated with infantile inguinal hernia, hypospadias, and limb hypoplasia *Maternal considerations* • Third-trimester use is associated with maternal liver toxicity	• Safe during lactation • Minimally transferred through breast milk. Absorption of tetracyclines is further limited by calcium binding in breast milk (86)

(Continued)

TABLE 7.1 (Continued)
Therapeutics for Acne during Pregnancy and Lactation

Agent	Pregnancy (Maternal and Fetal Considerations)	Lactation
Trimethoprim/Sulphonamides	• Indication: moderate-severe acne • Historic labelling 'C' • If utilised, ☑ second trimester *Fetal considerations* • First-trimester use of trimethoprim/sulfamethoxazole is associated with neural tube defects due to folate antagonism, increased risk of miscarriage, preterm birth, low birth weight, and cardiovascular defects (37) • Associated with neonatal hyperbilirubinemia during third trimester (16) *Maternal considerations* • With sulphonamides, there is theoretical risk of severe drug eruptions such as Stevens-Johnson syndrome (SJS) and toxic epidermolytic necrosis (TEN) and risk of agranulocytosis and other blood dyscrasias (77)	• Safe during lactation of healthy full-term infants • Minimally transferred through breast milk • Sulphonamides exacerbate hyperbilirubinemia by displacing bilirubin from albumin—to avoid in breastfed infants who are premature, G6PD deficient, or hyperbilirubinemic (83)
Isotretinoin	• Indications: severe acne • Historic labelling 'X' • Contraindicated in pregnancy • Those planning to conceive should wait at least 1 month after discontinuing isotretinoin before attempting to conceive. Studies reflect no evidence of increased risk of teratogenicity if conception occurs at least one menstrual cycle after stopping isotretinoin (87) • Isotretinoin use during pregnancy is associated with major fetal abnormalities, spontaneous abortions, premature births, and low IQ scores • Embryopathy reported in single doses	• Avoid in lactation (88) • Isotretinoin is excreted into breast milk because of its high lipid solubility (37)
Spironolactone	• Indication: moderate-severe acne • Historic labelling 'C' • Avoid during pregnancy *Fetal considerations* Spironolactone crosses the placenta and in utero exposure could cause feminisation and hypospadias of male fetus (62) *Maternal considerations* • Despite spironolactone having a theoretical risk of hyperkalaemia, multiple studies have shown that routine potassium monitoring is unnecessary for healthy women taking spironolactone for acne (89)	• Spironolactone is considered acceptable during lactation • Minimal transfer to breast milk and no associated adverse effects or electrolyte changes in breastfed infants (90)

(Continued)

TABLE 7.1 (*Continued*)

Therapeutics for Acne during Pregnancy and Lactation

Agent	Pregnancy (Maternal and Fetal Considerations)	Lactation
	ORAL (Contd)	
Corticosteroids	• May possibly be indicated for treatment-resistant or severe fulminant acne • Historic labelling 'C' • If utilised, ☑first trimester ☑second trimester ☑third trimester • When prescribed, short courses of oral corticosteroids or intralesional corticosteroids have been used • Oral prednisolone limited to <20 mg/day for a maximum duration of 1 month is thought to be safe during pregnancy in the second or third trimester (91) *Fetal considerations* • First-trimester use of oral prednisolone associated with orofacial clefts (92) • Some studies report that higher doses of prednisone associated with theoretical risks of premature labour, intrauterine growth restriction. However, in many of these studies, the studied pregnancies were also complicated by autoimmune disease (including rheumatoid arthritis, inflammatory bowel disease, and systemic lupus erythematosus) (93,94) *Maternal considerations* • Studies report risk of gestational diabetes and pre-eclampsia/eclampsia (95,96)	• Safe during lactation • Low levels of transfer of corticosteroids across breast milk • To minimise exposure, mothers are advised to wait 4 hours after taking oral corticosteroids before breastfeeding (83)
	OTHERS	
Laser and light therapies	• Not a mainstay treatment option for acne • Indication: Considered in cases of refractory acne • Options: Narrowband-ultraviolet B phototherapy (NBUVB), photodynamic therapy (PDT), Nd:YAG laser, pulse-dye laser regarded as safe during pregnancy • NBUVB: some studies have demonstrated reduction of folic acid with high cumulative NBUVB doses, raising concern for risk of neural tube defects. Physicians may consider appropriate folic acid supplementation, working with the obstetricians • PDT: Conflicting data on Aminolaevulinic acid (ALA), a topical photosensitiser commonly used with PDT (97,98). May avoid during pregnancy	• Safe during lactation • Minimal systemic absorption during procedures (76)

TABLE 7.2

Current Rosacea Therapeutics

Agent	Pregnancy	Lactation
	TOPICAL	
Azelaic acid	• Indication: inflammatory papules and pustules for mild-moderate rosacea • Historic labelling 'B' • ☑First trimester ☑second trimester ☑third trimester (62) *Fetal considerations* None significant *Maternal considerations* Adverse events were transient, mild-to-moderate intensity, with burning, stinging or irritation most commonly reported	• Considered safe in breastfeeding • Minimal systemic absorption after topical application • Moreover, azelaic acid is found in natural foods, and bloodstream and breast milk normally, hence azelaic acid is considered a low risk to the nursing infant (64) • Extra precautions to avoid application of azelaic acid to the breast or nipple and ensure that the infant's skin does not come into direct contact with the areas of skin that have been treated
Brimonidine	• Indication: persistent erythema in rosacea • Historic labelling 'B' • ☑First trimester ☑second trimester ☑early third trimester • Erythema can be reduced within 30 minutes reaching a peak at 3–6 hours, after which the effect diminishes and erythema returns to baseline *Fetal considerations* In the late third trimester and during lactation, experts may recommend avoidance of brimonidine as it penetrates the blood–brain barrier easily and can result in neonatal central nervous system depression and fetal apnoea (99) *Maternal considerations* Most adverse events were mild and transient. These include worsening of erythema, flushing, pruritus, and skin irritation	• Brimonidine poses substantial risk to the newborn • It has been reported to cause central nervous system depression and apnoea • The drug penetrates the blood–brain barrier and can cross the placenta and possibly excreted into breast milk, posing a real risk of apnoea or hypotension in infants • Experts recommend that if brimonidine is used during pregnancy, it should be discontinued before labour and during breastfeeding to prevent potential fetal apnoea in the infant

(Continued)

TABLE 7.2 (*Continued*)
Current Rosacea Therapeutics

Agent	Pregnancy	Lactation
	TOPICAL (Contd)	
Oxymetazoline	• Indication: persistent erythema in rosacea • No available data on oxymetazoline topical use in pregnant women to inform a drug-associated risk for major birth defects and miscarriage *Fetal considerations* • Use of oxymetazoline intranasal decongestant in pregnant women was historically labelled Category 'C'. Studies showed a potential association between second-trimester exposure to oxymetazoline (with no prior exposure in the first trimester) and renal collecting system anomalies (100) *Maternal considerations* Most adverse events were mild and transient. These include application-site dermatitis, pruritus, and erythema, worsening of inflammatory lesions and headaches	• Unknown if distributed in human breast milk • Likely minimal systemic absorption from topical use • Oxymetazoline was detected in breast milk of lactating rats when administered subcutaneously in previous studies (101) • To consider the developmental and health benefits of breastfeeding along with the mother's clinical need for the drug, and any potential adverse effects on the breastfed infant from the drug or from the underlying maternal condition
Ivermectin	• Indication: inflammatory lesions in rosacea • Historic labelling 'C' • Experts recommend to avoid during pregnancy if safer alternatives exist (102) *Fetal considerations* Inadvertent treatment of mothers with oral ivermectin during pregnancy has not been shown to lead to fetal issues (103). However, the manufacturer recommends to avoid *Maternal considerations* Most adverse events were mild and included skin burning, pruritus, and dry skin. In general, there is lack of safety data regarding its use in pregnancy	• Considered safe in lactation • No data are available on ivermectin excretion into breast milk after topical administration, but amounts should be less than after oral administration (104) • Avoid application to the breast area where the infant might directly ingest the drug

(Continued)

TABLE 7.2 (Continued)

Current Rosacea Therapeutics

Agent	Pregnancy	Lactation
Metronidazole	• Indication: inflammatory pustules and papules of rosacea • Historic labelling 'B' • ☑First trimester ☑second trimester ☑third trimester *Fetal considerations* Animal studies with topical formulations have not been reported Animal studies with the oral formulation have failed to reveal evidence of impaired fertility, teratogenicity, or fetal harm at higher doses; however, some intrauterine deaths were observed in mice when the drug was administered intraperitoneally (71) *Maternal considerations* Adverse events with topical form were mild, consisting of pruritus, skin irritation, and dry skin	• Overall safe for lactation *Maternal considerations* Few cases of diarrhoea, Candida infections, and lactose intolerance in breastfed infants have been reported in mothers taking oral metronidazole (72) *Infant considerations* Systemic absorption is negligible, and no adverse fetal effects have been reported with topical metronidazole use (37)
Cyclosporine	• Indicated for ocular rosacea • Historic labelling 'C' • ☑First trimester ☑second trimester ☑third trimester • Applied as topical eye drops • Cyclosporine 0·05% ophthalmic emulsion shown to be more beneficial than artificial tears (low-certainty evidence) (105) *Fetal considerations* • Reported in some studies to be associated with reduced fetal weight, skeletal retardation, and low birth weight (106) *Maternal considerations* • No specific pregnancy exposure data, however, topical administration of cyclosporine is associated with non-significant systemic absorption • Systematic reviews cite risk of pre-eclampsia with oral cyclosporine use (particularly with additional comorbid of older maternal age, pre-existing hypertension) (107)	• Systemic absorption from the eye is limited; hence ophthalmic cyclosporine would not be expected to cause any adverse effects in breastfed infants (108) • To substantially diminish the amount of drug that reaches the breast milk after using eye drops, the lactating individual may place pressure over the tear duct by the corner of the eye for 1 minute or more, then remove the excess solution with an absorbent tissue (108)

(Continued)

TABLE 7.2 (Continued)

Current Rosacea Therapeutics

Agent	Pregnancy	Lactation
	ORAL	
Macrolides (i.e. azithromycin)	• Indication: pustules and papules in rosacea • Historic labelling 'B' • ☑First trimester ☑second trimester ☑third trimester • Studies have shown that azithromycin may be as effective as 100 mg doxycycline. However, the evidence for the efficacy and safety is of very low certainty for azithromycin (105) *Fetal considerations* • No conclusive evidence on adverse fetal outcomes *Maternal considerations* • Contraindicated for individuals with history of cholestatic jaundice/hepatic dysfunction with prior use of azithromycin	• Safe in lactation • Low levels of azithromycin transmitted in breast milk • Unconfirmed epidemiologic evidence indicates that the risk of infantile hypertrophic pyloric stenosis might be increased by maternal use of macrolide antibiotics during the first two weeks of breastfeeding, however this was refuted by two meta-analyses which failed to demonstrate a relationship between maternal macrolide use during breastfeeding and infantile hypertrophic pyloric stenosis (109) • Monitor the infant for possible effects on the gastrointestinal flora, such as vomiting, diarrhoea, candidiasis (thrush, diaper rash) (110)
Tetracyclines (i.e. doxycycline)	• Indication: pustules and papules in rosacea. In particular, oral doxycycline can be considered for phymatous rosacea. • Historic labelling 'D' • If utilised, ☑first trimester • First trimester use not associated with increased risk of congenital malformations *Fetal considerations* • However, after the 15th week of gestation, there is risk of permanent fetal teeth discoloration and bone growth inhibition • Tetracyclines may also be associated with infantile inguinal hernia, hypospadias, and limb hypoplasia *Maternal considerations* • Third-trimester use is associated with maternal liver toxicity • Serious adverse events have been reported in rare cases with minocycline, such as autoimmune hepatitis, lupus erythematosus, and hyperpigmentation of the skin and tissues (111)	• Safe during lactation • Minimally transferred through breast milk. Absorption of tetracyclines is further limited by calcium binding in breast milk (86)

(Continued)

TABLE 7.2 (*Continued*)
Current Rosacea Therapeutics

Agent	Pregnancy	Lactation
Isotretinoin	• Indication: severe acne • Historic labelling 'X' • Contraindicated in pregnancy • Those planning to conceive should wait at least 1 month after discontinuing isotretinoin before attempting to conceive. Studies reflect no evidence of increased risk of teratogenicity if conception occurs at least one menstrual cycle after stopping isotretinoin (87) • Isotretinoin use during pregnancy is associated with major fetal abnormalities, spontaneous abortions, premature births, and low IQ scores • Embryopathy reported in single doses	• Avoid in lactation (88) • Isotretinoin is excreted into breast milk because of its high lipid solubility (37)
Corticosteroids	• May possibly be indicated for treatment of rosacea fulminans • Historic labelling 'C' • If utilised, ☑second trimester ☑third trimester • When prescribed, a short course of oral corticosteroids or intralesional corticosteroids have been used • Oral prednisolone limited to <20 mg/day for a maximum duration of 1 month is thought to be safe during pregnancy in the second or third trimester (91) *Fetal considerations* • First-trimester use of oral prednisolone associated with orofacial clefts • Some studies report that higher doses of prednisone associated with theoretical risks of premature labour, intrauterine growth restriction. However, in many of these studies, the studied pregnancies were also complicated by autoimmune disease (including rheumatoid arthritis, inflammatory bowel disease, and systemic lupus erythematosus) (93,94) *Maternal considerations* • Studies report risk of gestational diabetes and pre-eclampsia/eclampsia (95,96)	• Safe during lactation • Low levels of corticosteroids transfer to breast milk • To minimise exposure, mothers are advised to wait 4 hours after taking oral corticosteroids before breastfeeding (83)

(*Continued*)

TABLE 7.2 (*Continued*)

Current Rosacea Therapeutics

Agent	Pregnancy	Lactation
	ORAL (Contd)	
Beta-blockers	• Indication: for flushing in rosacea • When utilised, commonly used beta-blockers include propranolol and carvedilol • Historic labelling 'C' for above beta-blockers *Fetal considerations* Conflicting evidence on beta-blockers on safety to fetus. Beta-blockers can cross the placenta and potentially can cause physiological changes in the fetus. Although a previous meta-analysis (112) reported an association between β-blocker exposure and fetal congenital cardiovascular defects, several other studies did not find these associations (113,114) *Maternal considerations* • Cardiovascular: bradycardia, hypotension, decreased atrioventricular conduction • Pulmonary: exacerbation of existing reactive airway disease, bronchospasm • Metabolic: hypoglycaemia regarded as very rare and especially only in at-risk patients. Increased triglyceride levels • Absolute contraindications to beta-blockers include uncompensated congestive heart failure, cardiogenic shock, severe sinus bradycardia, severe heart block, severe hyperactive airway disease, severe depression, active Raynaud's disease, and hypersensitivity to beta-blockers (115) Overall, it is reasonable for use during pregnancy and patients should be counselled appropriately. Involvement of the obstetrics team to monitor fetal growth during pregnancy is also essential	• Propranol, carvedilol: safe for lactation • Transmitted levels of propranolol are low in breast milk • Studies during breastfeeding have found no adverse reactions in breastfed infants clearly attributable to propranolol • No special precautions are required
	OTHERS	
Laser and light therapies	• Indication: For erythema and mainly telangiectasia • ☑First trimester ☑second trimester ☑third trimester • Options: Photodynamic therapy (PDT), intense pulsed light (IPL), pulse-dye laser regarded as safe during pregnancy • NBUVB: some studies have demonstrated reduction of folic acid with high cumulative NBUVB doses, raising concern for risk of neural tube defects. Physicians may consider appropriate folic acid supplementation, working with the obstetricians • PDT: Conflicting data on aminolaevulinic acid (ALA), a topical photosensitiser commonly used with PDT (97,98). Although there are case reports of safe use in pregnancy (98), physicians may choose to avoid during pregnancy	• Safe during lactation • Minimal systemic absorption of light during procedures (76)

(Continued)

TABLE 7.2 (*Continued*)

Current Rosacea Therapeutics

Agent	Pregnancy	Lactation
Injection therapy (including botulinum toxin injections, IL-17 inhibitors)	*Botulinum toxin injections* • Indication: For erythema • Historic labelling 'C' • Intradermal injections of botulinum toxin significantly reduced erythema, oedema, telangiectasias, and flushing (116) *Fetal considerations* No evidence of birth defects or infantile botulism in the neonates was noted in any case *Maternal considerations* Information about exposure to botulinum toxin in human pregnancy is limited to case reports and a survey. Several cases of botulinum poisoning reported in second/third trimester (117) *IL-17 inhibitors* • Indication: IL-17 inhibitors such as secukinumab have been tried in severe, treatment-resistant papulopustular rosacea • Historic labelling—None • Exploratory studies have examined the utility of IL-17 inhibitors (118) *Fetal considerations* Secukinumab has been shown to cross the placenta in animal studies but failed to reveal evidence of fetotoxicity or teratogenicity when administered throughout organogenesis and late gestation up to 150 mg/kg/week; however, it may compromise the immunity of the fetus and neonate. There are no controlled data in human pregnancy	• Safe in lactation • Amount of secukinumab transmitted in breast milk is likely to be very low (119) • However, some experts advise waiting for at least 2 weeks postpartum to resume therapy to minimise transfer to the infant (120)

7.1.5 Real-World Trends in Acne Prescriptions for Expectant Individuals

A retrospective study in the US analysed prescriptions trends amongst 115 pregnancy-related encounters out of 4,050 total patient encounters with a diagnosis of acne vulgaris (36). The authors found that individuals who were intending to conceive or were currently pregnant or breastfeeding were exclusively prescribed medications from the historic categories 'B' and 'C'. Azelaic acid, clindamycin, and BPO were most commonly prescribed. Medications including retinoids, spironolactone, and dapsone were more frequently prescribed for the study's non-pregnant individuals, compared to pregnant individuals—suggesting substantial recognition of potential teratogenic side effects and practitioner adjustment of acne treatment regimes.

7.1.6 Therapeutic Options for Acne during Pregnancy and Lactation

It is reasonable to adopt a step-wise approach when considering therapeutics for acne during pregnancy to minimise risk. Physicians may start with topical treatments for mild-to-moderate acne, adding systemic therapies (including antibiotics) for moderate-to-severe acne, and reserving oral corticosteroids or procedural treatments for fulminant or refractory cases. For treating moderate-severe acne in pregnancy, studies recommend that order of preference of recommended oral antibiotics be: penicillins/aminopenicillins, followed by cephalosporins and macrolides (37,38). To reduce antibiotic resistance, oral antibiotics should not be used as monotherapy and advised for combination use with topical BPO/azelaic acid. Table 7.2 summarises current acne therapeutics with considerations for the pregnant and lactating individual.

7.2 ROSACEA

7.2.1 Introduction

Rosacea is a common inflammatory skin disorder that is characterised by facial flushing and facial erythema and can be accompanied by acneiform eruptions. Its pathogenesis is multifactorial, including abnormalities in innate immunity, inflammatory reactions to cutaneous microorganisms (increased colonisation by *Demodex* mites), ultraviolet damage, and vascular dysfunction (39). Hormonal changes and genetic factors are contributory (39).

Historically, four distinct subtypes of rosacea were recognised. These subtypes exhibit different disease courses and patterns of clinical behaviour. Untreated erythematotelangiectatic rosacea manifests with persistent facial erythema, sensitive skin, and intolerance to temperature fluctuations. The course of papulopustular rosacea (PPR) is characterised by episodic crops of inflammatory lesions with persistent perilesional erythema even after the inflammatory pustules and papules subside. Rhinophyma is chronic and progressively leads to varying degrees of nasal deformity if left untreated. Ocular rosacea runs a chronic course with episodic exacerbations. Untreated patients experience eye dryness and redness and may be more prone to secondary bacterial infections, conjunctival fibrosis, punctate keratitis, and corneal revascularisation (40). Recent guidelines (2019) by the US National Rosacea Society Expert Committee (NRSEC) advocate for a shift of rosacea classification from subtype to phenotype to better represent patients who were exhibited signs and symptoms which span across different subtypes (41).

7.2.2 Disease Progression of Rosacea during Pregnancy

During pregnancy, authors hypothesise that hormonal changes may increase the vascularity of the skin, sebhorrea, and dermal oedema, exacerbating rosacea or leading to de-novo development of rosacea (42). Oestrogen has been reported to cause dilation of spiral arterioles and is associated with angiogenesis and may contribute to overall vascular changes and facial flushing seen in rosacea. Progesterone (in the form of a progesterone-releasing intrauterine contraceptive device) has been previously suggested to be associated with rosacea, although the exact mechanisms are less clear. In particular, rosacea fulminans (RF), a severe form of rosacea characterised by rapid onset of marked facial erythema with nodular abscesses and indurated haemorrhagic plaques, may arise immediately following pregnancy and is associated with poor obstetrics outcomes such as intrauterine death (43), termination of pregnancy (43), and ocular perforation (44). In RF, there is absence of comedones and acneiform lesions over the trunk. Lesions consist of superficial papulopustules or nodules with cyanotic erythema. Very rarely, RF can be complicated by concomitant herpes infection and is termed rosacea fulminans herpeticum (45).

Whilst the emergence of rosacea fulminans during pregnancy has been relatively well documented, improvement of papulopustular rosacea (PPR) during pregnancy is scarcely documented. Shangraw et al. reported a single case of a multiparous 35-year-old female who prior to pregnancy had subclinical rosacea and demonstrated patterns of improvement during her pregnancies, with re-occurrence postpartum (46). Th1/Th17 cytokines are thought to be the main mediators of the inflammation in rosacea (39). Improvements in PPR as pregnancy progresses could be possibly explained by shift from Th1- to a Th2-predominant lymphocyte population that occurs during the second trimester (46). Other authors regard the clinical course of rosacea as unpredictable during pregnancy (47).

7.2.3 Pathophysiological Targets for Rosacea Management

The targets for rosacea management can be subdivided by its various pathophysiological aetiologies. The pathogenesis of rosacea may be divided into 2 broad, but overlapping domains of skin barrier dysfunction and environmental/genetic triggers. The commonly associated pathways are those that include components of the cathelicidin family (and post cleavage pro-inflammatory fragments which drive downstream inflammation), transient receptor potential channels (TRP), mast cells and the NOD-LRR-pyrin domain-containing protein (NLRP3) inflammasome. Mast cell activation and degranulation is thought to contribute towards erythrotelangiectatic, phymatous, and papulopustular rosacea phenotypes. Angiogenic chemokines include VEGF contribute to increase vascularity and flushing in rosacea patients. NLRP3 are involved in innate and inflammatory signaling and functions through various cytokines, such as IL-1 β and IL-18.

7.2.3.1 Targeting Vascular Changes in the Skin

Persistent erythema and telangiectasias can be treated medically and/or procedurally. Medical therapy entails the use of alpha-adrenergic vasoconstrictors which may be effective in temporarily reducing erythema. Brimonidine (an alpha-2 adrenergic receptor agonist) and oxymetazoline (a selective alpha-1-adrenergic receptor agonist) are two molecules which act similarly, even though their precise target is different. When applied, both cause local vasoconstriction within 30 minutes, an effect which may persist throughout the day. They do not target telangiectasias. In addition, brimonidine exerts an additional anti-inflammatory effect via mast cells (48).

Historically, electrocoagulation was used to treat telangiectasias but has limited utility against erythema. In comparison, pulsed-dye lasers (PDLw), potassium titanyl phosphate lasers, and intense pulsed light (IPL) are effective in treating the vascular aspect of rosacea—targeting both erythema and telangiectasia. Studies reveal that a combination of lasers may yield optimised results. In practice, the choice of laser therapy is influenced by the physician's degree of experience and availability of equipment and infrastructure. Medical therapy may also be combined with procedural treatments.

7.2.3.2 Targeting Flushing

Modifications of diet with avoidance of triggers (such as alcohol) are non-pharmacological means to address flushing. Laser therapy, as discussed, may also aid in reducing flushing by reducing the diameter of the vessels affected and the number of telangiectasias (49). Alpha adrenergic receptor agonists such as brimonidine and oxymetazoline can reduce flushing (50). Multiple case series and case reports describe the use of beta-blockers to treat flushing. A meta-analysis on beta-blocker use summarises that erythema and flushing improved in rosacea patients after initiation of oral β-blockers (51). Currently, the evidence is highest for carvedilol and propranolol, two nonselective β-blockers. Owing to the side effects of beta-blockers such as bradycardia, hypotension, and bronchospasm, with contraindications for patients with reactive airway disease, congestive cardiac failure, and various heart blocks, it is important to monitor patients who are started on these medications closely for blood pressure and heart rate. Clonidine and rilmenidine, other systemic medications attempted historically have now fallen out of favour (51). In recent years, botulinum toxin has also been used in small case series, but the overall level of evidence remains low. Combination therapy with botulinum toxin with PDL being efficacious for facial flushing has also been documented (52).

7.2.3.3 Targeting Innate Immunity

Innate immunity and its different mechanisms (activation, enzyme activity, production of proinflammatory mediators) constitute clear treatment targets in rosacea. The endothelial cells lining the microvascular system actively participate in regulating blood flow, protein uptake, and local inflammation (53). In rosacea skin, LL-37, a cathelicidin antimicrobial peptide, is over-expressed, promoting vascular proliferation in vivo. Drugs against rosacea such as doxycycline can decrease the production of pro-inflammatory mediators, including interleukin 8 (IL-8) and LL-37, and decrease toll-like receptor (TLR) activation. Mast cells, as part of innate immunity, may also play a role in both classic rosacea and its oedematous form, Morbihan disease. Hence, omalizumab, which acts by stabilising mast cells, decreasing Fc receptors on the cell surface, and binding circulating IgE, has been shown to be effective against Morbihan disease (54).

7.2.3.4 Targeting *Demodex* and Its Microbiota

Multiple studies demonstrate that *Demodex* (*D. folliculorum* and/or *D. brevis*) are present in higher load in rosacea patients compared to age- and sex-matched controls. The density *D. folliculorum* was also found to be higher in lesional areas than in non-lesional skin in the same patient. Agents against *Demodex* include anti-parasitic agent ivermectin (55), permethrin, and in a more recent retrospective study (56), benzyl benzoate and crotamiton (both of which are considered off-label use). Despite its apparent contribution to rosacea, the exact physiopathological role of *Demodex* remains partly unexplained. This is because certain drugs with no antiparasitic effect are in fact able to improve rosacea, and conversely, anti-parasitic products that decrease the *D. folliculorum* population do not always result in significant improvement in rosacea compared with placebo. This may be explained by the influence of microbiota around *Demodex*. Studies show that bacteria hosted by *D. folliculorum* (i.e. the microbiota particular to *Demodex*) are of numerous types—hence antibiotics such as tetracyclines may instead have an effect on this microbiota (57). The evidence on gut microbiota influencing rosacea is mixed, and no consensus exists at present. There is a lack of supporting evidence that preserving the gut microbiota may constitute a protective factor in rosacea, pending further research (58).

7.2.3.5 Targeting Sebaceous Glands

Studies have shown that sebaceous secretion anomalies occur in rosacea. These include the composition of saturated and unsaturated fatty acids. Tetracyclines like doxycycline can regulate differentiation of sebocytes: and decreases sebocyte proliferation. Doxycycline also increases the lipid content of sebocytes by upregulating peroxisome proliferator-activated receptor γ (59). Finally, isotretinoin exerts an anti-inflammatory role in resistant rosacea, via modulation of TLR-2, and also acts directly on sebaceous glands. As such, isotretinoin appears to be the treatment of choice in early rhinophyma and has been documented to be efficacious in Morbihan disease (60).

7.2.3.6 Targeting Environmental Factors

Several environmental factors are implicated in rosacea. The role of alcohol in rosacea is supported by mixed evidence, with several recent studies arguing for a link between alcohol and rosacea, with a dose-response effect. However, results were discordant and often depended on the populations studied (49). Coffee (and more likely caffeine intake) was shown to decrease the risk of rosacea, in proportion to daily intake. Smoking reduction may help with decreasing the pustular lesion load in rosacea and may improve rhinophyma (60).

Amongst the environmental factors influencing rosacea, UV exposure plays the most important role. UV exposure increases the innate immune-type inflammatory response in relation to endothelial cells. LL-37 is thought to increase sensitivity to UVB and modulates interactions with dermal vessels. Hence avoidance of excessive sun exposure and use of sunscreens has generally been recommended (49).

7.2.4 Therapeutic Options for Rosacea during Pregnancy and Lactation

Therapeutics for rosacea should be selected based on phenotyping. The shift of rosacea classification from subtyping to phenotyping emphasises the specific presentation and concerns of the individual patient, individualising therapy as part of a patient centric approach. Pregnant and lactating individuals struggling with the various phenotypes of rosacea can consider a combination of skin care/cosmetic treatments, topical therapies, oral therapies, laser/light-based therapies, and injection therapies. Table 7.2 summarises current rosacea therapeutics with considerations for the pregnant and lactating individual.

7.3 CONCLUSION

Both acne vulgaris and rosacea are chronic skin disorders that may affect women throughout pregnancy and in the postpartum period. In both conditions, exacerbations can be attributed to hormonal fluctuations and physiological changes that occur in the different phases of pregnancy. As randomised controlled trials for the treatment of acne or rosacea during pregnancy do not exist, treatment regimens are best tailored to the pregnant/lactating individual. Physicians should communicate clearly with patients to formulate acceptable treatment plans that take into consideration risks to the individual and fetus/infant.

REFERENCES

1. Lynn DD, Umari T, Dunnick CA, Dellavalle RP. The epidemiology of acne vulgaris in late adolescence. *Adolesc Health Med Ther.* 2016;7:13–25.
2. Gollnick H, Cunliffe W, Berson D, et al. Management of acne: A report from a Global Alliance to Improve Outcomes in Acne. *J Am Acad Dermatol.* 2003;49(1 Suppl):S1–37.
3. Geraghty LN, Pomeranz MK. Physiologic changes and dermatoses of pregnancy. *Int J Dermatol.* 2011;50(7):771–782.
4. Li CX, You ZX, Lin YX, et al. Skin microbiome differences relate to the grade of acne vulgaris. *J Dermatol.* 2019;46(9):787–790.
5. Huang C, Zhuo F, Han B, et al. The updates and implications of cutaneous microbiota in acne. *Cell Biosci.* 2023;13(1):113.
6. Dréno B. What is new in the pathophysiology of acne, an overview. *J Eur Acad Dermatol Venereol.* 2017; 31(Suppl 5):8–12.
7. Hoefel IDR, Weber MB, Manzoni APD, et al. Striae gravidarum, acne, facial spots, and hair disorders: Risk factors in a study with 1284 puerperal patients. *J Pregnancy.* 2020;2020:8036109.
8. Yang CC, Huang YT, Yu CH, et al. Inflammatory facial acne during uncomplicated pregnancy and postpartum in adult women: A preliminary hospital-based prospective observational study of 35 cases from Taiwan. *J Eur Acad Dermatol Venereol.* 2016;30(10):1787–1789.
9. Dréno B, Blouin E, Moyse D, et al. Acne in pregnant women: A French survey. *Acta Derm Venereol.* 2014;94(1):82–83.
10. Kutlu Ö, Karadağ AS, Ünal E, et al. Acne in pregnancy: A prospective multicenter, cross-sectional study of 295 patients in Turkey. *Int J Dermatol.* 2020;59(9):1098–1105.
11. O'Leary P, Boyne P, Flett P, et al. Longitudinal assessment of changes in reproductive hormones during normal pregnancy. *Clin Chem.* 1991;37(5):667–672.

12. Schock H, Zeleniuch-Jacquotte A, Lundin E, et al. Hormone concentrations throughout uncomplicated pregnancies: A longitudinal study. *BMC Pregnancy Childbirth.* 2016;16(1):146.

13. Kletzky OA, Marrs RP, Howard WF, et al. Prolactin synthesis and release during pregnancy and puerperium. *Am J Obstet Gynecol.* 1980;136(4):545–550.

14. Theofanakis C, Drakakis P, Besharat A, Loutradis D. Human chorionic gonadotropin: The pregnancy hormone and more. *Int J Mol Sci.* 2017;18(5).

15. Meulenberg PM, Hofman JA. Maternal testosterone and fetal sex. *J Steroid Biochem Mol Biol.* 1991;39(1):51–54.

16. Chien AL, Qi J, Rainer B, Sachs DL, Helfrich YR. Treatment of acne in pregnancy. *J Am Board Fam Med.* 2016;29(2):254–262.

17. Shaw JC, White LE. Persistent acne in adult women. *Arch Dermatol.* 2001;137(9):1252–1253.

18. Kanda N, Watanabe S. Regulatory roles of sex hormones in cutaneous biology and immunology. *J Dermatol Sci.* 2005;38(1):1–7.

19. Thiboutot D. Acne: Hormonal concepts and therapy. *Clin Dermatol.* 2004;22(5):419–428.

20. Kuijper EA, Ket JC, Caanen MR, Lambalk CB. Reproductive hormone concentrations in pregnancy and neonates: A systematic review. *Reprod Biomed Online.* 2013;27(1):33–63.

21. Thiboutot DM, Dréno B, Abanmi A, et al. Practical management of acne for clinicians: An international consensus from the Global Alliance to Improve Outcomes in Acne. *J Am Acad Dermatol.* 2018;78(2 Suppl 1):S1–S23.e1.

22. Nast A, Dréno B, Bettoli V, et al. European evidence-based (S3) guideline for the treatment of acne—update 2016—short version. *J Eur Acad Dermatol Venereol.* 2016;30(8):1261–1268.

23. Kurokawa I, Danby FW, Ju Q, et al. New developments in our understanding of acne pathogenesis and treatment. *Exp Dermatol.* 2009;18(10):821–832.

24. Kurokawa I, Layton AM, Ogawa R. Updated treatment for acne: Targeted therapy based on pathogenesis. *Dermatol Ther.* 2021;11(4):1129–1139.

25. Knutson DD. Ultrastructural observations in acne vulgaris: The normal sebaceous follicle and acne lesions. *J Invest Dermatol.* 1974;62(3):288–307.

26. Beylot C, Auffret N, Poli F, et al. Propionibacterium acnes: An update on its role in the pathogenesis of acne. *J Eur Acad Dermatol Venereol.* 2014;28(3):271–278.

27. Hebert A, Thiboutot D, Stein Gold L, et al. Efficacy and safety of topical clascoterone cream, 1%, for treatment in patients with facial acne: Two phase 3 randomized clinical trials. *JAMA Dermatol.* 2020;156(6):621–630.

28. Zimmerman Y, Eijkemans MJ, Coelingh Bennink HJ, et al. The effect of combined oral contraception on testosterone levels in healthy women: A systematic review and meta-analysis. *Hum Reprod Update.* 2014;20(1):76–105.

29. Layton AM, Eady EA, Whitehouse H, et al. Oral spironolactone for acne vulgaris in adult females: A hybrid systematic review. *Am J Clin Dermatol.* 2017;18(2):169–191.

30. Naik PP. Trifarotene: A novel therapeutic option for acne. *Dermatol Res Pract.* 2022;2022:1504303.

31. Zuliani T, Khammari A, Chaussy H, et al. Ex vivo demonstration of a synergistic effect of Adapalene and benzoyl peroxide on inflammatory acne lesions. *Exp Dermatol.* 2011;20(10):850–853.

32. Dispenza MC, Wolpert EB, Gilliland KL, et al. Systemic isotretinoin therapy normalizes exaggerated TLR-2-mediated innate immune responses in acne patients. *J Invest Dermatol.* 2012;132(9):2198–2205.

33. Burkhart CN, Burkhart CG. Microbiology's principle of biofilms as a major factor in the pathogenesis of acne vulgaris. *Int J Dermatol.* 2003;42(12):925–927.

34. Leachman SA, Reed BR. The use of dermatologic drugs in pregnancy and lactation. *Dermatol Clin.* 2006;24(2):167–197, vi.

35. Leek JC, Arif H. Pregnancy medications. *StatPearls.* Treasure Island (FL) ineligible companies. Disclosure: Hasan Arif declares no relevant financial relationships with ineligible companies.: StatPearls Publishing; 2023.

36. Garg SP, Alvi S, Kundu RV. Analyzing trends in treatment of acne vulgaris in pregnancy: A retrospective study. *Int J Womens Dermatol.* 2023;9(1):e076.

37. Ly S, Kamal K, Manjaly P, et al. Treatment of acne vulgaris during pregnancy and lactation: A narrative review. *Dermatol Ther (Heidelb).* 2023;13(1):115–130.

38. Awan SZ, Lu J. Management of severe acne during pregnancy: A case report and review of the literature. *Int J Womens Dermatol.* 2017;3(3):145–150.

39. Buhl T, Sulk M, Nowak P, et al. Molecular and morphological characterization of inflammatory infiltrate in rosacea reveals activation of Th1/Th17 pathways. *J Invest Dermatol.* 2015;135(9):2198–2208.

40. Saá FL, Cremona F, Chiaradia P. Association between skin findings and ocular signs in rosacea. *Turk J Ophthalmol.* 2021;51(6):338–343.

41. Tan J, Almeida LM, Bewley A, et al. Updating the diagnosis, classification and assessment of rosacea: Recommendations from the global ROSacea COnsensus (ROSCO) panel. *Br J Dermatol.* 2017;176(2):431–438.
42. Demir O, Tas IS, Gunay B, Ugurlucan FG. A rare dermatologic disease in pregnancy: Rosacea fulminans—case report and review of the literature. *Open Access Maced J Med Sci.* 2018;6(8):1438–1441.
43. Jarrett R, Gonsalves R, Anstey AV. Differing obstetric outcomes of rosacea fulminans in pregnancy: Report of three cases with review of pathogenesis and management. *Clin Exp Dermatol.* 2010;35(8):888–891.
44. de Morais e Silva FA, Bonassi M, Steiner D, da Cunha TV. Rosacea fulminans in pregnancy with ocular perforation. *J Dtsch Dermatol Ges.* 2011;9(7):542–543.
45. Tisack A, Singh RK, Kohen L. Rosacea fulminans herpeticum: Rosacea fulminans with superimposed herpetic infection. *JAAD Case Rep.* 2021;11:106–108.
46. Papulopustular rosacea improvement in pregnancy: A case report. *J Am Acad Dermatol.* 2017;76(6):AB187.
47. Nasca MR, Giuffrida G, Micali G. The influence of pregnancy on the clinical evolution and prognosis of pre-existing inflammatory and autoimmune skin disorders and their management. *Dermatology.* 2021;237(5):771–785.
48. Bertino B, Blanchet-Réthoré S, Thibaut de Ménonville S, et al. Brimonidine displays anti-inflammatory properties in the skin through the modulation of the vascular barrier function. *Exp Dermatol.* 2018;27(12):1378–1387.
49. Cribier B. Rosacea: Treatment targets based on new physiopathology data. *Ann Dermatol Venereol.* 2022;149(2):99–107.
50. Shanler SD, Ondo AL. Successful treatment of the erythema and flushing of rosacea using a topically applied selective alpha1-adrenergic receptor agonist, oxymetazoline. *Arch Dermatol.* 2007;143(11):1369–1371.
51. Logger JGM, Olydam JI, Driessen RJB. Use of beta-blockers for rosacea-associated facial erythema and flushing: A systematic review and update on proposed mode of action. *J Am Acad Dermatol.* 2020;83(4):1088–1097.
52. Al-Niaimi F, Glagoleva E, Araviiskaia E. Pulsed dye laser followed by intradermal botulinum toxin type-A in the treatment of rosacea-associated erythema and flushing. *Dermatol Ther.* 2020;33(6):e13976.
53. Michiels C. Endothelial cell functions. *J Cellular Physiology.* 2003;196(3):430–443.
54. Kafi P, Edén I, Swartling C. Morbihan syndrome successfully treated with omalizumab. *Acta Derm Venereol.* 2019;99(7):677–678.
55. Ebbelaar CCF, Venema AW, Van Dijk MR. Topical ivermectin in the treatment of papulopustular rosacea: A systematic review of evidence and clinical guideline recommendations. *Dermatol Ther (Heidelb).* 2018;8(3):379–387.
56. Forton FMN, De Maertelaer V. Treatment of rosacea and demodicosis with benzyl benzoate: Effects of different doses on Demodex density and clinical symptoms. *J Eur Acad Dermatol Venereol.* 2020;34(2):365–369.
57. Murillo N, Aubert J, Raoult D. Microbiota of Demodex mites from rosacea patients and controls. *Microb Pathog.* 2014;71–72:37–40.
58. Szántó M, Dózsa A, Antal D, et al. Targeting the gut-skin axis-Probiotics as new tools for skin disorder management? *Exp Dermatol.* 2019;28(11):1210–1218.
59. Zouboulis CC, Raghallaigh SN, Schmitz G, Powell FC. The pro-differentiation effect of doxycycline on human SZ95 sebocytes. *Dermatology.* 2021;237(5):792–796.
60. Ismail D, Asfour L, Madan V. Rhinophyma in women: A case series. *Lasers Med Sci.* 2021;36(6):1283–1287.
61. Kircik LH. Efficacy and safety of azelaic acid (AzA) gel 15% in the treatment of post-inflammatory hyperpigmentation and acne: A 16-week, baseline-controlled study. *J Drugs Dermatol.* 2011;10(6):586–590.
62. Kong YL, Tey HL. Treatment of acne vulgaris during pregnancy and lactation. *Drugs.* 2013;73(8):779–787.
63. Dréno B, Layton A, Zouboulis CC, et al. Adult female acne: A new paradigm. *J Eur Acad Dermatol Venereol.* 2013;27(9):1063–1070.
64. Akhavan A, Bershad S. Topical acne drugs: Review of clinical properties, systemic exposure, and safety. *Am J Clin Dermatol.* 2003;4(7):473–492.
65. Gurwith MJ, Rabin HR, Love K. Diarrhea associated with clindamycin and ampicillin therapy: Preliminary results of a cooperative study. *J Infect Dis.* 1977;135(Suppl):S104–S110.
66. Alkhawaja E, Hammadi S, Abdelmalek M, et al. Antibiotic resistant Cutibacterium acnes among acne patients in Jordan: A cross sectional study. *BMC Dermatol.* 2020;20(1):17.
67. Källén BA, Otterblad Olausson P, Danielsson BR. Is erythromycin therapy teratogenic in humans? *Reprod Toxicol.* 2005;20(2):209–214.

68. Abdellatif M, Ghozy S, Kamel MG, et al. Association between exposure to macrolides and the development of infantile hypertrophic pyloric stenosis: A systematic review and meta-analysis. *Eur J Pediatr.* 2019;178(3):301–314.
69. Goldstein LH, Berlin M, Tsur L, et al. The safety of macrolides during lactation. *Breastfeed Med.* 2009;4(4):197–200.
70. AAP Committee on Drugs. Transfer of drugs and other chemicals into human milk. *Pediatrics.* 2001;108(3):776–789.
71. Muanda FT, Sheehy O, Bérard A. Use of antibiotics during pregnancy and the risk of major congenital malformations: A population based cohort study. *Br J Clin Pharmacol.* 2017;83(11):2557–2571.
72. Hernández Ceruelos A, Romero-Quezada LC, Ruvalcaba Ledezma JC, López Contreras L. Therapeutic uses of metronidazole and its side effects: An update. *Eur Rev Med Pharmacol Sci.* 2019;23(1):397–401.
73. Kozer E, Nikfar S, Costei A, et al. Aspirin consumption during the first trimester of pregnancy and congenital anomalies: A meta-analysis. *Am J Obstet Gynecol.* 2002;187(6):1623–1630.
74. Sun S, Qian H, Li C, et al. Effect of low dose aspirin application during pregnancy on fetal congenital anomalies. *BMC Pregnancy Childbirth.* 2022;22(1):802.
75. Kristensen DM, Hass U, Lesné L, et al. Intrauterine exposure to mild analgesics is a risk factor for development of male reproductive disorders in human and rat. *Hum Reprod.* 2011;26(1):235–244.
76. Trivedi MK, Kroumpouzos G, Murase JE. A review of the safety of cosmetic procedures during pregnancy and lactation. *Int J Womens Dermatol.* 2017;3(1):6–10.
77. Fritsch PO, Sidoroff A. Drug-induced Stevens-Johnson syndrome/toxic epidermal necrolysis. *Am J Clin Dermatol.* 2000;1(6):349–360.
78. Vally H, Misso NL. Adverse reactions to the sulphite additives. *Gastroenterol Hepatol Bed Bench.* 2012;5(1):16–23.
79. Lee HY, Ithnin A, Azma RZ, et al. Glucose-6-phosphate dehydrogenase deficiency and neonatal hyperbilirubinemia: Insights on pathophysiology, diagnosis, and gene variants in disease heterogeneity. *Front Pediatr.* 2022;10:875877.
80. Autret E, Berjot M, Jonville-Béra AP, et al. Anophthalmia and agenesis of optic chiasma associated with adapalene gel in early pregnancy. *Lancet.* 1997;350(9074):339.
81. Loureiro KD, Kao KK, Jones KL, et al. Minor malformations characteristic of the retinoic acid embryopathy and other birth outcomes in children of women exposed to topical tretinoin during early pregnancy. *Am J Med Genet A.* 2005;136(2):117–121.
82. Han G, Wu JJ, Del Rosso JQ. Use of topical tazarotene for the treatment of acne vulgaris in pregnancy: A literature review. *J Clin Aesthet Dermatol.* 2020;13(9):E59–E65.
83. Butler DC, Heller MM, Murase JE. Safety of dermatologic medications in pregnancy and lactation: Part II. Lactation. *J Am Acad Dermatol.* 2014;70(3):417.e1–10; quiz 27.
84. Kalabalik-Hoganson J, Frey KM, Ozdener-Poyraz AE, Slugocki M. Clascoterone: A novel topical androgen receptor inhibitor for the treatment of acne. *Ann Pharmacother.* 2021;55(10):1290–1296.
85. Daniel S, Doron M, Fishman B, et al. The safety of amoxicillin and clavulanic acid use during the first trimester of pregnancy. *Br J Clin Pharmacol.* 2019;85(12):2856–2863.
86. Hale EK, Pomeranz MK. Dermatologic agents during pregnancy and lactation: An update and clinical review. *Int J Dermatol.* 2002;41(4):197–203.
87. Pugashetti R, Shinkai K. Treatment of acne vulgaris in pregnant patients. *Dermatol Ther.* 2013;26(4):302–311.
88. Koh YP, Tian EA, Oon HH. New changes in pregnancy and lactation labelling: Review of dermatologic drugs. *Int J Women's Dermatol.* 2019;5(4):216–226.
89. Plovanich M, Weng QY, Mostaghimi A. Low usefulness of potassium monitoring among healthy young women taking spironolactone for acne. *JAMA Dermatol.* 2015;151(9):941–944.
90. Phelps DL, Karim A. Spironolactone: Relationship between concentrations of dethioacetylated metabolite in human serum and milk. *J Pharm Sci.* 1977;66(8):1203.
91. Bandoli G, Palmsten K, Forbess Smith CJ, Chambers CD. A review of systemic corticosteroid use in pregnancy and the risk of select pregnancy and birth outcomes. *Rheum Dis Clin North Am.* 2017;43(3):489–502.
92. Hviid A, Mølgaard-Nielsen D. Corticosteroid use during pregnancy and risk of orofacial clefts. *CMAJ.* 2011;183(7):796–804.
93. Rom AL, Wu CS, Olsen J, et al. Fetal growth and preterm birth in children exposed to maternal or paternal rheumatoid arthritis: A nationwide cohort study. *Arthritis Rheumatol.* 2014;66(12):3265–3273.
94. Bröms G, Granath F, Linder M, et al. Birth outcomes in women with inflammatory bowel disease: Effects of disease activity and drug exposure. *Inflamm Bowel Dis.* 2014;20(6):1091–1098.

95. Park-Wyllie L, Mazzotta P, Pastuszak A, et al. Birth defects after maternal exposure to corticosteroids: Prospective cohort study and meta-analysis of epidemiological studies. *Teratology*. 2000;62(6):385–392.

96. Leung YP, Kaplan GG, Coward S, et al. Intrapartum corticosteroid use significantly increases the risk of gestational diabetes in women with inflammatory bowel disease. *J Crohns Colitis*. 2015;9(3):223–230.

97. Yang Y, Zhang Y, Zou X, et al. Perspective clinical study on effect of 5-aminolevulinic acid photodynamic therapy (ALA-PDT) in treating condylomata acuminata in pregnancy. *Photodiagnosis Photodyn Ther*. 2019;25:63–65.

98. Yang YG, Zou XB, Zhao H, et al. Photodynamic therapy of condyloma acuminata in pregnant women. *Chin Med J (Engl)*. 2012;125(16):2925–2928.

99. Razeghinejad MR, Nowroozzadeh MH. Anti-glaucoma medication exposure in pregnancy: An observational study and literature review. *Clin Exp Optom*. 2010;93(6):458–465.

100. Yau WP, Mitchell AA, Lin KJ, et al. Use of decongestants during pregnancy and the risk of birth defects. *Am J Epidemiol*. 2013;178(2):198–208.

101. Accessdata.fda.gov FaDA-. KOVANAZE (tetracaine HCl and oxymetazoline HCl) Nasal Spray.

102. Nicolas P, Maia MF, Bassat Q, et al. Safety of oral ivermectin during pregnancy: A systematic review and meta-analysis. Lancet Glob Health. 2020;8(1):e92–e100.

103. Chippaux JP, Gardon-Wendel N, Gardon J, Ernould JC. Absence of any adverse effect of inadvertent ivermectin treatment during pregnancy. *Trans R Soc Trop Med Hyg*. 1993;87(3):318.

104. Thomas C, Coates SJ, Engelman D, et al. Ectoparasites: Scabies. *J Am Acad Dermatol*. 2020;82(3): 533–548.

105. van Zuuren EJ, Fedorowicz Z, Tan J, et al. Interventions for rosacea based on the phenotype approach: An updated systematic review including GRADE assessments. *Br J Dermatol*. 2019;181(1):65–79.

106. Ponticelli C, Moroni G. Fetal toxicity of immunosuppressive drugs in pregnancy. *J Clin Med*. 2018;7(12).

107. Akiyama S, Hamdeh S, Murakami N, et al. Pregnancy and neonatal outcomes in women receiving calcineurin inhibitors: A systematic review and meta-analysis. *Br J Clin Pharmacol*. 2022;88(9):3950–3961.

108. *Drugs and Lactation Database (LactMed®)* [Internet]. Bethesda, MD: National Institute of Child Health and Human Development; 2006. Cyclosporine [Updated 2023 Apr 15]. Available from: www.ncbi.nlm. nih.gov/books/NBK501683/.

109. Almaramhy HH, Al-Zalabani AH. The association of prenatal and postnatal macrolide exposure with subsequent development of infantile hypertrophic pyloric stenosis: A systematic review and meta-analysis. *Ital J Pediatr*. 2019;45(1):20.

110. *Drugs and Lactation Database (LactMed®)* [Internet]. Bethesda, MD: National Institute of Child Health and Human Development; 2006. Azithromycin [Updated 2021 Jul 19]. Available from: www.ncbi.nlm. nih.gov/books/NBK501200/.

111. van Zuuren EJ. Rosacea. *N Engl J Med*. 2017;377(18):1754–1764.

112. Yakoob MY, Bateman BT, Ho E, et al. The risk of congenital malformations associated with exposure to β-blockers early in pregnancy: A meta-analysis. *Hypertension*. 2013;62(2):375–381.

113. Duan L, Ng A, Chen W, et al. β-blocker exposure in pregnancy and risk of fetal cardiac anomalies. *JAMA Intern Med*. 2017;177(6):885–887.

114. Bateman BT, Heide-Jorgenson U, Einarsdottir K, et al. β-blocker use in pregnancy and the risk for congenital malformations. *Annals Internl Med*. 2018;169(10):665–673.

115. Clanner-Engelshofen BM, Bernhard D, Dargatz S, et al. S2k guideline: Rosacea. *JDDG: J Dtsch Dermatol Ges*. 2022;20(8):1147–1165.

116. Bharti J, Sonthalia S, Jakhar D. Mesotherapy with botulinum toxin for the treatment of refractory vascular and papulopustular rosacea. *J Am Acad Dermatol*. 2023;88(6):e295–e296.

117. Robin L, Herman D, Redett R. Botulism in a pregnant woman. *N Engl J Med*. 1996;335(11):823–824.

118. Kumar AM, Chiou AS, Shih YH, et al. An exploratory, open-label, investigator-initiated study of interleukin-17 blockade in patients with moderate-to-severe papulopustular rosacea. *Br J Dermatol*. 2020;183(5):942–943.

119. Russell MD, Dey M, Flint J, et al. British Society for Rheumatology guideline on prescribing drugs in pregnancy and breastfeeding: Immunomodulatory anti-rheumatic drugs and corticosteroids. *Rheumatology (Oxford)*. 2023;62(4):e48–e88.

120. Krysko KM, Dobson R, Alroughani R, et al. Family planning considerations in people with multiple sclerosis. *Lancet Neurol*. 2023;22(4):350–366.

8 Melanocytic Nevi and Melanoma in Pregnancy

Yasmeen Jabeen Bhat and Kurat Sajad

8.1 INTRODUCTION

Melanocytic nevi are benign neoplasms resulting from the proliferation of melanocytes, the normal pigment-producing cells that constitutively colonise the epidermis.[1] These are primarily of cosmetic significance. However, in certain circumstances the presence of atypical nevi is a marker for an increased risk of developing malignant melanoma, which is the most common malignancy diagnosed in women during childbearing age, making it the most common malignancy to occur during pregnancy.[2] The relation between pregnancy, melanocytic nevi, and malignant melanoma is ambiguous.

There are marked changes in the level of sex hormones during pregnancy. The potential adverse effect of pregnancy-associated hormones and exogenous hormones on melanocytic nevi and malignant melanoma has been a concern among clinicians for many years. The significance of this issue has increased due to delayed childbearing in women in their 30s and 40s, when the likelihood of diagnosing melanoma during pregnancy is enhanced.[3]

Thus, it becomes imperative to study the effect of pregnancy on melanocytic nevi and melanoma to help in counselling and guiding women about the development, progression, and prognosis of melanoma.

8.2 PREGNANCY AND BENIGN MELANOCYTIC NEVI

8.2.1 Effect of Pregnancy on the Colour of Nevi

Hyperpigmentation occurring in pregnancy is attributed to increased levels of beta and alfa melanocyte-stimulating hormone, oestrogen, progesterone, and beta-endorphin that cause increased melanocyte stimulation.[4] The molecular pathways are not well understood, but the altered hormonal state of pregnancy may have distinct effects on melanocytic nevi.[5]

According to the older literature, the melanocytic nevi darken during pregnancy in response to hormonal changes.[6,7] However, there is insufficient evidence to support the notion that moles darken during pregnancy. In some reports patients experienced lightening of a giant congenital nevus and satellite nevi during pregnancy, followed by some, but not full, repigmentation after delivery.[8] It was documented using photographs taken before, during, and after the pregnancies. In a study using in vivo spectrophotometry, the changes in the pigmentation of melanocytic nevi in pregnant females were statistically insignificant when compared to the non-pregnant control group.

8.2.2 Effect of Pregnancy on the Size of Nevi

Mostly the changes in the size of nevi occur on the front of the body, likely because of stretching of the skin during pregnancy. However, nevi on locations unaffected by skin stretching during pregnancy have not shown any significant change in size. Common consensus from various studies indicate that the normal stretching and expansion of the skin of the breasts and abdomen might

DOI: 10.1201/9781003449690-8

explain much of the growth seen in these nevi during pregnancy whereas the nevi on the backs or lower extremities of pregnant women have not shown any significant changes in size over the course of pregnancy (Table 8.1).[8,9]

The other clinical changes which were reported include new onset of pruritus and pain, the development of new lesions, hair growth in existing lesions, or crust formation.

8.2.3 DERMOSCOPIC CHANGES IN MELANOCYTIC NEVI IN PREGNANCY

The dermoscopic changes in the melanocytic nevi of women, especially those located on the breast and abdomen, are transient. These changes often reflect stretching of the skin and do not necessarily suggest melanoma.

According to various studies, only the nevi on the breasts and abdomen grow in size. The lesions with a reticular pattern show enlargement, where the pigment network simply became clearer and more widely meshed. The lesions with a globular pattern showed an increased number of brown globules on the periphery.[11] There was no change in shape in either pattern. These changes occur due to the thinning and expanding of the skin in pregnancy, where deep nests of nevi may be pushed closer to the surface, causing them to appear as junctional nests. Thickening of pigment network lines was observed in some nevi.

Some studies also suggested that the number of vessels increased between the first and third trimesters but normalised after delivery.[13] The authors opined that the dermoscopic changes seen in pregnancy are same as typical vascular changes seen elsewhere on the skin during pregnancy and were caused by increased blood volume and vessel proliferation. However, none of these changes were suggestive of melanoma (Table 8.2).

8.2.4 HISTOLOGIC CHANGES IN MELANOCYTIC NEVI IN PREGNANCY

Biopsy specimens should be obtained promptly from any changing mole that would raise concern for malignancy. These procedures can be performed safely during pregnancy. Lidocaine does not cross the placenta;[16] thus it has been classified as Category B by the US Food and Drug Administration (FDA) and can be used safely during pregnancy. The addition of epinephrine to lidocaine provides an advantage, in that its vasoconstrictive effects can reduce peak serum levels of lidocaine in the mother and thus decrease its placental transfer to the fetus.[17]

Various studies have described histologic differences in biopsy specimens obtained from nevi in pregnant women. The nevi from pregnant women had slightly higher atypia scores than those from nonpregnant female controls.

In one study it was found that 83% of nevi excised from pregnant patients exhibited clusters of melanocytes with a specific appearance, which they termed "superficial micronodules of pregnancy". This appearance was described as "rounded clusters of 3 to 20 large epithelioid melanocytes with prominent nucleoli, abundant pale eosinophilic cytoplasm, and occasional fine melanosomes".

TABLE 8.1
Summary of Studies of Changes in the Size of Nevi during Pregnancy

Study	Findings during Pregnancy	Locations
Grin et al.[9]	No significant change in size	Back
Akturk et al.[10]	Increase in diameter	Changes most significant on abdomen and breast
Strumia et al.[11]	Some changes in diameter	Only appreciable on abdomen and breast
Pennoyer et al.[12]	No significant change in size	Back
Zampino et al.[13]	No significant change in size	Back

TABLE 8.2

Summary of Studies of Dermoscopic Changes in Nevi during Pregnancy

Study	Locations Assessed	Stages Compared	Changes Noted during Pregnancy	Postpartum Status
Akturk et al.[10]	All	First and third trimesters	New dot development in 6 of 82 nevi Increased TDS	Not assessed Not assessed
Strumia et al.[11]	All	Second and third trimesters	Pigment network became clearer and more widely meshed with growth Increased number of brown globules on the periphery with growth	Not assessed Not assessed
Zampino et al.[13]	Back	First and third trimesters	Increased number of vessels Decrease in pigmentation and prominence of pigment network Increased TDS	Normalised within 6 months after delivery Progressive through 6 months after delivery Decreased within 6 months after delivery
Gunduz et al.[14]	Back, face, and neck	First and third trimesters	Thickening of pigment network lines in 2 of 21 nevi Brown globules and black dots increased in number, colour, and size in 2 of 21 nevi Increased TDS	Not assessed Not assessed Returned to first trimester score by 6 months*
Rubegni et al.[15]	Excluded breasts, abdomen, and acral	First and third trimesters	Increase in prominence and thickening of pigment network Darkening of globules in nevi with a globular pattern Decreased organisation of reticular pattern Less homogeneity in size and distribution of globules	Regressed within 12 months after delivery Regressed within 12 months after delivery Persisted 12 months after delivery Persisted 12 months after delivery

* 3/4 returned, 1 lost to follow-up.

TDS, Total dermoscopy score.

This was speculated to represent a histopathologic characteristic of nevi from pregnant women; however, this feature was present in some controls also.[19]

In addition, there was a significantly higher mitotic rate in these nevi. There was also a marginally higher Ki-67 proliferation index in nevi from pregnant patients compared with the control nevi. The authors inferred that there may be both increased melanocyte proliferation and cell cycle progression during pregnancy. Any histopathologic features consistent with melanoma should be viewed as melanoma and not attributed to pregnancy (Table 8.3).

8.3 PREGNANCY AND DYSPLASTIC NEVUS SYNDROME

Dysplastic nevus syndrome (DNS), also known as atypical mole syndrome, is a sporadic or hereditary disorder resulting in numerous clinically atypical nevi and an increased risk for developing malignant melanoma.

Patients are defined as having dysplastic nevi if they had clinically atypical nevi and histologically a dysplastic nevus. Clinical atypia consists of abnormal lesion morphology, with nevi (1) often larger than 5 mm in diameter, (2) having irregular outlines, and (3) exhibiting colour variegation (tan, brown, and red shades within the lesion, focal black pigment suggest melanoma). The

TABLE 8.3

Summary of Studies of Histologic Changes in Nevi during Pregnancy

Study	Histologic Changes
Foucar et al.[18]	No significant difference in overall atypia, though slightly more atypical than nonpregnant female controls and similar to male controls
	Pregnant women more atypical than controls, specifically in mitotic activity, lentiginous proliferation, other cytologic atypia, demarcation of melanocytes at lateral margins of lesion, and the presence of small nevus cells in lower dermis
Chan et al.[19]	Clustered melanocytes with specific appearance in 83% of nevi from pregnant patients
	Multinucleated melanocytes seen exclusively in controls
	Significantly higher mitotic rate and number of mitotic figures compared with age-matched controls and marginally higher Ki-67 proliferation index
Sanchez et al.[20]	No significant differences between pregnant women and age-matched female controls

number and distribution of lesions are variable (from a few to more than 100). The histologic criteria include: (1) absolute criteria—(a) nuclear atypia and (b) lymphocytic and mesenchymal response (lamellar fibroplasia) and (2) relative criteria—(a) lentiginous hyperplasia; (b) ellipsoid irregular nested hyperplasia; (c) epithelioid cells, singly and grouped; (d) small dermal melanocytic cells, with impairment of maturation and synthesis of pigment; and (e) prominent junctional component, often at the shoulders of the papular component where dysplasia is most evident.[21]

Clinical and histologic changes in nevi during pregnancy may occur in patients with DNS. According to various studies the rate of clinical change in these women was found to be 3.9 times higher when they were pregnant than when they were not. The biopsy specimens of the patients from these lesions during pregnancy were twice as likely to show histologic dysplastic changes.[22] These changes were independent of trimester of pregnancy, number of pregnancies, sex of the child, history of blistering burns, or the use of artificial UV light.

The rate of change in dysplastic nevi was same in in pregnant and nonpregnant women with familial dysplastic nevus syndrome (FDNS). In contrast, patients with sporadic dysplastic nevus syndrome (SNDS) had a high rate of changing dysplastic nevi while pregnant but a low rate of changing dysplastic nevi when they were not pregnant. This eightfold increase in the rate of changing dysplastic nevi in pregnancy in SDNS patients suggests that pregnancy may be a high-risk period for dysplastic nevus change in these patients, and this change might correlate with an increased risk of melanoma, although there are no studies done to confirm it.

Focal acantholytic dyskeratosis (FAD) and epidermolytic hyperkeratosis (EHK) are histologic findings often seen in nevi biopsies. The incidence of FAD and EHK have statistically increased within dysplastic nevi, suggesting that these histologic patterns reflect cellular epidermal damage and have potential diagnostic utility. SOX-10 and Melan-A melanocytic inmunostains provide positive results when used for staining tissue samples of dysplastic nevi in the area of FAD and EHK. However, a study has demonstrated that incidental FAD and EHK within dysplastic nevi biopsies are capable of aberrantly staining with melanocytic markers. These immunostains may be used to determine the degree of atypia in melanocytic neoplasms, suggesting that aberrant staining in FAD and EHK could lead to the misdiagnosis of dysplastic nevi as more severe processes. Thus, this study proposed that this aberrant melanocytic immunostaining in FAD and EHK may be a diagnostic pitfall when assessing dysplastic nevi.[23]

It is currently recommended that DNS patients be closely observed during times of increased hormonal activity.[24] Recent reports indicate that cutaneous photography provides an early melanoma detection method for DNS patients.[25]

8.4   PREGNANCY AND MELANOMA

Melanoma is a malignant tumour arising from melanocytes. It is a very deadly disease, accounting for 75% of skin cancer deaths, though it only accounts for 4% of skin cancer cases.[26] Malignant melanoma (MM) is the most common malignancy reported during pregnancy, one third of all new cases being diagnosed during childbearing age. Melanoma accounts for approximately 8% of maternal malignancies. Furthermore, if only metastases to the fetus are considered, the percentage resulting from melanoma rises to 43%. An incidence between 2.8 to 5.0 cases of melanoma per 100,000 pregnancies has been reported by earlier studies, and this number continues to increase as more women postpone childbearing.[27] The influence of pregnancy on the clinical course of malignant melanoma is controversial.

8.4.1   Clinical and Histological Features of Melanoma in Pregnancy

MMs diagnosed during pregnancy have shown an increased tumour thickness compared to nonpregnant controls.[28,29] The pregnancy-associated growth factor may accelerate tumour growth. However, the more likely explanation is delay in diagnosis due to the accepted fact that nevus change in pregnancy is physiological. Some studies have observed no significant difference in tumour depth overall in pregnant patients compared with nonpregnant controls, except for MMs diagnosed in the third trimester.[30]

According to various studies there was no significant difference between the groups for ulceration, mitotic rate, stage of disease, anatomic location of MM, histologic subtype, Clark level, regression, necrosis, or vascular invasion. The only difference noted was more marked inflammation around the tumour in the pregnancy associated MM group.[31] The recent controlled trials have shown no differences in MMs diagnosed during pregnancy from nonpregnant controls in anatomic location of primary lesions or histologic type.[28,32]

8.4.2   Immunologic Changes during Pregnancy

During pregnancy the cytotoxic adaptive immune responses are significantly diminished, innate immunity remains intact, and regulatory adaptive immunity is enhanced. The expansion of CD4+ CD25+ regulatory T cells (Tregs) are essential for allowing the fetus to survive. Tregs mediate tolerance in pregnancy as well as cancer.[33] These cells increase in cancer and may be implicated in impaired antitumor immunity, suppression of effector T lymphocyte proliferation, and increased tumour vascularity. Uterine natural killer cells (uNKs), found in the decidua of the pregnant uterus, are the most common immune cells found at the materno-fetal interface. These may play a role in inducing tolerance and angiogenesis in the decidua and placenta. A similar reduction in NK cell cytotoxic activity has been shown by certain malignancies.[33]

During the first two trimesters, the transition at the materno-fetal interface from the inflammatory T helper cell 1 (TH1)–predominant environment to the immunologically tolerant T helper cell 2 (TH2) environment parallels immunologic alterations seen in malignancies.[34] This TH2-driven environment favours tumour survival, and TH2 cytokines are elevated in patients with metastatic compared to resected MMs. However, there is no evidence to suggest that pregnancy induces specific immunologic changes that lead to the development or spread of MM. According to some studies the physiologic state of pregnancy and the immunosuppressed state that fosters the growth and tolerance of cancer cells is the same.

8.5   CLINICAL OR LABORATORY EVIDENCE DEPICTING A LINK BETWEEN HORMONES (OR OTHER GROWTH FACTORS) AND EITHER NEVI OR MELANOMA

According to earlier studies, MM is likely to be a hormonally responsive tumor.[35] The other evidence in favour of this is that skin hyperpigmentation occurs in in selected anatomic areas in pregnant females, the incidence of MM is low before puberty, evidence of receptors for oestrogen and progesterone in some MMs, and enhanced growth rate of some MMs in mice after administration of oestrogen. The recent data suggests no association between the two, as there is a lack of strong evidence for physiologic, hormone-induced changes in nevi during pregnancy, various studies showing no effect of pregnancy on the prognosis of MM, and epidemiologic evidence showing no effect of exogenous hormones (OCPs or HRT) on the risk of MM.[3]

As for laboratory evidence, the early studies showed that the specific binding of hormones to MMs in tissue culture was at a very low level.[36] Further studies utilising monoclonal antibody techniques failed to detect oestrogen receptors (now recognised as oestrogen receptor alpha (ERα) in benign nevi, dysplastic nevi, primary or metastatic MM, or pregnancy-associated MM.[37] ERb has been found as the predominant receptor in all of the melanocytic lesions studied. A strong correlation was found between ERb expression and the proximity of melanoma cells to keratinocytes; that is, expression was most intense in melanoma cells in the epidermis and in the papillary dermis close to the epidermis, compared with melanoma cells deeper in the dermis. This was demonstrated by greater expression of ERb in severely dysplastic nevi and lentigo malignas compared with thick nodular MMs with greater Breslow depth. These investigators concluded that oestrogen may indeed play a role in MM. There is no role of any specific growth factor in the growth or spread of MM, but placenta growth factor, a member of the platelet-derived growth factor family, has been found to be secreted by human melanoma cell lines.[38] A single study has observed proliferation in response to this factor. Thus, the evidence for a link between hormones and MM and/or nevi is possible, but certainly pregnancy-associated hormones have not been clearly established to affect the prognosis or risk for MM.

8.6 EVALUATION OF PATIENTS WITH MELANOMA IN PREGNANCY

The evaluation of the pregnant patient diagnosed with MM is the same as that recommended for the nonpregnant patient. There is significant controversy concerning the safety and timing of some of the diagnostic and staging procedures in pregnant females. Prompt biopsy of a suspected lesion should be performed with the patient under local anaesthesia, which is safe and should not be delayed due to pregnancy. Lidocaine, a Pregnancy Category B drug according to Food and Drug Administration (FDA) classification, is generally thought to be safe for local anaesthesia during pregnancy.[39] After establishing the histological diagnosis, Breslow depth and other important prognostic indicators will dictate further evaluation which needs to be done for appropriate staging of the patient.

A multidisciplinary approach is important even in the management of localised disease, since maternal fetal monitoring may be desirable during the performance of a biopsy.

If sentinel lymph node (SLN) mapping and biopsy is indicated, different surgeons and/or medical centres may perform this procedure differently, using a radioactive colloid, such as 99mTc labelled sulphur colloid, 1% isosulfan blue dye, or both.[40] There are different opinions regarding the use of these substances. Some clinicians prefer to avoid the use of radiocolloid during pregnancy, while others have pointed out that the average doses of radiation to which the fetus is exposed are well below the teratogenic threshold.[40] The primary safety concern for pregnant women is the risk of anaphylaxis to isosulfan blue dye, and therefore radiocolloid alone is used for SLN mapping and biopsy.[41] Some studies state that blue dye is contraindicated in pregnant patients. and some centres do not offer SLN biopsy and mapping to women under 30 weeks' gestation because of fear of any possible impact on fetal organogenesis, which becomes most critical at the end of the first trimester.

In the case of evaluation for distant metastases, the safety of selected imaging studies in the pregnant woman with MM is also controversial. While a chest x-ray examination may be performed safely if shielding is utilised, it is recommended that in early pregnancy, sonographic evaluation of the abdomen and liver is preferred over computed tomographic (CT) scanning with intravenous contrast, because of the absorbed fetal radiation dose.[42] Magnetic resonance imaging (MRI) is safer than CT scanning, but the former is not recommended during the first trimester because of the heating of tissues associated with radiofrequency fields used during MRI.[43]

8.7 PROGNOSIS OF MELANOMA IN PREGNANCY

8.7.1 PROGNOSIS FOR THE MOTHER

Since the 1950s, multiple case reports that have been published suggest a poor prognosis for women who were either diagnosed with MM during or soon after pregnancy.[44] It was suggested that this was such an ominous diagnosis that surgical sterilisation might be appropriate. The depth of the MM, which is the most important prognostic factor, was not considered by most of these studies. However, the published data since 1980s have now consistently observed no significant effect on survival in women diagnosed with localised MM (American Joint Committee on Cancer [AJCC] stage I or II) during pregnancy.[28,29] These studies utilised appropriate control groups and considered stage of disease and important prognostic factors such as tumour thickness.

Common consensus from various studies reported no significant difference in survival between pregnant and non-pregnant patients.[29] In two studies, the disease-free interval (DFI) was significantly shorter in the pregnant women compared with nonpregnant, with nodal metastases as the most frequent site of recurrence. Other studies showed no adverse effect of pregnancy on DFI.

8.7.2 PROGNOSIS FOR THE FETUS

The transplacental spread of MM with metastasis to the fetus is rare. The placental barrier against maternal cancer cells functions less effectively in cases of melanoma. It is estimated that only 25% of the fetuses are affected. The hematogenous spread to the placenta is observed only in women with widely metastatic MM. However, considering all types of cancer that occur during pregnancy, MM is the most common maternal malignancy to metastasise to the placenta.[45] The spread of MM to the placenta does not imply that metastasis to the fetus has occurred. According to reported cases of MM affecting the newborn or fetus, most of them died of metastatic MM, with time of death after delivery ranging from hours to 11 months. The skin and liver were the most common sites for MM in these cases. In general, the prognosis for the fetus depends on the stage of disease of the mother. Transplacental spread of MM to the fetus has been observed only in women with distant metastases; which occurs rarely even in these patients. However, spontaneous regression may occur after delivery. Therefore, therapeutic abortion is not recommended. A thorough gross and microscopic examination of the placenta for MM should be undertaken in women with advanced disease; if placental involvement is documented, close follow-up of the infant is necessary, including frequent skin examination by the dermatologist. Therefore, the presence of placental metastases is not necessarily an indication for treatment of the newborn.

8.7.3 PROGNOSIS OF MM DIAGNOSED BEFORE PREGNANCY

Earlier data published over the past 50 years have suggested either a very poor prognosis[35] or no effect[46] of a subsequent pregnancy after diagnosis with MM. However, in cases with adverse outcomes, hormonal stimulation during pregnancy was thought to cause growth and spread of MMs. Pregnancy within 5 years of diagnosis of MM was not found to significantly affect the prognosis. The counselling on the topic of future pregnancies should be based on established prognostic factors, such as tumour thickness and ulceration. Based on the time period of recurrence and not on the negative impact of a subsequent pregnancy on MM, it is often stated that a woman diagnosed with MM should wait 2 to 3 years to become pregnant.

8.7.4 PROGNOSIS OF MM DIAGNOSED AFTER PREGNANCY

Early studies have suggested either a favourable or absent effect upon prognosis. However, tumour thickness, the most important prognostic factor, has not been taken into consideration in these studies.[47] Some studies hypothesised that prior pregnancies may have a prognostically protective effect since some MM antigens resemble fetal antigens, and thus an immune response to MM may be enhanced.[47] According to recent studies, prior pregnancies do not appear to influence the survival of women diagnosed with localised melanoma. However, women who have had five or more pregnancies prior to diagnosis may have some survival advantage.

8.8 TREATMENT OF PATIENTS WITH MELANOMA IN PREGNANCY

The treatment is based on stage of disease. There exists controversy regarding the therapies for the fetus as well as the appropriate timing of these therapies during the pregnancy. If the procedure of choice indicated is a wide local excision, it can be safely performed under local anaesthesia. Maternal fetal monitoring may be desirable during wide local excision utilising lidocaine.[42] The addition of epinephrine (a Category C drug according to the FDA) to lidocaine for improved haemostasis and prolonged effect at the surgical site is controversial, as in animals it has the potential to decrease uterine blood flow.[48,49] It has to be used cautiously in pregnancy, at a concentration of 2.5 to 5.0 g/mL, or the equivalent of 1:400,000 or 1:200,000 concentration, respectively, when mixed with lidocaine if larger doses of lidocaine are anticipated.[48]

The treatment of pregnant women who have advanced metastatic MM with chemotherapy or interferon should be limited to exceptional cases.[49]

8.9 COUNSELLING PATIENTS WITH MELANOMA IN PREGNANCY

Counselling pertaining to future pregnancies and/or the use of oral contraceptives and hormone replacement therapy is important in patients diagnosed with melanoma in pregnancy. According to various studies, future pregnancies do not appear to affect the prognosis of the patient diagnosed as having localised MM.[28,29] The risk of recurrence based on the established prognostic factors, primarily tumour thickness, presence or absence of ulceration, and stage of disease as determined by the AJCC, determines the delay in the next pregnancy. In general, a patient with a "thin" MM, where the risk of recurrence is unlikely, need not delay pregnancy.

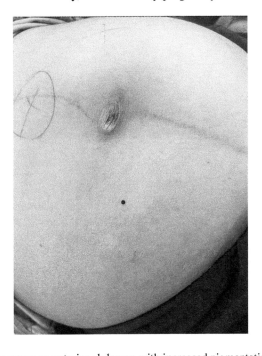

FIGURE 8.1   Melanocytic nevus on anterior abdomen with increased pigmentation.

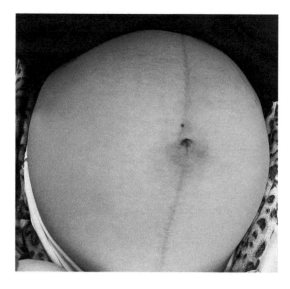

FIGURE 8.2   Melanocytic nevus in the midline with increased pigmentation.

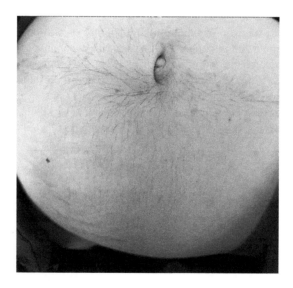

FIGURE 8.3   Melanocytic nevus on anterior abdomen with increase in diameter.

For patients with a high risk or recurrence, the recommendation is to wait for 2 to 3 years, which in general is based on the time period within which recurrence is most likely. These decisions need to be made on an individual basis, where prognosis for the mother, age of the mother, her fertility status, and family support are all considered. Most of the studies published over the past 30 years have not shown an association between exposure to OCPs and risk for MM. There is no significant association between hormonal replacement therapy (HRT) and risk for MM.[50] Therefore, these exogenous hormones are not contraindicated if a woman diagnosed and treated for MM has a subsequent need for either OCPs or HRT and reasonable alternative therapies do not exist.

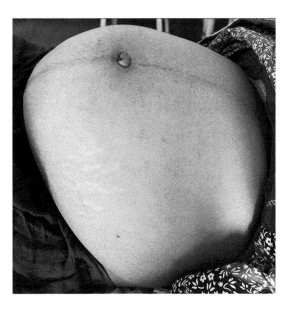

FIGURE 8.4   Melanocytic nevus on the left flank with no chages in colour or diameter.

REFERENCES

1. Damsky WE, Bosenberg M. Melonocytic nevi and melanoma: unraveling a complex relationship. *Oncogene*. 2017;36(42):5771–5792.
2. Lee YY, Roberts CL, Dobbins T, et al. Incidence and outcomes of pregnancy-associated cancer in Australia, 1994–2008: a population-based linkage study. *BJOG*. 2012;119:1572–1582.
3. Driscoll MS, Grant-Kels JM. Hormones, nevi, and melanoma: an approach to the patient. *J Am Acad Dermatol*. 2007;57(6):919–931;quiz 932–936.
4. Tyler KH. Physiological skin changes during pregnancy. *Clin Obstet Gynecol*. 2015;58:119–124.
5. James WD, Berger T, Elston D, eds. *Andrews' diseases of the skin: clinical dermatology*. Philadelphia: W.B. Saunders; 2015.
6. Winton GB, Lewis CW. Dermatoses of pregnancy. *J Am Acad Dermatol*. 1982;6:977–998.
7. Wong RC, Ellis CN. Physiologic skin changes in pregnancy. *J Am Acad Dermatol*. 1984;10:929–940.
8. Nading MA, Nanney LB, Ellis DL. Pregnancy and estrogen receptor b expression in a large congenital nevus. *Arch Dermatol*. 2009;145:691–694.
9. Grin CM, Rojas AI, Grant-Kels JM. Does pregnancy alter melanocytic nevi? *J Cutan Pathol*. 2001;28:389–392.
10. Akturk AS, Bilen N, Bayramgurler D, et al. Dermoscopy is a suitable method for the observation of the pregnancy-related changes in melanocytic nevi. *J Eur Acad Dermatol Venereol*. 2007;21:1086–1090.
11. Strumia R. Digital epiluminescence microscopy in nevi during pregnancy. *Dermatology*. 2002;205: 186–187.
12. Pennoyer JW, Grin CM, Driscoll MS, et al. Changes in size of melanocytic nevi during pregnancy. *J Am Acad Dermatol*. 1997;36:378–382.
13. Zampino MR, Corazza M, Constantino D, et al. Are melanocytic nevi influenced by pregnancy? A dermoscopic evaluation. *Dermatol Surg*. 2006;32:1497–1504.
14. Gunduz K, Koltan S, Sahin MT, E Filiz E. Analysis of melanocytic naevi by dermoscopy during pregnancy. *J Eur Acad Dermatol Venereol*. 2003;17:349–351.
15. Rubegni P, Sbano P, Burroni M, et al. Melanocytic skin lesions and pregnancy: digital dermoscopy analysis. *Skin Res Technol*. 2007;13:143–147.
16. Lawrence C. Drug management in skin surgery. *Drugs*. 1996;52:805–817.
17. Gormley DE. Cutaneous surgery and the pregnant patient. *J Am Acad Dermatol*. 1990;23:269–279.

18. Foucar E, Bentley TJ, Laube DW, Rosai J. A histopathologic evaluation of nevocellular nevi in pregnancy. *Arch Dermatol.* 1985;121:350–354.
19. Chan MP, Chan MM, Tahan SR. Melanocytic nevi in pregnancy: histologic features and Ki-67 proliferation index. *J Cutan Pathol.* 2010;37:843–851.
20. Sanchez JL, Figueroa LD, Rodriguez E. Behavior of melanocytic nevi during pregnancy. *Am J Dermatopathol.* 1983;6:89–91.
21. Elder DE, Green MR, Guerry DIV, et al. The dysplastic nevus syndrome: our definition. *Am J Dermatopathol.* 1982;4:455–460.
22. Ellis DL. Pregnancy and sex steroid hormone effects on nevi of patients with the dysplastic nevus syndrome. *J Am Acad Dermatol.* 1991;25:467–482.
23. Erickson K, RohrB. 34997 Melanocytic staining of focal acantholytic dyskeratosis and epidermolytic hyperkeratosis within dysplastic nevi. *J Am Acad Dermatol.* 2022;87(3):Ab80.
24. Greene MH, Clark WH Jr, Tucker MA, et al. Acquired precursors of cutaneous malignant melanoma: the familial dysplastic nevus syndrome. *N Engl J Med.* 1985;312:91–97.
25. Rigel DS, Rivers JK, Kopf AW, et al. Dysplastic nevi: markers for increased risk for melanoma. *Cancer.* 1989;63:386–389.
26. Davis LE, Shalin SC, Tackett AJ. Current state of melanoma diagnosis and treatment. *Cancer Biol Ther.* 2019;20(11):1366–1379.
27. Dillman RO, Vandermolen LA, Barth NM, Bransford KJ. Malignant melanoma and pregnancy ten questions. *West J Med.* 1996;164:156–161.
28. Reintgen DS, McCarty KS, Vollmer R, et al. Malignant melanoma and pregnancy. *Cancer.* 1985;55:1340–1344.
29. MacKie RM, Bufalino R, Morabito A, et al. Lack of effect of pregnancy on outcome of melanoma. *Lancet.* 1991;337:653–655.
30. Lens MB, Rosdahl I, Ahlbom A, et al. Effect of pregnancy on survival in women with cutaneous malignant melanomas. *J Clin Oncol.* 2004;22:4369–4375.
31. Fabian M, Toth V, Somlai B, et al. Retrospective analysis of clinicopathologic characteristics of pregnancy associated melanoma. *Pathol Oncol Res.* 2015;21:1265–1271.
32. Riberti C, Margola G, Bertani A. Malignant melanoma: the adverse effect of pregnancy. *Br J Plast Surg.* 1981;34:338–339.
33. Holtan SG, Creedon DJ, Haluska P, Markovic SN. Cancer and pregnancy: parallels in growth, invasion, and immune modulation and implications for cancer therapeutic agents. *Mayo Clin Proc.* 2009;84:985–1000.
34. Nevala WK, Vachon CM, Leontovich AA, et al. Evidence of systemic Th2-driven chronic inflammation in patients with metastatic melanoma. *Clin Canc Res.* 2009;15:1931–1939.
35. Pack GT, Scharnagel IM. The prognosis for malignant melanoma in the pregnant woman. *Cancer.* 1951;4:324–334.
36. Cohen C, DeRose PB, Campbell WG, et al. Estrogen receptor status in malignant melanoma. *Am J Dermatopathol.* 1990;12:562–564.
37. Lecavalier MA, From L, Gaid N. Absence of estrogen receptors in dysplastic nevi and malignant melanoma. *J Am Acad Dermatol.* 1990;23:242–246.
38. Graeven U, Rodeck U, Karpinski S, et al. Expression patterns of placenta growth factor in human melanocytic cell lines. *J Invest Dermatol.* 2000;114:118–123.
39. Sweeney SM, Maloney ME. Pregnancy and dermatologic surgery. *Dermatol Clin.* 2006;24:205–214.
40. Mondi MM, Cuena RE, Ollila DW, et al. Sentinel lymph node biopsy during pregnancy: initial clinical experience. *Ann Surg Oncol.* 2006 [E-pub ahead of print].
41. Schwartz JL, Mozurkewich EL, Johnson TM. Current management of patients with melanoma who are pregnant, want toget pregnant, or do not want to get pregnant. *Cancer.* 2003;97:2130–2133.
42. Shapiro RL. Surgical approaches to malignant melanoma: practical guidelines. *Dermatol Clin.* 2002;20:681–699.
43. Campbell FA, Campbell C. Magnetic resonance imaging for Stage IV melanoma during pregnancy. *Arch Dermatol.* 2006;142:393.
44. Byrd BF, McGanity WJ. The effect of pregnancy on the clinical course of malignant melanoma. *South Med J.* 1954;47:196–200.
45. Anderson JF, Kent S, Machin G. Maternal malignant melanoma with placental metastasis: a case report with literature review. *Pediatric Pathol.* 1989;9:35–42.
46. McManamny DS, Moss ALH, Pocock PV, Briggs JC. Melanoma and pregnancy: a long-term follow-up. *Br J Obstet Gynaecol.* 1989;96:1419–1423.

47. Hersey P, Morgan G, Stone DE, et al. Previous pregnancy as a protective factor against death from melanoma. *Lancet.* 1977;1:451–452.
48. Rosenberg PH, Veering BT, Urmey WF. Maximum recommended doses of local anesthetics: a multifactorial concept. *Reg Anesth Pain Med.* 2004;29:564–567.
49. Beyeler M, Hafner J, Beinder E, et al. Special considerations for Stage IV melanoma during pregnancy. *Arch Dermatol.* 2005;141:1077–1078.
50. Holman CDJ, Armstrong BK, Heenan PJ. Cutaneous malignant melanoma in females: exogenous sex hormones and reproductive factors. *Br J Cancer.* 1984;50(5):673–680.

9 Common Infections and Infestations during Pregnancy

Arunima Dhabal and Indrashis Podder

9.1 INTRODUCTION

Pregnancy is a physiologic state in females associated with profound alterations in the endocrine, vascular, metabolic, and immunological systems.[1] Immune alterations are necessary to prevent fetal rejection by host immune cells. There is a shift towards T-helper Type 2 immunity associated with predominance of anti-inflammatory cytokines (e.g., IL-4, IL-10, IL-13) due to high levels of circulating oestrogen.[2] These changes increase the susceptibility of pregnant women to various infections and infestations and additionally alter the lesional morphology, clinical course, and severity of infectious diseases. Certain infections in pregnancy may be associated with serious consequences such as congenital malformations in the growing fetus due to transplacental transfer. Management of infections in pregnancy often requires special considerations, as certain medications are contraindicated in pregnant women.[3]

This chapter briefly discusses some of the common cutaneous infections and infestations encountered in pregnant women along with their recommended treatment options. Sexually transmitted infections are not discussed, as they have been covered elsewhere.

9.2 BACTERIAL INFECTIONS

9.2.1 STAPHYLOCOCCAL AND STREPTOCOCCAL INFECTIONS

Pyogenic infections such as impetigo, furunculosis, abscesses, and cellulitis are commonly seen in pregnancy. Methicillin-resistant *Staphylococcus aureus* (MRSA) is often implicated in bullous impetigo, furuncles, and abscesses, whereas cellulitis is more commonly caused by *Streptococcus pyogenes*. Cervicofacial cellulitis originating from dental plaques or odontogenic procedures have been reported during pregnancy and are associated with high morbidity and mortality due to persistent threat to airways and risk of fetal hypoxia.[4] Cellulitis associated with community-acquired MRSA usually involves the gluteal and vulvovaginal areas and results in abscess formation.[5] Pregnant patients are also at increased risk for invasive Group A Streptococcal infection, in the form of cellulitis, necrotising fasciitis, toxic shock syndrome, sepsis, and endomyometritis. These account for approximately 50% of sepsis-related fatalities during pregnancy in the UK.[6] Additionally, Group B Streptococcal (*S. agalactiae*) vaginal colonisation during pregnancy may result in premature rupture of membranes, leading to fetal morbidity and mortality. Therefore, pregnant women are routinely screened for Group B Streptococci in the United States, Canada, and Australia.[7]

Treatment—Staphylococcal infections in pregnancy are treated with topical mupirocin and oral first-generation cephalosporins or dicloxacillin, while the first-line treatment for Streptococcal infection is oral or intravenous penicillin. MRSA infections are best treated by clindamycin, as sulphonamides and tetracyclines are contraindicated in late pregnancy.[5]

DOI: 10.1201/9781003449690-9

9.2.2 LISTERIOSIS

Listeriosis is a food-borne disease caused by *Listeria monocytogenes*. It is encountered 20 times more frequently in pregnant women than in the general population, due to reduced cell-mediated immunity.[8] Cutaneous lesions are relatively uncommon in listeriosis. In pregnancy, it manifests as an indeterminate febrile illness or flu-like syndrome, usually mild, and may be rarely associated with purpuric rash. However, transplacental fetal transmission may result in abortion, stillbirth, or premature labour.[7]

Diagnosis of listerial infection is established by blood culture or, less frequently, amniotic or cerebrospinal fluid culture.

Treatment—The treatment of choice is ampicillin at a dose of 2 g every 6 to 8 hours for at least 3–4 weeks. This dosage is essential for adequate intracellular penetration and transplacental passage in adequate concentration. Erythromycin may be used as an alternative in patients allergic to penicillin.[8]

9.2.3 BACTERIAL VAGINOSIS

Bacterial vaginosis is the most commonly diagnosed vaginal infection in pregnancy, affecting 10–30% pregnant women.[9] It occurs due to an imbalance in the composition of normal vaginal flora caused by hormonal changes, leading to reduced acid-producing lactobacilli and an overgrowth of anaerobic bacteria. Vaginal douching, history of sexually transmitted infections, and HIV-positive status are its important risk-factors.[10] Patients may be asymptomatic or present with abnormal grey to white foul-smelling vaginal discharge. Although symptoms are mild and easily treatable, in untreated cases, it can lead to premature labour and fetal complications.

Diagnosis is established by a higher-than-normal vaginal pH (>4.5), clue cells on wet mount of vaginal discharge, and a positive whiff test (fishy odour on addition of potassium hydroxide solution to vaginal discharge).

Treatment—The recommended treatment regimen is metronidazole 500 mg or clindamycin 300 mg twice daily for 7 days. Topical formulations may also be used, but clindamycin cream is contra-indicated in the third trimester.[9]

9.3 MYCOBACTERIAL INFECTIONS

An intact cell-mediated immune response is essential for prevention and dissemination of myco-bacterial infection. Thus, depressed cell-mediated immunity in pregnancy, along with nutritional and hormonal changes, predispose pregnant women to these infections. Additionally, these diseases often have an altered course during pregnancy.

9.3.1 LEPROSY

In 20 to 30% of women, signs and symptoms of leprosy develop for the first time during pregnancy.[11] This is possibly due to subclinical infections becoming apparent as a result of increased bacillary load in a relatively immunosuppressed state. There is frequent worsening of disease, with progression towards the lepromatous spectrum. The bacteriological index may increase maximally in the third trimester, although this is usually transient, with reduction to the pre-pregnancy levels after delivery.[12] Relapse may also occur due to multiplication of persisters, especially in the third trimester.

Lepra reactions also present differently in pregnant women. Type 1 reactions, which are associated with an improvement in cell-mediated immunity, are less frequent during pregnancy and more frequent in the postpartum period. When they do occur in pregnancy, cutaneous symptoms like lesional erythema and oedema are mild, and neuritis is rare. Type 2 reactions, on the other hand, are more frequent and severe during pregnancy due to increased bacillary load. Leprosy-associated neuritis in pregnancy is primarily a result of increased bacillary load causing neural granuloma.[12]

The effects of leprosy on pregnancy include possible transplacental transmission of infection, which may rarely lead to prematurity or fetal loss. Intrauterine growth retardation has also been reported due to smaller placental size and inadequate fetoplacental perfusion in pregnant women with lepromatous leprosy.[12]

Treatment—The treatment of leprosy in pregnancy is similar to other patients, irrespective of the trimester. Patients on multi-drug therapy with dapsone, rifampicin, and clofazimine who become pregnant should continue the treatment for the duration recommended. Reactions in pregnancy are usually treated with oral corticosteroids, as other anti-reaction drugs like thalidomide, methotrexate, cyclosporine, and azathioprine are contraindicated.[12]

9.3.2 CUTANEOUS TUBERCULOSIS

Although pulmonary tuberculosis may occur in endemic areas, cutaneous tuberculosis has been rarely reported in pregnant women. It may present as jelly-like nodules, which can ulcerate and cause extensive scarring. Other manifestations include papules, vesicles, and necrotic lesions with local lymphadenopathy.[13]

The treatment includes a standard duration anti-tubercular drug regimen, as with other variants of tuberculosis, in all affected pregnant women.

9.4 VIRAL INFECTIONS

The severity of many viral infections reportedly increase during pregnancy due to immunological alterations. Placental response to viruses has also been suggested to play a key role in their severity.[9] In addition, prenatal and perinatal transmission of viral infections often have severe detrimental effects on the newborn. Common cutaneous viral infections affecting pregnant women include herpes simplex, varicella zoster, rubella, and viral warts.

9.4.1 HERPES SIMPLEX INFECTIONS

Infection with herpes simplex virus (HSV) 1 and 2 is common in the reproductive age group. While HSV-1 predominates in orofacial lesions, genital lesions are more common with HSV-2. Genital herpes shows a high prevalence in the pregnant population.[14] Primary infection during pregnancy is associated with increased severity and a potentially fatal course, owing to a higher risk of viral dissemination leading to hepatitis, encephalitis, and coagulopathy.[3,9] Recurrences are also more frequent in pregnant women.[9]

HSV is a component of the "TORCH" complex, which also include toxoplasmosis, rubella, and cytomegalovirus infections.[5] These infections affecting the mother at any time during pregnancy may be transmitted to the fetus, leading to complications like microcephaly, hepatosplenomegaly, thrombocytopenia, sensorineural deafness, and chorioretinitis. In addition, disseminated and genital HSV infections are also associated with spontaneous abortion, intrauterine growth retardation, preterm labour, and congenital and neonatal herpes infections.[14]

Treatment—Active HSV infections in pregnancy are usually treated with the standard regimen of acyclovir. Data on use of valacyclovir and famciclovir in pregnant women are limited, but they are Category B drugs and considered safe.[5] As perinatal transmission of HSV occurs most commonly in the intrapartum period, prophylactic suppressive therapy should be started from 36 weeks of gestation in patients with recurrent infections to reduce the risk of viral shedding at delivery.[5] The presence of active genital lesions during delivery is an indication for caesarean section.

9.4.2 Varicella and Herpes Zoster

Primary varicella zoster virus (VZV) infection is relatively uncommon in pregnancy, as most patients develop anti-VZV antibodies following infection in childhood. However, it may occur in seronegative pregnant patients and tends to have a more severe course, especially when it develops in late pregnancy. The risk of complications like pneumonia, hepatitis, and encephalitis correlates with the severity of the exanthem and may occur within 3–5 days of rash onset. Primary VZV infection in pregnancy may also be life threatening, with an estimated 10% mortality rate.[15]

The risk of transplacental infection is about 25%, with highest risk in the early second trimester. However, clinical manifestations in the form of fetal malformations, known as congenital varicella syndrome, develop in only 1–2% of these cases.[3] Spontaneous abortion may occur in few cases. On the other hand, perinatal VZV infection, especially between 5–7 days before and 2–7 days after delivery, carries 20–50% risk of neonatal varicella.[15]

Herpes zoster, caused by reactivation of latent VZV following previous primary infection, may occur during pregnancy due to the immunocompromised state. However, due to the presence of antibodies, there are no significant risks of dissemination in the mother or transplacental transmission.[16]

Treatment—VZV infection in pregnancy is treated based on the disease severity and gestational age. Uncomplicated primary infections occurring beyond 20 weeks of pregnancy are treated with oral acyclovir 800 mg 5 times daily for 7 days. Intravenous acyclovir 10 mg/kg/day is indicated in case of persistent fever, haemorrhagic rash and complications like pneumonia. Caesarean delivery should be done in such cases to avoid maternal respiratory insufficiency and consequent risk to the fetus.[3]

In patients that develop varicella before 20 weeks of gestation, in addition to the previous treatment, fetal monitoring by high-resolution ultrasound, magnetic resonance imaging, and analysis of fetal VZV IgM antibodies is essential. Significant fetal anomalies in serial tests may necessitate termination of pregnancy.[3]

Tocolysis or delaying of delivery has been recommended in perinatal VZV infection to allow more time for transplacental passage of protective maternal antibodies to the fetus. In addition, the newborn should receive passive immunisation with varicella zoster immunoglobulin (VZIG) immediately after delivery.[3]

For herpes zoster in pregnancy, specific antiviral therapy is generally not required, except in case of herpes zoster oticus, herpes zoster ophthalmicus, haemorrhagic lesions, mucosal involvement, or disseminated herpes zoster.[16]

9.4.3 Rubella

Rubella, or German measles, is a viral infection typically seen in children. Although the incidence has decreased in most countries due to vaccination campaigns, in developing countries rubella viruses have been found to circulate in young children. Thus, susceptible pregnant women in these countries are at higher risk of acquiring the infection.[17]

The clinical presentation in pregnancy is not significantly different from other patients, with more than half cases being asymptomatic. Clinically apparent cases show mild prodromal symptoms, followed by a maculopapular rash. Polyarthritis and polyarthralgia are common complications in pregnancy, while encephalitis, thrombocytopenia, and Guillain-Barre Syndrome have been reported very rarely.[18]

Infection in the first trimester commonly leads to spontaneous abortion, intrauterine fetal death, or congenital rubella syndrome, where the newborn presents with microcephaly, cataract, deafness, and cardiac abnormalities. Therefore, patients presenting within 18 weeks of gestation should be subjected to detailed ultrasound examination for fetal anomalies and serology from amniotic fluid. Termination of pregnancy should be considered in case of gross fetal abnormalities.[17]

9.4.4 Condyloma Acuminata

Genital warts are usually caused by human papilloma virus (HPV) 6, 11, 16, and 18 infection. Reduced cell-mediated immunity and increased vascularity of the genital tract during pregnancy leads to increased activation and infectivity of HPV. This results in rapid growth of existing lesions along with appearance of new lesions, especially between 12 and 14 weeks of gestation. Lesions may also become more friable, leading to frequent bleeding. In rare cases, they may become large enough to cause obstruction of the birth canal.[3]

Vertical transmission of HPV 6, 11, 16 or 18 during pregnancy or delivery may result in the development of anogenital, oral or conjunctival warts in the neonate. HPV 6 and 11 are also known to cause juvenile laryngeal papillomatosis following perinatal transmission.[3] Genital warts may also cause bacterial trapping, leading to chorioamnionitis and premature rupture of membranes following ascending infection.[19] In addition, HPV 16 and 18 have been found to be associated with preterm birth and placental abnormalities.[20]

Treatment—Cryotherapy is regarded as the first-line treatment of genital warts during pregnancy. Other surgical methods of destruction which can also be used include electrocautery, excision, and CO_2 laser ablation.[3] Among non-surgical modalities, chemical destruction with trichloroacetic acid is considered safe, while all other topical agents like podophyllin, imiquimod, and cantharidin are contraindicated in pregnancy.[5] Caesarean delivery is recommended in patients with large lesions due to risk of excessive bleeding, although it has not shown a significant protective role in preventing vertical transmission of HPV.[3]

9.5 FUNGAL INFECTIONS

9.5.1 Vulvovaginal Candidiasis

Pregnancy is one of the most important predisposing factors for vulvovaginal candidiasis (VVC), which affects up to 50% of pregnant women. This is attributed to a fall in pH due to high oestrogen levels; a raised glycogen content in the vaginal mucosa, associated with enhanced adherence of yeasts to the mucosal cells; and a decline in the growth of protective commensal bacteria during pregnancy.[3,9] Among the causative agents, *Candida albicans* comprises 80% of all cases, although organisms like *C. tropicalis, C. glabrata*, and *C. parapsilosis* are also commonly isolated.[3]

The risk of acquiring VVC and severity of the infection increases with gestational age. Patients are often asymptomatic in early pregnancy but usually present with vulvovaginal irritation and discharge in late pregnancy. Maternal VVC is also associated with fetal risks. Preterm delivery and low birth weight have been associated with recurrent VVC in early pregnancy. Ascending infection can lead to congenital candidiasis, characterised by generalised papulopustular eruption, pneumonia, or sepsis in the neonate shortly after birth. On the other hand, perinatal transmission during delivery through an infected birth canal leads to neonatal candidiasis, which is generally limited to the skin and mucosa of the newborn.[3]

Treatment—Topical azoles are the first-line treatment of VVC in pregnancy. They should be continued for 2 weeks, as clinical response is slower and there is a higher risk of recurrences during pregnancy.[3] Preliminary evidence has shown that clotrimazole can also prevent preterm birth in patients with asymptomatic infection.[21] Other topical agents, which can also be used in pregnant women are nystatin and amphotericin B. Oral antifungals are usually not recommended, especially in the first trimester, due to potential fetal risks.[5] However, in severe primary infections with pronounced inflammation in late pregnancy, fluconazole may be used in doses of 150 mg/day for 7–14 days.[3] It has not shown any increased risk of fetal complications in this dose, although higher doses (400–800 mg/day) for longer duration have been reported to cause birth defects.[9,22]

9.5.2 DERMATOPHYTOSIS

Superficial fungal infections caused by dermatophytes are one of the most common infections world-wide. Over the past few years, the prevalence of these infections has been increasing further across the world and has reached epidemic proportions in tropical and developing countries like India. Pregnant women are particularly at risk due to immune suppression, weight gain, and increased sweating caused by hormonal changes, which facilitate fungal growth.[23] Lesions involving the groins (tinea cruris) and feet (tinea pedis) are relatively more common in pregnancy, although any body part may be affected.

Treatment—Topical azole antifungals are the first choice of treatment of tinea infections in any stage of pregnancy as systemic absorption is minimal. Among azoles, clotrimazole is the preferred drug as it is Pregnancy Category B, whereas miconazole and econazole are categorised as C and preferably avoided.[24] Other topical agents that are considered safe include oxiconazole, terbinafine, naftifine, and ciclopirox. Whitfield's ointment, containing salicylic and benzoic acid, is a Category C drug due to risk of systemic absorption of salicylic acid. However, it may be considered in localised hyperkeratotic lesions, especially if benefits outweigh the risks.[23] Systemic drugs are indicated only in cases of bullous lesions, kerion, Majocchi's granuloma, recurrent and extensive infections, and in immunocompromised patients.[5] In all other cases, systemic drugs should be deferred until delivery or lactation. Terbinafine is the only oral antifungal included in pregnancy Category B. However, due to limited data on placental transfer of the drug, it is best avoided in the first and second tri-mesters. Oral fluconazole, itraconazole, and griseofulvin are categorised as C and therefore not recommended, especially in early pregnancy, due to the risk of congenital defects in the fetus.[5,24]

As pharmaceutical options are limited in pregnancy, patients should be counselled properly regarding general measures and personal hygiene. Loose cotton clothes and daily washing of under-garments should be encouraged, and patients should be advised to avoid occlusive garments and footwear and sharing of personal items. Absorbent antifungal dusting powders may be used as adjuvant options, and affected family members should be treated simultaneously.[23,24]

9.5.3 *PITYRIASIS VERSICOLOR AND PITYROSPORUM FOLLICULITIS*

Pregnancy is associated with an increased incidence of pityriasis versicolor and pityrosporum fol-liculitis, both of which are caused by the dimorphic fungus, *Malassezia furfur*.[1] This has been attributed to the increased adrenocortical function and depressed cell-mediated immunity associ-ated with pregnancy. In addition, increased activity of sebaceous glands produces a favourable micro-environment for the growth and proliferation of the lipophilic fungi.[25]

Treatment—Localised lesions in pregnant women are usually treated with topical clotrimazole or allylamines. For widespread lesions, topical benzoyl peroxide and zinc pyrithione soap are con-sidered safe and effective alternatives.[5] Treatment with systemic drugs should be deferred until the completion of pregnancy and lactation as the infection is usually asymptomatic and does not pose any serious risk to the mother or fetus.

9.6 PARASITIC INFESTATIONS

9.6.1 SCABIES

Scabies, caused by the *Sarcoptes scabiei* mite, is the most common parasitic disease in pregnant women, accounting for 2–6% of all skin disorders occurring in pregnancy.[3] As in non-pregnant women, it presents with intensely pruritic generalised papules and excoriations, which may be com-plicated by secondary bacterial infections. Crusted scabies is rare in immunocompetent patients. Maternal scabies has not been linked to any adverse effects on the fetus.[3] Scabies in pregnancy should be differentiated from specific dermatoses of pregnancy, which have a similar presenta-tion. Demonstration of jet-with-contrail sign on dermoscopy or mites, eggs, and faecal pellets on microscopy of skin scrapings may help to confirm the diagnosis in doubtful cases. A similar history in close contacts also serves as an important clue.

Treatment—The treatment of choice in pregnant patients is permethrin 5% cream, which is a Category B drug. Alternatively, other topical scabicides like 6–10% precipitated sulphur, 10% crotamiton, and 25% benzyl benzoate may be used, but these are considered less effective than permethrin. Lindane is contraindicated in pregnancy due to potential neurotoxicity in the mother and risk of fetal neural tube defects and mental retardation.[5] Oral ivermectin is a Category C drug and should be used only in immunosuppressed patients with crusted scabies. It has been found to have teratogenic effects in high doses in animal studies, although no adverse outcomes have been reported in humans.[26]

9.6.2 Pediculosis Capitis

Head louse infestation may occur during pregnancy as a result of inadequate hair hygiene. As in case of non-pregnant women, permethrin 1% lotion is the first-line treatment for pediculosis capitis in pregnancy.[5] Newer anti-lice agents include benzyl alcohol 5% (Category C) and spinosad (Category B). Benzyl alcohol paralyses the lice, causing their respiratory spiracles to open and get plugged by inert ingredients, leading to death by asphyxiation. Spinosad is a neurotoxic insecticide derived from the fermentation of filamentous bacteria, *Saccharopolyspora spinosa*. It is available as a suspension, which also contains benzyl alcohol. Current literature concerning efficacy and safety of these drugs is scarce, so permethrin remains the first choice.[5,27]

REFERENCES

1. Kroumpouzos G, Cohen LM. Dermatoses of pregnancy. *J Am Acad Dermatol.* 2001;45:1–19.
2. Yip L, McCluskey J, Sinclair R. Immunological aspects of pregnancy. *Clin Dermatol.* 2006;24(2):84–87.
3. Müllegger RR, Häring NS, Glatz M. Skin infections in pregnancy. *Clin Dermatol.* 2016;34(3):368–377.
4. Omeje KU, Omeje IJ, Agbara R. Severe cervicofacial cellulitis in pregnancy: A review of 18 cases. *Iran J Otorhinolaryngol.* 2020;32(109):93–100.
5. Elston CA, Elston DM. Treatment of common skin infections and infestations during pregnancy. *Dermatol Ther.* 2013;26(4):312–320.
6. Cantwell R, Clutton-Brock T, Cooper G, et al. Saving mothers' lives: Reviewing maternal deaths to make motherhood safer: 2006–2008. The eighth report of the confidential enquiries into maternal deaths in the United Kingdom [published correction appears in BJOG. 2015 Apr;122(5):e1] [published correction appears in BJOG. 2015 Apr;122(5):e1]. *BJOG.* 2011;118(Suppl 1):1–203.
7. Hay RJ, Morris-Jones R. Bacterial infections. In: Griffiths C, Barker J, Bleiker T, eds. *Rook's Textbook of Dermatology*, 9th edn. West Sussex: John Wiley & Sons, Ltd; 2016:26.1–26.87.
8. Janakiraman V. Listeriosis in pregnancy: Diagnosis, treatment, and prevention. *Rev Obstet Gynecol.* 2008;1(4):179–185.
9. Ledan S. Infectious diseases in pregnancy. *USPharm.* 2020;45(9):22–26.
10. Shaffi AF, Balandya B, Majigo M, et al. Predictors of bacterial vaginosis among pregnant women attending antenatal clinic at tertiary care hospital in Tanzania: A cross sectional study. *East Afr Health Res J.* 2021;5(1):59–68.
11. Lockwood DN, Sinha HH. Pregnancy and leprosy: A comprehensive literature review. *Int J Lepr Other Mycobact Dis.* 1999;67:6–12.
12. Khanna N. Leprosy and pregnancy. In: Kumar B, Kar HK, eds. *IAL Textbook of Leprosy*, 2nd edn. New Delhi: Jaypee Brothers Medical Publishers; 2017:352–359.
13. Datta S, Spencer J. Cutaneous tuberculosis in pregnancy. *J Obstet Gynaecol.* 2004;24:455.
14. Straface G, Selmin A, Zanardo V, et al. Herpes simplex virus infection in pregnancy. *Infect Dis Obstet Gynecol.* 2012;2012:385697.
15. Sauerbrei A, Wutzler P. Herpes simplex and varicella-zoster virus infections during pregnancy: Current concepts of prevention, diagnosis and therapy. Part 2: Varicella-zoster virus infections. *Med Microbiol Immunol.* 2007;196:95–102.
16. Smith CK, Arvin AM. Varicella in the foetus and newborn. *Semin Fetal Neonatal Med.* 2009;14:209–217.
17. Bouthry E, Picone O, Hamdi G, et al. Rubella and pregnancy: Diagnosis, management and outcomes. *Prenat Diagn.* 2014;34:1246–1253.

18. Figueiredo CA, Klautau GB, Afonso AMS, et al. Isolation and genotype analysis of rubella virus from a case of Guillain–Barré syndrome. *J Clin Virol.* 2008;43:343–345.

19. Khan F, Mays R, Brooks J. Viral and sexually transmitted disease. In: Kroumpouzos G, ed. *Text Atlas of Obstetric Dermatology.* Philadelphia: Lippincott Williams & Wilkins; 2013:126–140.

20. Zuo Z, Goel S, Carter JE. Association of cervical cytology and HPV DNA status during pregnancy with placental abnormalities and preterm birth. *Am J Clin Pathol.* 2011;136:260–265.

21. Roberts CL, Algert CS, Rickard KL, et al. Treatment of vaginal candidiasis for the prevention of preterm birth: A systematic review and meta-analysis. *Syst Rev.* 2015;4:31.

22. Norgaard M, Pedersen L, Gislum M, et al. Maternal use of fluconazole andrisk of congenital malformations: A Danish population-based cohort study. *J Antimicrob Chemother.* 2008;62(1):172–176.

23. Prabhu SS, Sankineni P. Managing dermatophytoses in pregnancy, lactation, and children. *Clin Dermatol Rev.* 2017;1(Suppl 1):S34–S37.

24. Kaul S, Yadav S, Dogra S. Treatment of dermatophytosis in elderly, children, and pregnant women. *Indian Dermatol Online J.* 2017;8(5):310–318.

25. Zampino MR, Osti F, Corazza M, Virgili A. Prevalence of pityriasis versicolor in a group of Italian pregnant women. *J Eur Acad Dermatol Venereol.* 2007;21(9):1249–1252.

26. Chippaux JP, Gardon-Wendel N, Gardon J, et al. Absence of any adverse effect of inadvertent ivermectin treatment during pregnancy. *Trans R Soc Trop Med Hyg.* 1993;87:318.

27. Patel VM, Lambert WC, Schwartz RA. Safety of topical medications for scabies and lice in pregnancy. *Indian J Dermatol.* 2016;61(6):583–587.

10 Connective Tissue Diseases and Pregnancy

Shital Poojary and Anmol Bhargava

10.1 INTRODUCTION

10.1.1 BACKGROUND INFORMATION ON CONNECTIVE TISSUE DISEASES

Connective tissue diseases (CTDs) encompass a diverse group of disorders characterised by abnormalities in the connective tissues, which provide structural support and maintain the integrity of various organs and systems in the body. Examples of CTDs include systemic lupus erythematosus, rheumatoid arthritis, and scleroderma. These conditions result from immune dysregulation and can affect multiple organ systems, leading to a range of symptoms and complications.

Pregnancy can pose unique challenges for women with CTDs, as the physiological changes and immune adaptations that occur during pregnancy can influence disease activity and progression. It is crucial to understand the impact of CTDs on pregnancy outcomes to optimise maternal and fetal health. Women with CTDs may face an increased risk of adverse pregnancy outcomes, such as miscarriage, preterm birth, and intrauterine growth restriction. Understanding these risks can guide healthcare professionals in providing appropriate care and interventions.

This chapter provides a comprehensive overview of the relationship between CTDs and pregnancy. It aims to examine the influence of CTDs on pregnancy outcomes, explore the management strategies for pregnant women with CTDs, and discuss the long-term implications for both the mother and the child. Additionally, the chapter will highlight specific considerations and complications associated with different types of CTDs during pregnancy.

10.2 DEFINITION AND CLASSIFICATION OF CTDs

Connective tissue disorders can be classified as follows:

1. *Autoimmune Connective Tissue Disorders*
   - Systemic lupus erythematosus (SLE)
   - Dermatomyositis
   - Rheumatoid arthritis (RA)
   - Sjögren's syndrome
   - Systemic sclerosis (scleroderma)

2. *Vasculitis-Associated Connective Tissue Disorders*
   - Polyarteritis nodosa (PAN)
   - Takayasu arteritis
   - Granulomatosis with polyangiitis (GPA, formerly Wegener's granulomatosis)
   - Churg–Strauss syndrome (CSS, eosinophilic granulomatosis with polyangiitis)

DOI: 10.1201/9781003449690-10

3. *Other Connective Tissue Disorders*
   - Myositis
   - Mixed connective tissue disease (MCTD)
   - Undifferentiated connective tissue disease (UCTD)

10.3 PREGNANCY AND CONNECTIVE TISSUE DISEASES

10.3.1 EPIDEMIOLOGY OF CTDS AND PREGNANCY

The epidemiology of CTD in pregnancy is not well established, as most studies are based on small cohorts or case reports. However, some general trends can be observed. For example, SLE is more prevalent among women of African, Asian, or Hispanic origin and affects about 0.1% of pregnancies. Antiphospholipid antibody syndrome is associated with recurrent miscarriages, fetal growth restriction, and pre-eclampsia and affects about 1–5% of pregnancies. Rheumatoid arthritis affects about 0.5–1% of pregnancies and tends to improve during pregnancy but flare up postpartum. Scleroderma is rare in pregnancy, affecting about 0.01% of pregnancies, and can cause severe complications such as renal crisis, pulmonary hypertension, and fetal death.[1]

10.3.2 PATHOGENESIS OF COMPLICATIONS

The following factors may play a role in antenatal and perinatal pregnancy complications associated with CTDs:

1. Inadequate invasion of trophoblastic tissue has been observed in uterine artery Doppler studies in patients with connective tissue diseases.
2. Role of antibodies: Antibodies can directly affect pregnancy outcomes. ANA and other antibodies can contribute to adverse pregnancy outcomes in the following ways:
   - Adversely affect oocyte quality and embryo development, thereby reducing the implantation rates.[2]
   - Activation of the complement cascade.

These factors cause an impaired uterine perfusion, suboptimal endometrial receptivity, endothelial dysfunction,[3] and cytokine imbalance,[4] ultimately causing defective placentation.

Fibrin Deposition and Massive Perivillous Fibrin Deposition in the Placenta (MPVFD): MPVFD is a rare and serious condition of unknown aetiology, although autoimmune mechanisms have been suspected. Incidence is estimated between 0.028 and 0.5%, with risk factors including infection, autoimmune disease, and thrombophilia. Autoimmune conditions that have been associated with MPVFD include SLE, antiphospholipid antibody syndrome, systemic sclerosis, and inflammatory myopathy. The condition is characterised by diffuse fibrin deposition within the intervillous space and is associated with prematurity, intrauterine growth restriction (IUGR), and intrauterine fetal demise (IUFD).

10.3.3 EFFECT OF PREGNANCY ON CTDS

- *Lupus Erythematosus*: SLE usually does not worsen during pregnancy, especially for patients on immunosuppressive therapy. The chances of a flare are further lowered with remission or minimal disease activity in the 6–12 months prior to conception. The risk factors for a flare are active disease at conception and active lupus nephritis. Lupus flares during pregnancy and postpartum are usually non-severe, involving articular, dermatological, and haematological systems, although severe flares with major organ involvement may occur. Facial flushing or hyperpigmentation of normal pregnancy may look like a lupus malar rash. HELLP syndrome, characterised by a low platelet count, increased liver function tests, haemolysis, abdominal pain, and eclampsia, which includes seizures and rarely stroke, can also be mistaken for active SLE or vasculitis.

- *Sjögren Syndrome*: Frequent gum swelling and bleeding may exacerbate oral and dental issues in Sjögren's syndrome patients. There are no large-scale studies evaluating the impact of pregnancy on Sjögren's syndrome. Case reports have shown occasional complications like acute renal failure due to mesangial proliferative glomerulonephritis and pericarditis. While there is insufficient data to conclude how pregnancy impacts disease activity during pregnancy, it is probably best to use the approach applied to other rheumatologic disorders that disease should be in remission at the time of conception.

- *Mixed Connective Tissue Disease*: A recent review described a 26.7% risk of disease relapse during pregnancy, similar to that of other autoimmune diseases.[5] The limited data available on the effect of pregnancy on MCTD suggests that there is a small risk of disease flare during pregnancy.

- *Undifferentiated Connective Tissue Disorder*: UCTD is defined as the presence of the following criteria:

  1. Signs and symptoms indicative of a connective tissue disorder but not meeting the required criteria to diagnose a specific CTD
  2. Positive antinuclear antibodies on two separate measurements

     - Thirty percent of patients with UCTD eventually develop a specific CTD, while 20–87% persist in the undifferentiated state.[6–10]
     - Among the UCTD patients who evolve to CTDs, SLE is the most common.[6]
     - Pregnancy and puerperium may trigger disease flares and evolution to a definite CTD.[11,12] The risk of flare was found to be higher in women with anti-ds DNA antibodies and higher disease activity; therefore, assessment of autoantibody profile and disease activity prior to conception is important.

- *Antiphospholipid Antibody Syndrome*: Pregnancy induces a prothrombotic state based on changes in both procoagulant and fibrinolytic systems; this, together with mechanical factors such as venous stasis, compression by the gravid uterus, or bed rest, leads to an increased thromboembolic disease risk in women with antiphospholipid antibodies and active inflammatory disease.

- *Rheumatoid Arthritis and Other Chronic Inflammatory Arthritides*: Rheumatoid arthritis is an autoimmune, chronic inflammatory disorder of unknown aetiology occurring in approximately 0.5–1% of the population worldwide. The majority of patients improve during pregnancy, with a decrease in disease activity. About 20% of patients go into remission by the third trimester, followed by a postpartum flare within 3–4 months.[13] Women with positive rheumatoid factor (RF) and anti-cyclic citrullinated peptide (anti-CCP) are less likely to improve during pregnancy.[14] Barret et al. found that the disease response to one pregnancy was predictive of the response in a subsequent pregnancy. [15] Amelioration of RA in the pregnancy was associated with an increased number of Treg cells that induced a pronounced anti-inflammatory cytokine milieu. Psoriatic arthritis also tends to improve in most patients, while the clinical course of ankylosing spondylitis (AS) remains unaltered or worsens during pregnancy. Approximately 20% of AS patients improve from spinal and extraspinal symptoms during pregnancy.[16,17] These patients most often have a history of arthritis in joints other than the spine or psoriasis or IBD associated with their AS. Fifty to 80% of AS patients experience aggravation of symptoms 4–12 weeks after delivery, and disease activity returns as a rule to the pre-pregnancy pattern during the year following delivery.

- *Systemic Sclerosis*: Pregnancy does not affect disease activity in most patients. One third of patients experience either improvement or worsening in disease. Raynaud's phenomenon generally improves because of the physiological vasodilation of pregnancy, whereas gastroesophageal reflux disease symptoms worsen. Skin involvement usually remains stable or improves but may worsen postpartum. It is unlikely that pregnancy increases the risk of developing renal crisis; however, literature on this specific subject is lacking. Recent onset of disease (last 4 years) and diffuse type of scleroderma with anti-Scl-70 or anti-RNA-polymerase-III antibodies are risk factors for worsening of disease activity in pregnancy.

- *Vasculitis*: Among primary vasculitides, young women in the reproductive age group are mainly affected by Takayasu arteritis (TAK), polyarteritis nodosa (PAN), ANCA-associated vasculitis (AAV), immune-complex small-vessel vasculitis (IgA vasculitis), and Behçet's disease (BD).[18] Th-2 cytokine polarisation during pregnancy may explain the improvement of primarily Th1-mediated vasculitides (mainly Takayasu arteritis and Behçet disease) and the worsening of Th2-driven ones, such as granulomatosis with polyangiitis (Wegener's granulomatosis) or eosinophilic granulomatosis with polyangiitis (Churg–Strauss syndrome). Pregnancy is not recognised as a trigger for the development of vasculitis. However, vasculitis can present itself for the first time during pregnancy, and in such cases PAN and microscopic polyangiitis (MPA) are shown to have the worst prognosis. Risk of flare during pregnancy is higher in patients with active or recently diagnosed vasculitis. The risk of flare also depends on the type of vasculitis, with retinal vasculitis, small-vessel vasculitis, and necrotising vasculitis associated with a higher risk of flare.[19,20] Physiologic palmar erythema associated with pregnancy may be mistaken for cutaneous vasculitis.

- *Myositis*: The idiopathic inflammatory myopathies (IIM) are a group of rare autoimmune conditions that share the common theme of an immune-mediated attack on skeletal muscle with resulting clinical weakness. The group includes dermatomyositis (DM), polymyositis (PM), juvenile myositis (JM), inclusion body myositis (IBM), cancer-associated myositis, overlap myositis, and necrotising autoimmune myopathy (NAM). There are reports of new-onset inflammatory myopathy presenting shortly after pregnancy,[21–28] ranging from 4 days to 3 months postpartum. Authors argue that this high percentage of patients who develop disease temporally close to pregnancy suggests that the association is not coincidental, though larger studies with conclusive evidence are lacking. Over 60% of inflammatory myositis in pregnancy has occurred in patients with pre-existing myositis. Of these, 44% were complicated by flare during the pregnancy.

10.3.4 INFLUENCE OF CTDS ON PREGNANCY

- *Lupus Erythematosus*: There is a higher risk of complicated pregnancies in SLE in all patients in the form of hypertension, pre-eclampsia, and thrombotic complications. Risk factors are chronic hypertension, lupus nephritis, and women taking high-dose oral steroids. Prognosis is relatively favourable if disease activity is minimal in the 6 months prior to conception.

- *Mixed Connective Tissue Disorder*: There is an increased risk of pre-eclampsia, venous thromboembolism (VTE), and maternal mortality comparable to other CTDs.

- *Undifferentiated Connective Tissue Disorder*: There is a possible increased risk of pre-eclampsia, gestational hypertension, and gestational diabetes in pregnant patients with UCTD; therefore, these possible complications should be watched out for.

- *Antiphospholipid Syndrome*: Antiphospholipid syndrome is an autoimmune disorder characterised by thrombosis (venous, arterial, and microvascular) and pregnancy complications. The condition is associated with a spectrum of autoantibodies directed against the cellular phospholipid component (hence the term "antiphospholipid antibodies" or APA), most commonly lupus anticoagulant, anticardiolipin, and anti-β2 glycoprotein I (anti-B2GPI). In addition to the detection of APA on at least two occasions more than 12 weeks apart, APLS is defined by any one of the following adverse pregnancy outcomes:

1. One or more unexplained deaths of a normal fetus after the 10th week of gestation
2. Three or more unexplained consecutive spontaneous miscarriages before the 10th week of gestation (with maternal anatomical and parental chromosomal causes excluded)
3. One or more preterm births of a normal fetus before the 34th week of gestation because of eclampsia or recognised features of placental insufficiency

- Other complications include catastrophic APLS, thrombosis, and HELLP syndrome (haemolysis, elevated liver enzymes, low platelet count). The term "primary APLS" is used when the condition occurs in the absence of any other related disease. The term "secondary APLS" is used when the condition occurs in the context of other autoimmune diseases, such as systemic lupus erythematosus and other autoimmune diseases such as rheumatoid arthritis, Sjögren syndrome, and systemic sclerosis.

- **Rheumatoid Arthritis and Other Chronic Inflammatory Arthritides**: There is an increased risk of hypertensive pregnancy disorders, including pre-eclampsia. Involvement of the cervical spine with cervical instability in RA is rare, but when atlanto-axial subluxation is present, cervical cord damage is a risk during delivery. It is important to know of this deformity before considering general anaesthesia for a surgical delivery. Cervical radiographs or MR examination in RA patients before a planned pregnancy is recommended to exclude atlanto-axial subluxation. In pregnant women with AS, sometimes the anaesthesiologist will not give epidural anaesthesia because they fear problems with positioning the epidural catheter in case of ankylosis of the lumbar spine. Sometimes calcification of the posterior, longitudinal ligament inhibits spreading of the anaesthetic solution by the epidural route; then intrathecal anaesthesia may be necessary.[29]

- **Systemic Sclerosis**: Systemic sclerosis increases the risk of hypertensive pregnancy disorders, including pre-eclampsia.

- **Vasculitis**: Hypertensive disorders are associated with up to 20% of these pregnancies.[30,31] Higher rates of hypertension and pre-eclampsia are seen in patients with Takayasu arteritis (TAK), which are risk factors for poor outcomes.[19,32]

10.3.5 IMPACT OF CTDs ON PREGNANCY OUTCOMES

- **Lupus Erythematosus**: There is an increased risk of obstetric complications like preterm birth, intrauterine growth restriction, fetal loss, and neonatal lupus erythematosus.
  Risk factors for poor pregnancy outcomes in LE:[33,34]

  - African and Hispanic descent
  - Chronic hypertension and antihypertensive use at baseline
  - Renal impairment
  - Active disease or flare in 6 months leading up to conception
  - Non-reversible organ damage
  - Hypocomplementemia
  - Thrombocytopenia
  - Presence of the lupus anticoagulant
  - Secondary antiphospholipid syndrome

    - Active lupus nephritis poses the greatest risk to pregnancy outcomes, with a history of lupus nephritis posing a risk of 8–36% of non-elective pregnancy loss.

Favourable prognostic indicators are SLE in remission without major organ involvement, minimal disease activity in the 6 months prior to conception, and cutaneous lupus erythematosus only.[35] The increased risk of fetal death may be because of immune complex deposition on the trophoblast basement membrane or the transplacental passage of antiphospholipid antibodies.

- *Sjögren Syndrome*: Patients with primary or secondary SS and anti-Ro/La antibodies have an increased risk of neonatal lupus. There is an increased risk of low birth weight and increased chances of delivery by caesarean section or vacuum extraction than in the background population.[36]

- *Neonatal LE*: Neonatal lupus erythematosus (NLE) is a type of lupus erythematosus caused by the transplacental passage of maternal antibodies. The most frequent clinical manifestations are cutaneous lesions and congenital heart block (CHB). The presence of the Ro/SS-A antibody is strongly associated with NLE, being present in 82–100% of infants and 92–100% of mothers. La/SS-B antibodies are less frequent (in 50% of NLE infants and 60% of mothers, usually in association with Ro/SSA antibodies). These antibodies have also been shown to bind to Ro/SS-A and La/SS-B antigen in human fetal cardiac-conducting tissue, thereby causing conduction abnormalities. However, these antibodies are not specific for NLE, also occurring in Sjögren syndrome, SLE, RA, SSc, and healthy asymptomatic carriers (11%). The onset may be up to 12–16 weeks postpartum. The clinical presentation may be either cutaneous or cardiac, although rarely other systems may be involved early. Cutaneous manifestations are seen in approximately half of the neonates in the form of an erythematous, slightly scaly, photosensitive rash on the face and periorbital skin (raccoon sign/owl eye/eye mask), scalp, trunk, extremities, neck, and intertriginous areas. Other manifestations include vitiligo-like lesions, morphea-like lesions, and papules on the feet. Complete heart block is the most common cardiac manifestation and affects approximately 2% of babies born to anti-Ro and/or anti-La-positive mothers. This risk increases to 18% if the mother has already had a child affected by CHB and up to 50% if she has had two affected children.[37] Other manifestations include pericardial effusions, pleural effusions, ascites, intrauterine growth retardation, hydrops fetalis, and dilated cardiomyopathy. Haematological abnormalities like transient thrombocytopenia, neutropenia, haemolytic anaemia, and aplastic anaemia have also been reported. Hepatic involvement may occur in the form of neonatal hepatitis and hepatosplenomegaly. The rash usually resolves without scarring by 12 months of age. The heart block is permanent and usually requires a permanent pacemaker. Rare complications of NLE include pneumonitis, haemochromatosis, aseptic meningitis, myelopathy, transient myasthenia gravis, spastic paraparesis and chondrodysplasia punctata, and hydrocephalus. Investigations include skin biopsy to confirm the diagnosis, antibody testing for both child and mother, and investigations to screen for cardiac involvement. Management of skin disease includes photoprotection, low potent steroids, and antimalarials. Oral steroids or antimalarials given to the mother in the first 16 weeks of pregnancy may prevent conduction defects. Pacemaker insertion is the definitive management for CHB.

  - Long-term follow-up of both infant and mother is recommended to screen for development of autoimmune CTDs in the future.

- *Mixed Connective Tissue Disorder*: Fetal complications include an increased risk of prematurity, IUGR, and perinatal mortality, comparable to other CTDs. The rate of complications (both maternal and fetal) has been shown to be directly influenced by disease activity.[5] There is an increased risk of neonatal lupus in pregnant women with MCTD (28%), more commonly in women with anti-Ro/La antibodies but also in women with anti-U1 RNP antibodies only, though less commonly. The data is inconsistent as to whether MCTD diagnosed prior to pregnancy causes higher rates of fetal loss. Due to the limited information in the literature, it is impossible to conclude whether MCTD increases the risk of other pregnancy complications such as pre-eclampsia, prematurity, and SGA infants. Thus, one can reassure patients that the existing information suggests that pregnancy outcome in women with MCTD appears to be good.

- ***Undifferentiated Connective Tissue Disorder***: There is an increased risk of pregnancy complications like preterm birth, small for gestational age infants, fetal growth retardation, intrahepatic cholestasis of pregnancy, preterm premature rupture of the membranes, and miscarriage. This prevalence of complications was higher in the subgroup of patients with certain antibody profiles like anti-Ro (SSA) antibodies and antiphospholipid antibodies. Hence screening of antibody profile in patients with UCTD should be done prior to pregnancy.

- ***Antiphospholipid Antibodies and Antiphospholipid Syndrome***: Antiphospholipid antibodies are found in APLS, SLE, and other CTDs and in the general population (1–5%) and are a major risk factor for poor obstetric outcome. Lupus anticoagulant (LAC), among the three APAs, is the primary predictor of poor pregnancy outcomes in women. Other predictors for poor pregnancy outcomes include IgG anticardiolipin antibodies at ≥40 units/ml, SLE, and a history of thrombosis and history of prior fetal loss.[38] The poor obstetric outcomes associated with APLS include spontaneous miscarriages, preterm birth, IUGR, fetal distress, and premature rupture of membranes.

- Women with lupus anticoagulant antibodies and thrombotic antiphospholipid syndrome have the worst obstetric outcomes. Untreated APS may lead to an increased rate of fetal loss in 45–90% of pregnancies, which falls to 30% with adequate treatment. Despite treatment, around 30% of APLS pregnancies will still result in pregnancy loss.

- ***Rheumatoid Arthritis and Other Chronic Inflammatory Arthritides***: For women with well-controlled RA, pregnancy outcomes are comparable to the general obstetric population, whereas higher levels of RA disease activity are associated with increased risk of less favourable pregnancy outcomes like preterm birth, IUGR, low birth weight, premature rupture of membranes, and caesarean section. Studies have shown an increased relative risk of spontaneous abortion among patients with RA. Perinatal morbidity and mortality is slightly increased in arthritic patients, especially RA. RA can also indirectly affect the pregnancy outcome, as hypertensive disorders may be more frequent in women with RA, which are often related to preterm deliveries and intrauterine growth restriction. Patients with ankylosing spondylitis show no increase in adverse pregnancy outcomes compared to healthy women. Compared to healthy women, elective CS is more frequently performed in patients with AS.

- ***Systemic Sclerosis***: There is an increased risk of preterm delivery, intrauterine growth restriction, and longer hospitalisation. Women with long-standing diffuse scleroderma also have an increased risk of miscarriage. Women with limited scleroderma generally have better pregnancy outcomes compared to diffuse disease.

- ***Vasculitis***: The incidence of fetal complications seems to be higher in mothers with more severe disease and with a higher number of damaged vessels. A minimal disease activity in the last 6 months leading up to conception is ideal for favourable outcomes. There is an increased risk of preterm birth, low birth weight, IUGR, caesarean deliveries, and less commonly miscarriages. In children of mothers with ANCA-associated vasculitides, two cases of microscopic polyangiitis-like syndrome were described in newborns, potentially due to the passage of maternal ANCA through the placenta. It has been suggested that maternal treatment with immunosuppressive therapy may prevent the onset of this syndrome in the child. Several cases of transient neonatal Behçet's disease have been reported, probably due to diffusion of lesional lymphocytes in the placenta, but more data is needed.

- *Myositis*: There is a paucity of data on inflammatory myositis and pregnancy, probably since onset of disease typically occurs after the reproductive years. Available literature shows a possible link between disease activity, especially during early pregnancy, and adverse pregnancy outcomes. As one might expect, the absence of disease activity during pregnancy appears to be associated with a higher percentage of favourable outcomes. Also, earlier the disease presents during pregnancy, the greater the likelihood of a poor outcome. The main complications, albeit seen rarely, are preterm delivery and small for gestational age neonate. More recent studies on inflammatory myopathies and pregnancy did not appear to be associated with adverse maternal or fetal outcomes. In general, neonatal outcome is good and is complicated primarily by the sequelae associated with preterm delivery or small size for gestational age. Moreover, there does not appear to be support for the idea that the outcome of one pregnancy is predictive of subsequent pregnancies in women with inflammatory myopathies.

10.3.6 SPECIAL CONSIDERATIONS RELATED TO CONTRACEPTION IN CTD PATIENTS

Special considerations pertain to the use of contraceptives in rheumatic disease. In APA-positive patients, considering their increased risk of thrombotic complications, hormonal contraceptives are avoided. Similarly, in SLE patients, irrespective of APA status, the latest research suggests that use of hormonal contraceptives, particularly the newer third-generation pill, patch, and vaginal rings, carries an increased thrombotic risk and is therefore best avoided.[38]

For APA-negative patients, combined and progestin-only contraceptives can be used. DMPA by intramuscular injection is also an effective and long-lasting option, though long-term use is associated with osteoporosis and therefore needs to be used with caution in patients with high cumulative corticosteroid exposure.

The non-hormone-containing copper-IUD, which lasts for 10 years, has no restriction for use in SLE patients (with positive or unknown APA status). However, due to increased menstrual bleeding, it is not recommended for patients with severe thrombocytopenia.

10.4 MANAGEMENT OF CONNECTIVE TISSUE DISEASES DURING PREGNANCY

10.4.1 PRECONCEPTION COUNSELLING AND PLANNING

Considering a higher maternal and fetal risk, pregnant women with connective tissue disorder should be referred to a high-risk pregnancy centre for preconception counselling and obstetric care. Patients should be counselled about their individual risk profile and morbidity and mortality risks to mother and fetus. The preconception workup should include the following points:

- Previous obstetric and medical history
- Current disease activity
- Last flare date
- Chronic organ damage
- Recent serological profile
- Baseline blood pressure, urinalysis, and renal function
- Current medications

- *Medication adjustments*: For patients on a potentially teratogenic drug, it is recommended to switch to a safer alternative at least 3 months prior (ideally 6 months) to conception to monitor new flares or adverse effects from the change in drug regimen. Medications for which a washout period is indicated prior to pregnancy are methotrexate, mycophenolate mofetil (MMF), and leflunomide (1–3 months is sufficient for most medications used for rheumatic diseases). Non-rheumatology medications should also be assessed and modified if required. Angiotensin-converting enzyme inhibitors may be changed to pregnancy-safe substitutes several weeks before attempting to conceive. Warfarin should be changed to heparin prior to conception. When this switch is not possible prior to conception, it must be made prior to the sixth week of pregnancy to avoid warfarin embryopathy.

- *Preconceptional risk stratification*: On the basis of these factors, severity of disease and potential risk of disease flare or poor outcomes must be assessed. Risk of complications like pre-eclampsia, gestational diabetes, and venous thromboembolism (VTE) should be estimated, and appropriate management should be outlined.

- *Assessment of disease activity*: Since preconceptional disease activity has a significant impact on pregnancy outcomes in almost all CTDs (especially SLE and vasculitis), an assessment of the same prior to conception is recommended. In women with high disease activity, achieving optimum control in the months leading up to conception is essential. Ideally, patients should have a minimal disease activity 6 months leading to conception for more favourable outcomes.

- *Assessment of antibody profile*: Anti-Ro/SSA and anti-La/SSB antibodies, antiphospholipid antibodies and anti-dsDNA antibodies were found to be associated with pregnancy complications and should therefore be assessed prior to pregnancy. Additionally, antithyroperoxidase (anti-TPO) and antithyroglobulin (anti-TG) antibodies should be screened for, as they are associated with increased risk of pregnancy loss, congenital heart block, and other complications of pregnancy. RA patients without RF or ACPA are the most likely to remain inactive during pregnancy. Baseline antibody profiles in women with systemic sclerosis may assist clinicians in making the diagnosis of renal crisis. Presence of anti-RNA polymerase III antibodies even in low titres should alert the clinician to the possibility of renal crisis. In case of positivity of these antibodies, patients should be counselled regarding the risks and possible complications and appropriate fetal monitoring to be done as per guidelines. (See section on monitoring disease activity and other investigations during pregnancy.)

- *Timing of pregnancy and contraception*: Conception must ideally be planned during a period of minimal disease activity. For women with active disease, such as lupus nephritis, 6 months or more of inactive disease is desirable before conception and is associated with more favourable maternal and fetal outcomes.

- *Impact of CTDs on fertility*: Fertility in women with CTD is generally not affected, although patients with chronic kidney disease (CKD stage 3–5, with an estimated glomerular filtration rate (eEGR) of <50 ml/min), amenorrhoea because of previous high cumulative doses of cyclophosphamide, or active disease may have reduced fertility.

  - The risk of infertility with cyclophosphamide is related to greater age at administration as well as higher cumulative dose. For women under treatment regimens with gonadotoxic agents, such as cyclophosphamide, some special considerations are noteworthy. Minimising cumulative exposure is the goal, which is found to be lower with IV regimens compared to daily oral regimens. The "Euro-lupus" regimen, a low-dose IV CYC regimen consisting of six 500-mg CYC pulses every 2 weeks, followed by maintenance therapy with azathioprine (AZA), results in substantially lower cumulative doses compared to the standard 6 month courses. Induction with mycophenolate mofetil is another alternative for induction therapy for mild lupus nephritis. However, standard CYC induction is indicated for patients with severe lupus nephritis with renal insufficiency or those who have not responded to MMF.

- Another useful approach is use of adjunctive GnRH-analogues during CYC therapy, as it is shown to have ovarian protective effects.
- Women planning for assisted reproductive techniques should be counselled about risk of disease flare and thromboembolic events. For such cases, identification of high-risk pregnancy factors, pre-cycle counselling, adequate thromboprophylaxis, and close surveillance are necessary.

- *Screening of systemic involvement*: A complete screening to look for systemic involvement/complications and their extent should be done prior to planning conception to rule out relative contraindications to pregnancy and as a baseline evaluation.

- *Relative contraindications for pregnancy in women with CTDs*:[5]

  1. Severe CTD flare or stroke in last 6 months
  2. Pulmonary hypertension
  3. Severe restrictive lung disease (FVC < 1L)
  4. Heart failure with LVEF < 40%, cardiomyopathy or severe valvular disease
  5. Uncontrolled hypertension
  6. CKD stage 4 or 5 (eGFR < 30 ml/min)
  7. History of severe early-onset pre-eclampsia despite treatment with aspirin and heparin
  8. Recent arterial thrombosis, particularly cerebral vascular accident (CVA)

  Therefore, patients with connective tissue diseases, especially systemic sclerosis and mixed CTD, should have baseline echocardiograms and pulmonary function tests done to rule out relative contraindications prior to conceiving.

10.4.2 MULTIDISCIPLINARY APPROACH TO CARE (INVOLVEMENT OF RHEUMATOLOGISTS, OBSTETRICIANS, AND OTHER SPECIALISTS)

It is important that a multidisciplinary team consisting of a dermatologist, rheumatologist, obstetrician, neonatologist, and specialist management for individual systems involved be involved in management and treatment decisions.

10.4.3 TREATMENT

10.4.3.1 Medication Considerations

As a general rule, untreated disease in pregnancy is associated with risks to the mother and child, and evidence suggests the importance of continuing medications that prevent active disease and that do not harm the baby throughout pregnancy.

Table 10.1 outlines the commonly used drugs in management of CTDs and their safety in pregnancy and breastfeeding.

1. **NSAIDs** can be associated with renal and cardiac failure, hypertension, and fluid overload in the mother and oligohydramnios and renal impairment in the fetus if used for long periods. NSAIDs should be withheld towards the end of pregnancy (>30–32 weeks) because of an increased risk of early closure of the baby's ductus arteriosus and increased risk of maternal bleeding and of asthma in the child. There is insufficient data to make recommendations about selective COX II inhibitors, and they should therefore be avoided in pregnancy.

2. **Corticosteroids**: At doses of ≤20 mg, approximately 10% of non-fluorinated glucocorticoids cross into the fetal circulation and are therefore considered safe. However, minimum required maintenance doses (prednisone <7.5 mg/day) for shortest duration possible, along with steroid-sparing agents, are recommended.[39] According to some guidelines,

TABLE 10.1

Commonly Used Drugs in the Management of CTDs and Their Safety in Pregnancy and Breastfeeding

Drug	FDA Category	Safety in Pregnancy and Possible Maternal Risks	Possible Risks: Fetal	Breastfeeding
NSAIDs and aspirin	< 30 weeks: B >30 weeks: D Cox II inhibitors are Category C	• Safe • Risk of reduced fertility	• Safe before 28 weeks and intermittent use • Premature closure of ductus arteriosus after 28 weeks • Possible increased risk of miscarriage	• Compatible
Hydroxychloroquine	C	• Safe	• Safe	• Compatible
Glucocorticoids	C	• Safe • Possible side effects: PROM, glucose intolerance, hypertension, osteoporosis	• SGA, adrenal hypoplasia, 3.4-fold risk of cleft palate • Fluorinated glucocorticoids promote lung maturity	• Compatible • doses > 20 mg/ day: avoid first 4 h following dose
Azathioprine	D	• Safe	• SGA, prematurity, IUGR	• Contraindicated
Sulfasalazine	B	• Safe • Folate supplementation 5 mg/day preconception and throughout pregnancy	• Safe	• Compatible
Cyclosporin	C	• Safe • Renal insufficiency	• SGA, prematurity, IUGR	• Contraindicated
Tacrolimus	C	• Safe	• SGA, prematurity, IUGR, transient hyperkalaemia in neonates	• Compatible
Mycophenolate mofetil	D	• Avoid in pregnancy	• Shortened digits and hypoplastic nails, auditory canal atresia, cleft lip and palate	• Contraindicated
Methotrexate	X	• Avoid in pregnancy	• Embryotoxic skeletal and facial malformations	• Contraindicated
Leflunomide	X	• Avoid in pregnancy	• Multiple congenital anomalies	• Contraindicated
Cyclophosphamide	D	• Avoid in pregnancy	• Micrognathia, hypertelorism ocular coloboma, SGA, limb abnormalities, coronary artery agenesis, tumours in offspring	• Contraindicated
Anti-tumour necrosis factor agents	B	• Safe in first and second trimesters	• Minimal placental transfer • Etanercept: VACTERL syndrome reported but unproven	• Currently contraindicated but little absorbed by infant's GI tract
Certolizumab	B	• Probably safe	—	• Currently contraindicated but little absorbed by infant's GI tract
Anakinra	B	• Unknown risk	—	• Contraindicated
Rituximab	C	• Unknown risk	—	• Contraindicated

(Continued)

TABLE 10.1 (*Continued*)
Commonly Used Drugs in Management of CTDs and Their Safety in Pregnancy and Breastfeeding

Drug	FDA Category	Safety in Pregnancy and Possible Maternal Risks	Possible Risks: Fetal	Breastfeeding
Abatacept	C	• Unknown risk	—	• Contraindicated
Tocilizumab	C	• Unknown risk	—	• Contraindicated
Belimumab	C	• Unknown risk	—	• Contraindicated
IVIG	C	• Safe • Risk of hepatitis C	• Risk of hepatitis C, SGA, autoantibodies	• Probably compatible
Endothelin receptor antagonists	X	• Avoid in pregnancy	—	• Contraindicated
Heparin	C	• Safe • Bleeding risk	• None	• Compatible
Colchicine	C	• Probably safe	• Limited studies	• Probably compatible
Warfarin	X	• Avoid in pregnancy	• Embryopathy, eye defects, deafness, congenital heart disease, hypoplasia of extremities, developmental retardation	• Compatible

stress doses of hydrocortisone at delivery are recommended in patients taking long-term therapy.[40]

- Apart from the well-known systemic side effects of glucocorticosteroids, use during the first trimester increases the risk of cleft palate formation by two- to threefold, with a baseline risk of approximately 1/1000 live births. Use in late pregnancy can be associated with premature rupture of membranes and small for gestational age births, and high or prolonged doses put the newborn at risk for adrenal insufficiency. In systemic sclerosis, corticosteroids for fetal lung maturation are avoided because they may precipitate a renal crisis. In case of renal crisis, management must be with angiotensin-converting enzyme inhibitors (ACEIs) despite the risks to the baby, as it is potentially lifesaving for the mother.

3. **Antimalarials (hydroxychloroquine and chloroquine)**: It is recommended that hydroxychloroquine be continued during pregnancy considering it's safe and there is evidence that it can reduce disease flares, improve birth outcomes, and decrease the risk of neonatal lupus and heart block in neonates of mothers with anti-Ro antibodies. While less is known about the effect of chloroquine, there is no evidence that it is unsafe to use in pregnancy and breastfeeding. Hydroxychloroquine, due to its anti-inflammatory, anti-thrombotic, pro-endothelial effects, can be considered for selected cases of APLA with previous thrombosis or previous ischemic placenta-mediated complications or after standard treatment failure with aspirin and a heparin agent.

4. **Steroid-sparing immunosuppressants**: Azathioprine is considered safe for use throughout pregnancy. For AZA, monitoring of 6-thioguanine nucleotide and 6-methylmercaptopurine levels can be considered during pregnancy, as thiopurine metabolism is altered during pregnancy. Potential rare side effects in the newborn are transient hypogammaglobulinemia

and pancytopenias, which usually normalise within 10 weeks of birth. Monitoring of complete blood count and vigilance for neonatal infection after in utero AZA exposure has been recommended. Recent data also suggests a potential association with developmental delays, but based on a risk–benefit ratio, AZA, if indicated, should not be stopped during pregnancy. Tacrolimus and cyclosporine have been shown to be safe during pregnancy; however, the lowest effective dose should be used, and levels must be monitored to avoid toxicity.

5. **Sulfasalazine**: In patients taking sulfasalazine, folate supplementation (5 mg/day) is recommended from 3 months before conception until at least the end of the first trimester to prevent neural tube defects. Active metabolites of sulfasalazine can cause hyperbilirubinemia in a G6PD-deficient or premature infant. Therefore, some recommend that breastfeeding while taking sulfasalazine be restricted to full-term, healthy infants.

6. **Biologics**: Even though the available data is too limited to claim safety of these drugs during gestation, the existing evidence suggests that the overall risk of anti-TNF agents is relatively low. Disseminated Bacillus Calmette–Guérin (BCG) infection has been reported in babies of mothers who received biologics during pregnancy, and therefore these women are advised to avoid live vaccines for their neonates until at least 7 months of age. Little data exists regarding the safety of other biologics during pregnancy and breastfeeding, and they are therefore not recommended. Anti-tumour necrosis factor (anti-TNF) agents and anakinra are classified as FDA Pregnancy Category B, while rituximab, abatacept, and tocilizumab are FDA Pregnancy Category C.

7. **Warfarin and other vitamin K antagonists** are teratogenic during organogenesis, and switching to low-molecular-weight heparin (LMWH) is recommended as soon as pregnancy is confirmed. In LE, treatment with prophylactic low molecular weight heparin (LMWH) and low-dose aspirin is recommended for women with antiphospholipid antibodies and a history of pregnancy complications or vascular thrombosis. In APLS, heparin with low-dose aspirin throughout pregnancy is started as soon as pregnancy is confirmed.

8. **Prevention of pre-eclampsia and related complications**: Low-dose aspirin (LDA) (75 mg/day) started before 16 weeks of gestation significantly reduces the risk of perinatal death, pre-eclampsia, and its complications in women with CTDs at risk for the previous complications (hypertension, renal insufficiency, and history of pre-eclampsia), and its maximum effect is likely when taken during afternoon or at bedtime.

   • Additionally, the intake of at least 1 g of calcium daily has been shown to dramatically reduce the risk of pre-eclampsia and associated complications.

9. **Methotrexate, leflunomide, mycophenolate mofetil, and cyclophosphamide** are contraindicated in pregnancy. It is therefore recommended that they be discontinued prior to conception (6 weeks in the case of mycophenolate mofetil and at least 3 months in the case of methotrexate). For leflunomide, it may take up to 2 years after cessation of treatment for metabolite levels to become non-detectable. Therefore, documentation of metabolite blood levels of <0.02 µg/mZZL is recommended prior to conception for women who have taken leflunomide in the last 2 years. A cholestyramine drug elimination procedure is recommended for women with detectable metabolite levels who are planning conception and those who become pregnant while on leflunomide.

10. **Role of vitamin D**: Vitamin D has been shown to have an immunomodulatory role in autoimmune diseases. It modulates differentiation and activation of CD4+ lymphocytes, increases the number and function of Treg cells, inhibits the differentiation of monocytes and dendritic cells, stimulates the function of Th2 cells, and reduces pro-inflammatory cytokines. Since T cells are shown to have a possible role in achieving and maintaining pregnancy, a link between vitamin D levels and pregnancy outcomes in women with autoimmune disease is possible. Therefore, screening and appropriate treatment for vitamin D deficiency in women at high risk of vitamin D deficiency, such as in those with autoimmune diseases, is recommended prior to conception.[41]

10.4.4 MONITORING DISEASE ACTIVITY AND OTHER INVESTIGATIONS DURING PREGNANCY

Rheumatologic evaluation should be carried out every 4–8 weeks, while obstetric clinical evaluations should be performed monthly.

- *Fetal monitoring*: The frequency of ultrasound scans with fetal biometry and Doppler assessment should be based on the autoantibody positivity, severity of disease, and Doppler pulsatility index of uterine arteries. In patients with APLS, current recommendations are to monitor for fetal distress during the third trimester utilising non-stress tests, umbilical artery Dopplers, or serial ultrasounds. A pregnant patient who is known to have Ro/SS-A or La/SS-B antibodies should be screened for fetal cardiac involvement through serial fetal echocardiograms beginning at 16–18 weeks. For high-risk patients (those with a previous child with NLE), echocardiograms are recommended weekly from weeks 18–26 and every 2 weeks until week 32. In all women with connective tissue disorders, uterine artery Doppler at 22–24 weeks of gestation is recommended because of its high negative predictive value for pre-eclampsia and IUGR.

- *Maternal monitoring for complications*: Monitoring for blood pressure and renal parameters during pregnancy is desirable in all patients of CTD, especially SLE patients and systemic sclerosis patients at risk for lupus nephritis and scleroderma renal crisis, respectively. Pre-eclampsia may be difficult to differentiate from flare of lupus nephritis or vasculitis, or scleroderma renal crisis in certain situations (Table 10.2). Both are associated with proteinuria and rising creatinine, but examination of

---

TABLE 10.2
Differentiating Pointers for Lupus Nephritis vs Pre-Eclampsia

Lupus Nephritis	Pre-Eclampsia
Onset: Can be in first 20 weeks of gestation	Onset: After 20 weeks of gestation
Typical features of pre-eclampsia are less common	Typical clinical features more common: Headache, visual disturbances, right upper quadrant tenderness
Urinary sediment: Active	Urinary sediment: Bland
Serum uric acid: May be normal	Serum uric acid: Increased
Usually not associated with haemolysis and elevated liver enzymes	Often associated with haemolysis and elevated liver enzymes
Associated with falling complement levels and rising antibody titres (anti-ds DNA)	Usually not associated with falling complement levels and rising antibody titres (anti-ds DNA)
Evidence of lupus flare in other organs	No evidence of lupus flare in other organs
Treatment of choice: IV corticosteroids	Definitive treatment is prompt delivery

urinary sediment will reveal activity in LN as opposed to a bland urinary sediment in pre-eclampsia. Serum uric acid may be elevated in pre-eclampsia and could provide another marker to help distinguish between the two processes. Onset of signs and symptoms within the first 20 weeks, high or increasing anti-ds DNA antibodies, or evidence of lupus flare in other organs are pointers for lupus nephritis. In patients with permanent proteinuria, this can increase throughout pregnancy (and can reach up to double the baseline) because of increased renal blood flow and does not necessarily indicate active nephritis.

- *Pregnancy physiology and laboratory markers*: Haemodilution of pregnancy leads to anae-mia and lowered platelet counts in many healthy patients, mimicking hematologic manifes-tations of connective tissue disease. Pregnancy-induced elevation in white blood cell count may be confusing in certain conditions such as vasculitides or adult-onset Stills disease. In pregnancy, erythrocyte sedimentation rate (ESR), CRP, and serum C3 and C4 levels usu-ally increase and are therefore not considered valid markers of disease activity, but relative variation rather than absolute levels may be more reliable.

- *Radiological imaging* should not be withheld in pregnant women if clinically indicated, although caution is recommended with the use of gadolinium contrast, as recent data shows an association with an increased risk of neonatal deaths and stillbirths.

10.5 POSTPARTUM MANAGEMENT AND LONG-TERM FOLLOW-UP

10.5.1 Postpartum Surveillance for Women with CTDs

There is a high risk of disease flare postpartum in CTDs (especially LE, RA, and Behçet's disease); therefore, close surveillance for 6 months after delivery is important. A plan should be in place before delivery regarding treatment for postpartum flare if and when it occurs. The risk of throm-boembolism is also increased postpartum; therefore, all women should have an assessment of VTE risk and receive thromboprophylaxis postpartum accordingly.

10.5.2 Breastfeeding Considerations

Breastfeeding is possible for many but not all patients. Patients with recurrence of active dis-ease should be treated with the most effective medication, which may preclude breastfeeding. Breastfeeding is probably safe with NSAIDs, low-dose glucocorticoids, cyclosporin, and HCQ is considered safe during lactation.

Caution regarding breastfeeding during therapy with AZA and sulfasalazine is recommended in thiopurine methyltransferase-deficient mothers and children and premature infants, respectively. A study showed that the majority of azathioprine is excreted within 4 h of ingestion; therefore, it is recommended that feeds be given at least 4 h post-maternal dose. Anti-TNF inhibitors are con-sidered safe, as their size reduces the likelihood of gut absorption. A general recommendation to reduce risk of exposure while nursing is to advise mothers to avoid feeding at the time of peak levels in the breast milk (4 hours after the dose). Refer to Table 10.1 for medications and breastfeeding considerations. Breastfeeding also may be a concern in patients with osteoporosis, as it may further lower bone density.

10.5.3 Resumption of Medications and Disease Management

Postpartum disease and flare management needs to be done aggressively with due breastfeeding considerations (see previous section on breastfeeding considerations). A common approach is to treat with low-dose corticosteroid while the mother weans the infant, with resumption of disease-modifying or immunosuppressive therapy after weaning.

Patients on prophylactic anticoagulation therapy during pregnancy (antiphospholipid syndrome or APA positive) are generally advised to continue anticoagulation for approximately 6 weeks postpartum to minimise risk of venous thrombosis; those requiring long-term anticoagulation can be switched back to warfarin postpartum, as this is compatible with breastfeeding.

10.5.4 LONG-TERM IMPLICATIONS FOR BOTH THE MOTHER AND THE CHILD

*   *Long-term sequelae of preterm birth*: Preterm birth can lead to long-term neurodevelopmental disabilities, especially in infants born with a very low birth weight (VLBW), predominantly cognitive deficits without major motor deficits. An increased prevalence of cognitive impairment, poorer educational achievement, and specific language difficulties has been repeatedly observed among school-age children after extremely preterm birth as compared with those born at full term. Other sequelae include periventricular leukomalacia, encephalopathy of prematurity, and retinopathy of prematurity.

*   *Long-term neurodevelopmental sequelae*: Maternal antibodies can cross the placenta after week 12 of gestation and potentially act on the developing fetus. Maternal APA could potentially react directly with fetal cerebral tissue (during the fetal period, the blood–brain barrier is still incomplete) and continue their pathogenic effect during the early life through microthrombosis and inflammatory reactions, leading to further disruption of the blood–brain barrier.

    *   A number of studies support a relationship between APA positivity and neurological manifestations such as migraine, epilepsy, and movement disorders in positive patients, but there are no data suggesting an increased risk of development of these disorders in the offspring of APA-positive patients. In children born to mothers with APA positivity and SLE, global intelligence capacity is unimpaired. However, an increased risk of language delay and learning disabilities (LDs) has been observed, which could be due to transplacental passage of maternal antibodies as well as other well-known risk factors (prematurity, genetic and environmental factors).

    *   Ideally, clinical follow-up of newborns of mothers with rheumatic diseases would include a neuropsychiatry expert's intervention to evaluate the child's development and identify any neurodevelopmental problems at an early stage. The first year of life represents a critical period for psychomotor development.

*   *Long-term sequelae of NLE*: Studies evaluating the long-term outcome of these children note no negative effects on neurodevelopment and suggest a normal quality of life.

*   *Sequelae due to transplacental passage of antibodies*: Transplacental passage of Ro/SS-A and La/SS-B antibodies can lead to development of NLE in the neonate, as explained in previous sections. Thyroid autoimmunity is often part of the picture of systemic autoimmune diseases. Transplacental passage of thyroid-stimulating immunoglobulin can result in thyrotoxicosis in the fetus after 20 weeks gestation. Both fetal hypo- and hyperthyroidism may occur, especially during the first trimester of gestation. Maternal hypothyroidism is associated with impaired fetal neurological development and delayed mental and motor development.

- *Sequelae due to medications*: Antenatal steroid administration has shown possible adverse short- and long-term outcomes in the form of neurodevelopmental and hearing impairments, but these results have been conflicting across studies and larger studies are needed to confirm them.

- *Psychosocial sequelae*: Another factor to be considered is the potential influence of the mother's chronic illness on psychological and behavioural aspects of her children. Several studies have focused on the impact of chronic illness on quality of life as well as on relationships with other family members, including the offspring. Generally, the presence of a chronic disease in the mother and the attendant emotional distress can interfere with parenthood.

Furthermore, maternal distress and depression during the pregnancy can produce a characteristic hormonal response with increased cortisol levels and decreased dopamine and serotonin levels, which can promote premature delivery of low birth weight babies. A similar effect may be seen with corticosteroid treatment in mothers with rheumatic diseases.

Overall, children born to mothers with rheumatic disease do not generally show a significantly increased risk of developing the autoimmune disease of their parents. In addition, offspring have uncomplicated growth and are usually healthy, with a normal intelligence level.

10.6   CONCLUSION/SUMMARY

Treating the pregnant rheumatology patient can be challenging but extremely rewarding. While not all medications can be used safely during pregnancy, most disease flares can be adequately managed during pregnancy. If possible, pregnancies should be planned so that the underlying rheumatologic disease is under good control and medications can be appropriately adjusted for safety. Ideally, pre-pregnancy evaluation with both the rheumatologist and, in cases of complicated disease, a maternal–fetal obstetrical specialist should be done. This preconception counselling is an ideal time to discuss and formulate a plan in case of flares.

REFERENCES

1. Ateka-Barrutia O, Nelson-Piercy C. Connective tissue disease in pregnancy. *Clin Med (Lond)*. 2013;13(6):580–584.
2. Ying Y, Zhong YP, Zhou CQ, et al. A further exploration of the impact of antinuclear antibodies on in vitro fertilization-embryo transfer outcome. *Am J Reprod Immunol*. 2013;70:221–229.
3. Laczik R, Soltesz P, Szodoray P, et al. Impaired endothelial function in patients with undifferentiated connective tissue disease: A follow-up study. *Rheumatology (Oxford)*. 2014;53(11):2035–2043.
4. Nakken B, Bodolay E, Szodoray P. Cytokine milieu in undifferentiated connective tissue disease: A comprehensive review. *Clin Rev Allergy Immunol*. 2015;49(2):152–162.
5. Tardif ML, Mahone M. Mixed connective tissue disease in pregnancy: A case series and systematic literature review. *Obstet Med*. 2019;12(1):31–37.
6. Mosca M, Tani C, Neri C, et al. Undifferentiated connective tissue diseases (UCTD). *Autoimmun Rev*. 2006;6(1):1–4.
7. Vaz CC, Couto M, Medeiros D, et al. Undifferentiated connective tissue disease: A seven-center cross-sectional study of 184 patients. *Clin Rheumatol*. 2009;28(8):915–921.
8. Conti V, Esposito A, Cagliuso M, et al. Undifferentiated connective tissue disease—an unsolved problem: Revision of literature and case studies. *Int J Immunopathol Pharmacol*. 2010;23:271–278.
9. Deane KD, El-Gabalawy H. Pathogenesis and prevention of rheumatic disease: Focus on preclinical RA and SLE. *Nat Rev Rheumatol*. 2014;10(4):212–228.
10. Pepmueller PH. Undifferentiated connective tissue disease, mixed connective tissue disease, and overlap syndromes in rheumatology. *Mo Med*. 2016;113(2):136–140.
11. Castellino G, Capucci R, Bernardi S, et al. Pregnancy in patients with undifferentiated connective tissue disease: A prospective case-control study. *Lupus*. 2011;20(12):1305–1311.

12. Yang S, Ni R, Lu Y, et al. A three-arm, multicenter, open-label randomized controlled trial of hydroxy-chloroquine and low-dose prednisone to treat recurrent pregnancy loss in women with undifferentiated connective tissue diseases: Protocol for the Immunosuppressant regimens for LIving FEtuses (ILIFE) trial. *Trials.* 2020;21(1):771.
13. de Man YA, Dolhain RJ, van de Geijn FE, et al. Disease activity of rheumatoid arthritis during pregnancy: Results from a nationwide prospective study. *Arthritis Rheum.* 2008;59:1241–1248.
14. de Man YA, Bakker-Jonges LE, Goorbergh CM, et al. Women with rheumatoid arthritis negative for anti-cyclic citrullinated peptide and rheumatoid factor are more likely to improve during pregnancy, whereas in autoantibody-positive women autoantibody levels are not influenced by pregnancy. *Ann Rheum Dis.* 2010;69:420–423.
15. Barrett JH, Brennan P, Fiddler M, et al. Does rheumatoid arthritis remit during pregnancy and relapse postpartum? Results from a nationwide study in the United Kingdom performed prospectively from late pregnancy. *Arthritis Rheum.* 1999;42:1219–1227.
16. Ostensen M, Husby G. A prospective clinical study of the effect of pregnancy on rheumatoid arthritis and ankylosing spondylitis. *Arthritis Rheum.* 1983;26:1155–1159.
17. Ostensen M, Romberg O, Husby G. Ankylosing spondylitis and motherhood. *Arthritis Rheum.* 1982;25:140–143.
18. Pagnoux C. Pregnancy and vasculitides. *Presse Med.* 2008;37(11):1657–1665.
19. Nguyen V, Wuebbolt D, Pagnoux C, et al. Pregnancy outcomes in women with primary systemic vasculitis: A retrospective study. *J Matern Fetal Neonatal Med.* 2019:1–7.
20. Pagnoux C, Le Guern V, Goffinet F, et al. Pregnancies in systemic necrotizing vasculitides: Report on 12 women and their 20 pregnancies. *Rheumatology (Oxford).* 2011;50(5):953–961.
21. Gutierrez G, Dagnino R, Mintz G. Polymyositis/dermatomyositis and pregnancy. *Arthritis Rheum.* 1984;27:291–294.
22. Ishii N, Ono H, Kawagushi T, et al. Dermatomyositis and pregnancy—case report and review of the literature. *Dermatologica.* 1991;183:146–149.
23. Steiner I, Averbuch-Heller L, Abramsky O, et al. Postpartum idiopathic polymyositis. *Lancet.* 1992;339:256.
24. Yassaee M, Kovarik CL, Werth VP. Pregnancy-associated dermatomyositis. *Arch Dermatol.* 2009;145(8):952–953.
25. Suwa A, Hirakata M, Tsuzaka K, et al. Spontaneous remission of dermatomyositis which developed one month after normal delivery. *Ryumachi.* 1992;32:73–79.
26. Kanoh H, Izumi T, Seishima M, et al. A case of dermatomyositis that developed after delivery: The involvement of pregnancy in the induction of dermatomyositis. *Br J Dermatol.* 1999;141:897–900.
27. Takei R, Suzuki S, Kijima K, et al. First presentation of polymyositis postpartum following intrauterine fetal death. *Arch Gynecol Obstet.* 2000;264:47.
28. Hung NA, Jackson B, Nicholson M, et al. Pregnancy-related polymyositis and massive perivillous fi brin deposition in the placenta: Are they related? *Arthritis Rheum.* 2006;55(1):154–156.
29. Hoffman SL, Zaphiratos V, Girard MA, et al. Failed epidural analgesia in a parturient with advanced ankylosing spondylitis: A novel explanation. *Can J Anaesth.* 2012;59:871–874.
30. Pagnoux C, Mahendira D, Laskin CA. Fertility and pregnancy in vasculitis. *Best Pract Res Clin Rheumatol.* 2013;27(1):79–94.
31. Chen JS, Roberts CL, Simpson JM, et al. Pregnancy outcomes in women with rare autoimmune diseases. *Arthritis Rheumatol.* 2015;67(12):3314–3323.
32. Machen L, Clowse ME. Vasculitis and pregnancy. *Rheum Dis Clin N Am.* 2017;43(2):239–247.
33. Clowse ME, Witter FR, Magder LC, et al. The impact of increased lupus activity on obstetrical outcomes. *Arthritis Rheum.* 2005;52:514–522.
34. Buyon JP, Kim MY, Guerra MM, et al. Predictors of pregnancy outcomes in patients with lupus: A cohort study. *Ann Intern Med.* 2015;163:153–163.
35. Ruiz-Irastorza G, Khamashta MA. Lupus and pregnancy: Integrating clues from the bench and bedside. *Eur J Clin Invest.* 2011;41:672–678.
36. Hussein SZ, Jacobsson LTH, Lindquist PG, et al. Pregnancy and fetal outcome in women with primary Sjögren's syndrome compared with women in the general population: A nested case-control study. *Rheumatology.* 2011;50:1612–1617.
37. Izmirly PM, Rivera TL, Buyon JP. Neonatal lupus syndromes. *Rheum Dis Clin N Am.* 2007;33:267–285.
38. Marder W, Littlejohn EA, Somers EC. Pregnancy and autoimmune connective tissue diseases [published correction appears in Best Pract Res Clin Rheumatol. 2020 Dec;34(6):101490]. *Best Pract Res Clin Rheumatol.* 2016;30(1):63–80.

39. Bramham K, Thomas M, Nelson-Piercy C, et al. First-trimester low-dose prednisolone in refractory antiphospholipid antibody-related pregnancy loss. *Blood*. 2011;117:6948–6951.
40. Cooper GS, Gilbert KM, Greidinger EL, et al. Recent advances and opportunities in research on lupus: Environmental influences and mechanisms of disease. *Environ Health Perspect*. 2008;116:695–702.
41. Cyprian F, Lefkou E, Varoudi K, et al. Immunomodulatory effects of vitamin D in pregnancy and beyond. *Front Immunol*. 2019;10:2739.

11 Sexually Transmitted Diseases in Pregnancy

Taru Garg and Apoorva Maheshwari

11.1 INTRODUCTION

Infections (bacterial, viral, fungal, parasitic) transmitted from an infected person to an uninfected person through sexual contact are called sexually transmitted diseases. Pregnancy is a physiological state. However, there are immunological, anatomical, physiological and microbiological alterations during pregnancy which may alter the presentation and course of these infections (Figure 11.1). Because of immunocompromised state during pregnancy, any infection contracted may have variable presentation compared to non-pregnant state and has potential for not only causing excessive maternal morbidity but also perinatal morbidity and mortality (Table 11.1). The impact of these depends on the time period when these infections are acquired. Prior to conception, these infections can affect the fertility; in pregnancy these may be responsible for abortion, still birth or infectious complications in the fetus or placenta and congenital infection, while in the postpartum period, these may be responsible for sepsis in mother or the neonate. Another point of consideration is the management of these infections during pregnancy, which may differ, as certain drugs may not be safe to use during pregnancy, and second, it is not only treatment of the mother to make her all right but also to prevent damage to the fetus.

Since STDs are widely preventable, it is imperative to not only offer STD prevention counselling, but also provide adequate early diagnosis and treatment in case the pregnant female or her partner exhibit symptoms of STDs. In this chapter, we will learn about clinical features, screening guidelines, diagnosis and treatment of frequently encountered STDs in pregnancy.

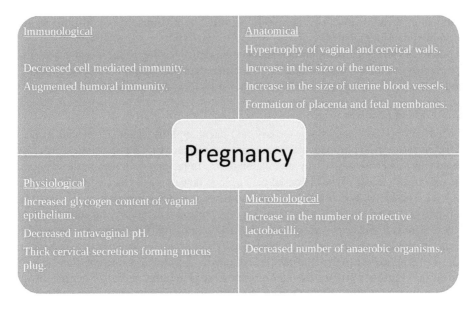

FIGURE 11.1   Physiological changes during pregnancy.

DOI: 10.1201/9781003449690-11

TABLE 11.1

Effects of STDs on Pregnancy and Fetus

	Effect on Pregnancy	Effect on Fetus
Syphilis	Larger chancre, multiple chancres.	Miscarriage, stillbirth, congenital syphilis (early and late), prematurity
Gonorrhoea	Pharyngeal and disseminated gonococcal infection, chorioamnionitis, prematurity, premature rupture of membrane, postpartum endometritis and salpingitis	Intrauterine growth retardation (IUGR), conjunctivitis, pharyngitis, proctitis, sepsis, death
Chlamydia	Chorioamnionitis, prematurity, premature rupture of membrane, postpartum endometritis and salpingitis	IUGR, conjunctivitis, pneumonia, low birth weight (LBW), sepsis
Bacterial vaginosis	Chorioamnionitis, premature rupture of membrane, spontaneous abortion,	LBW, sepsis, skin abscesses
Herpes simplex	Severe primary episode, frequent and more prolonged recurrences	Neurological involvement, ocular complications, scarring, TORCH syndrome
Viral warts	Larger, more numerous warts	Anogenital warts, juvenille laryngeal papillomatosis
Molluscum contagiosum	Larger, more numerous lesions	Congenital and neonatal molluscum contagiosum
Vulvovaginal candidiasis	Chorioamnionitis, prematurity, abortion	Congenital and neonatal candidiasis
Trichomoniasis	Chorioamnionitis, premature delivery, premature rupture of membrane, postpartum endometritis and salpingitis,	IUGR, LBW

11.2 BACTERIAL STDs

11.2.1 SYPHILIS IN PREGNANCY

Syphilis is a treponemal infection caused by *Treponema pallidum*. It adversely affects the pregnancy as well as its outcome. It is an important and widely known preventable cause of abortion, still birth and congenital infection. The WHO reported approximately 661,000 infants with congenital syphilis in 2016 globally.[1]

Apart from the physiological immunological compromise leading to increased susceptibility, the presence of other risk factors like multiple sexual partners, substance abuse, residence in high endemic areas and lack of condom use contributes to the increasing prevalence of syphilis in pregnancy.

11.2.1.1 Clinical Features

It is divided into primary, secondary, tertiary and latent syphilis. After an incubation period (IP) of 10–90 days, primary syphilis manifests as primary chancre, which is a painless, indurated ulcer with raised edges and base with clean granulation tissue. In pregnancy, however, the chancre may be multiple and larger because of the increased pelvic blood flow or maybe located so as to go unnoticed (Figure 11.2). The cervix is common site for chancre in pregnancy because of increased friability. This is usually accompanied by painless, firm, rubbery unilateral inguinal lymph nodes. It heals spontaneously over next 2–6 weeks.[2] Secondary syphilis presents itself in highly variegated form. The lesions may be papular, maculopapular, lichenoid, psoriasiform or follicular or may present as condyloma lata. The eruption is usually non-itchy and not easily discernible to the untrained eye.[3] Syphilis acquired during pregnancy progresses to the tertiary stage of gumma and cardiovascular involvement.

Outcomes in terms of fetal morbidity and mortality are dependent on the stage of infection, gestational age and adequacy of treatment. An early stage of disease in pregnancy causes a large number of treponemes crossing the placenta, hence a higher risk of fetal transmission than pregnancy

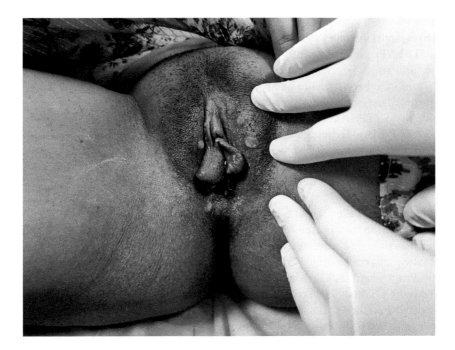

FIGURE 11.2   Multiple chances in a pregnant female.

occurring in tertiary or latent stages of syphilis. When acquired in the first trimester, placental infection and reduced blood flow may lead to stillbirth, spontaneous abortion, prematurity or intrauterine growth retardation (IUGR). Infection during the third trimester may result in congenital syphilis (CS). The risk of transmission from a mother with primary or secondary syphilis is 70–100%, 40% with early latent syphilis and approximately 10% with late latent syphilis. Thus, at an average, 50% of infected mothers transmit the infection to the fetus.[4]

11.2.1.2   Congenital Syphilis

It can be clinically divided into early and late CS, with a cutoff at 2 years of age. Early CS can present as pemphigus syphiliticus, papulosquamous eruption, snuffles, mucous patches, syphilitic alopecia, syphilitic onychia and systemic involvement depending on treponemal load. Late CS presents as interstitial keratitis, conductive deafness, gummatous periosteitis, parrot nodes, Clutton's joints and mucous patch.[4]

11.2.1.3   Diagnosis

All pregnant women should be tested during the first prenatal visit. Subsequently, they should be tested at 28 weeks and at the time of delivery if they have high risk factors for contracting STDs, live in an area with high syphilis prevalence, were not tested at first prenatal visit or had positive results during the first visit.[5]

Testing/diagnosis are done as for non-pregnant females. It can be done either by direct detection of the organism (by dark field microscopic examination and histopathological evaluation) or by direct detection of antigen [using enzyme immunoassay (EIA), direct fluorescent antibody for *T. pallidum* (DFA-TP) or polymerase chain reaction (PCR)] or by serological investigations. Dark field microscopy is the point-of-care (POC) test, allowing direct detection of *T. pallidum* from primary and secondary syphilis lesions, demonstrating its characteristic angular and bending motility. Direct fluorescent antibody staining of *T. pallidum* (DFA-TP) is more advantageous as it is more sensitive and specific than dark field microscopy and also can differentiate pathogenic from non-pathogenic treponemes. Seroconversion occurs in about 3–6 weeks after infection. Serological investigations may be non-treponemal, usually employed for screening purposes, and include vene-real disease research laboratory (VDRL), rapid plasma reagin test (RPR) and toluidine red unheated serum test (TRUST). Non-treponemal tests help to monitor treatment adequacy, as they provide quantitative titres which fall on appropriate treatment. The sensitivity and specificity of VDRL and RPR in chancre have been found to be about 62–78%. Treponemal tests are used as confirmatory tests and include fluorescent treponemal antibody absorption test (FTA-ABS), *T. pallidum* hem-agglutination assay (TPHA), *T. pallidum* particle agglutination (TPPA) and *T. pallidum* enzyme immunoassay (TP-EIA). Treponemal tests are qualitative and remain positive regardless of treat-ment. They are reported as reactive or non-reactive and thus cannot differentiate between recent or remote and treated or untreated infection. The WHO recommends dual rapid diagnostic testing for HIV and syphilis, as it aids in the timely diagnosis of two leading preventable causes of fetal morbidity and mortality.[6–11]

Pregnancy is one of the causes of biological false positives because of upregulation of humoral immunity. However, in the absence of adequate treatment history documentation, all seropositive pregnant females should be considered infected, regardless of titres.[12]

Congenital syphilis can be diagnosed antepartum with the help of ultrasonography. Skin thickening, placental thickening, hepatosplenomegaly, hydramnios and serous cavity effusions on ultrasound can help in diagnosing CS. Long bone radiography and detection of spirochetes in amniotic fluid further support the diagnosis. Chest radiographs, liver function tests, ophthalmologic and auditory tests along with neuroimaging and CSF evaluation should be performed in all newborns with suspected CS.[4]

11.2.1.4 Management

Patient should be treated with inj. benzathine penicillin G 2.4 million units intramuscular (IM) after sensitivity testing. Additional therapy in early syphilis, with repeat dose after 1 week, is con-sidered beneficial.[12] Pregnant women allergic to penicillin should be treated with erythromycin 500 mg orally four times a day for 15 days, and neonates should be treated for congenital syphilis.[13] However, according to CDC guidelines, pregnant women allergic to penicillin should be desensi-tised and treated with the mentioned dose of penicillin. All pregnant women undergoing treatment should be educated about Jarisch–Herxheimer reaction (fever, tachycardia, hypertension, worsen-ing of existing rash of secondary syphilis) and instructed to consult an obstetrician if they notice decreased fetal movements or premature contractions.

Follow-up must be done at 28–32 weeks of gestation and again at the time of delivery. However, if high risk factors like residence in high-prevalence geographic areas are present, then monthly follow-ups can be considered.

Newborns with proven or highly probable CS (nontreponemal serologic titre fourfold or higher than that of mother, positive dark field microscopy or physical examination consistent with CS) must be evaluated thoroughly and treated with intravenous aqueous crystalline penicillin G 100,000–150,000 units/kg/day, given as 50,000 units/kg/dose twice a day for first 7 days and then thrice a day for a total of 10 days.[12]

11.2.3 Gonorrhoea and Chlamydia in Pregnancy

Cervicitis and urethritis are caused by intracellular Gram-negative diplococci (ICGND), *Neisseria gonorrhoeae* or an intracellular obligate bacterium called *Chlamydia trachomatis*. Both these organisms present as cervicitis with/without urethritis and extragenital complications. According to a systematic review published in 2022, the global prevalence of gonorrhoea in pregnancy was 1.85%, with the highest number of cases in the African region.[14] The global prevalence of chlamydia in females of the reproductive age group was 3.8% in 2016.[15]

11.2.3.1 Clinical Features

Cervicitis primarily manifests as abnormal vaginal discharge. While profuse mucopurulent discharge is suggestive of gonorrhoea, scanty to moderate mucoid discharge is suggestive of chlamydial infection.

Cervical friability is seen in both. Vaginitis is usually not a feature. In the majority of cases, infection remains confined to the lower genital tract, as fetal membranes prevent ascension of the infection. However, infection may traverse to the fallopian tubes, ovaries and other pelvic organs, leading to pelvic inflammatory disease (PID), which is commoner and more severe in gonococcal infections than chlamydia. This usually occurs before 12 weeks of gestation, as chorion is yet to fuse with decidua by this time, resulting in pyosalpinx and, rarely, tubo-ovarian abscess. Pyosalpinx eventually leads to tubal adhesions and thus contributes to tubal factor infertility in subsequent attempts to conceive.[16]

Certain important clinical features of gonorrhoea in pregnancy include increased incidence of asymptomatic infection, pharyngeal and anal involvement and haematological dissemination, which may lead to disseminated gonococcal infection (DGI) characterised by arthritis, dermatitis, endocarditis, myocarditis, pericarditis, meningitis, pneumonitis, hepatitis and pyelonephritis.[14,15] Extragenital involvement in gonococcal and chlamydial infections in the form of ano-rectal and pharyngeal infection may occur due to peno-anal contact, fellatio and cunnilingus. Fitz-Hugh Curtis syndrome is perihepatitis, seen in patients of DGI or pelvic inflammatory disease. It is characterised by fever, nausea, vomiting and upper abdominal pain. Conjunctivitis can occur due to autoinoculation in both etiologies.[17,18]

Adverse pregnancy outcomes such as preterm delivery, premature rupture of membranes, chorioamnionitis and postpartum septicaemia are known. Vertical transmission of infection may lead to ophthalmia neonatorum, a mucopurulent and membranous conjunctivitis with severe repercussions, including blindness. Other complications in the newborn include intrauterine growth retardation (IUGR), low birth weight, pharyngitis, proctitis, sepsis and death.

11.2.3.2 Diagnosis

All pregnant women under the age of 25 years and older pregnant women with high risk factors for STD contraction should be tested for gonorrhoea and chlamydia during the first prenatal visit. Subsequent tests should be done in the third trimester if high-risk features persist.[5]

11.2.3.2.1 *Gonorrhoea*

Gram staining of the cervical discharge is the POC test, which demonstrates polymorphonuclear cells and ICGND. However, since a high proportion of infection is asymptomatic, and Gram stain is less sensitive in asymptomatic women than asymptomatic men, it is of less relevance. Culture helps in assessment of antibiotic resistance and has a sensitivity of about 70–90%. Culture reports are, however, unavailable before a minimum of 48 hours. NAAT techniques like PCR, strand displacement amplification (SDA) and transcription-mediated amplification (TMA) are the gold standard for diagnosis. Major advantages are provision of highly sensitive (almost 100%) and specific results within hours and the ability of the test to produce reproducible results even on non-invasive samples like urine and vaginal swabs, while the disadvantage is that antimicrobial resistance cannot be assessed.[19,20]

11.2.3.2.2 *Chlamydia*

NAAT is the gold standard for diagnosis, as it is not only highly sensitive, but co-infection with *N. gonorrhoeae* can also be detected. Rapid POC assays like the XPert and CT/NG assay (binx io) are available, the results of which can be obtained within 90 and 30 minutes, respectively. Other tests that can be performed if facilities are available include culture, serology, antigen detection and gene probe assays.[21,22]

11.2.3.3 Management

Treatment is based on isolation of ICGND from cervical or vaginal smears. Specimens should be sent for NAAT in all patients to confirm the diagnosis and to diagnose co-infection.

Gonococcal cervicitis should be treated with inj. ceftriaxone 500 mg IM single dose, which should be combined with azithromycin 1 gm single dose if chlamydial co-infection is diagnosed or cannot be ruled out.[23] According to syndromic management of cervicitis, all patients are to be treated with a cefixime 400-mg single tablet with azithromycin 1-gm single tablet. Test-of-cure should be performed in all patients at 3–4 weeks post-treatment in chlamydial infection, as severe sequelae can occur in mother and neonate if infection persists. Ophthalmia neonatorum and pneumonia must be treated with erythromycin base or ethylsuccinate 50 mg/kg/day, PO, divided into four doses, for 14 days.[13]

11.2.4 Bacterial Vaginosis in Pregnancy

Bacterial vaginosis is characterised by replacement of normal vaginal flora (lactobacilli) with characteristic anaerobes like *Gardnerella vaginalis* (*G. vaginalis*), *Atopobium vaginae*, *Leptotrichia amnionii*, *Sneathia* and *Megasphaera* species. It is usually considered a sexually enhanced disease and not sexually transmitted, as it is attributed to a shift in the normal vaginal microbiome. *Lactobacillus crispatus* is the most important species for maintaining vaginal health, and its predominance over other lactobacilli species has been known to be protective against microbiota shift.[24]

11.2.4.1 Clinical Features

Symptomatic women complain of malodourous vaginal discharge and pruritus. However, half the patients may be asymptomatic. Malodour is enhanced post-coitus as the alkaline pH of seminal fluid leads to increased production of amines like putrescine, cadaverine and trimethylamine by anaerobes. On examination, scanty to moderate grey homogenous discharge can be seen coating vaginal walls uniformly.

Various adverse pregnancy outcomes include preterm labour, premature rupture of membranes, preterm birth, spontaneous abortion, amniotic fluid infection, chorioamnionitis, deciduitis, postpartum wound infection and endometritis. These complications occur due to ascension of the anaerobes or due to production of prostaglandins (which induces preterm labour) and activation of metalloproteinases (which cause denaturation and rupture of membranes) in response to release of cytokines like IL-6 and IL-1.[24]

11.2.4.2 Diagnosis

Routine screening is not recommended in asymptomatic pregnant women in high or low risk for preterm delivery.[5] The diagnosis of BV is based on Amsel's criteria, which include homogenous, grey-white, thin discharge, uniformly coating the vaginal walls; vaginal pH >4.5; positive whiff test (fishy odour from vaginal discharge after addition of 10% KOH); and presence of clue cells, accounting for >20% of all epithelial cells in the smear. Atleast three out of these four should be present for the diagnosis of BV.[25] Nugent's criteria is considered the gold standard and takes into account the presence of lactobacilli, anaerobes and cocci in each field.[26] Culture is of limited value, as it represents the presence of organisms like *G. vaginalis,* which are normally encountered in vaginal flora.[27] Various commercially available molecular diagnostic tests such as OSOM BV Blue, Affirm VPIII and Aptima BV are now FDA approved. They provide quick results with high sensitivity and specificity.[28–30]

11.2.4.3 Management

Symptomatic BV in pregnancy should be treated with metronidazole 500 mg twice a day or 250 mg thrice a day for 7 days.[13,31] When treatment of asymptomatic BV in pregnant women with high risk for preterm delivery was studied, results documenting harm, no benefit and benefit were obtained. However, in women with low risk for preterm delivery, treatment of asymptomatic BV showed no benefit.[31]

Patients should be followed up after 7 days to document symptomatic cure and results of HIV and syphilis.[13]

11.2.5 Donovanosis in Pregnancy

The causative organism of donovanosis is *Klebsiella granulomatis,* which is an intracellular, Gram-negative coccobacilli.

11.2.5.1 Clinical Features

The commonest presentation is presence of beefy red, fleshy, exuberant and non-tender ulcers that bleed on touch. Hypertrophic ulcers with raised and irregular edges may be more common in pregnancy. Other variants of donovanosis include necrotic and sclerotic variant. Autoinoculation may lead to kissing or mirror lesions. In pregnancy, ulcers tend to proliferate and respond slowly to treatment. Because of pregnancy-induced immunosuppression, ulcers on the cervix may extend to pelvic structures and result in peri-partum haemorrhage due to the vascular nature of these ulcers. If vertical transmission occurs, it may lead to complications like ulcerative lesions, acute suppurative otitis media and lymphadenopathy.[32,33]

11.2.5.2 Diagnosis

A high degree of suspicion is necessary to evaluate donovanosis in non-endemic countries. Donovan bodies can be found on Giemsa staining of the ulcer exudate, which is a POC test. Histological examination can be performed where cytology has failed to reveal Donovan bodies. Bacteria can be found in Giemsa stained smears, both within and outside histiocytes. If facilities are available, ulcer exudate can be cultured on Hep-2 cells and human monocyte co-culture.[34] While PCR may be considered highly sensitive, no FDA-approved PCR test is available.

11.2.5.3 Treatment

Azithromycin should be given 1 gm weekly or 500 mg daily for 3 weeks and until all lesions have healed.[35]

11.2.6 Lymphogranuloma Venereum in Pregnancy

Lymphogranuloma venereum (LGV) is caused by *Chlamydia trachomatis* (*C. trachomatis*) serovar. L1, L2 or L3, which is an intracellular obligate organism.

There are three stages of the disease. The primary stage reflects the stage of genital ulceration, the secondary stage occurs due to involvement of draining lymph nodes (inguinal syndrome) and the tertiary stage is stage of genitoanorectal syndrome.[36]

For diagnosis, ulcer exudate and lymph node aspirate can be subjected to culture, NAAT and serology. Other tests like histological analysis of ulcer or bubo by Giemsa staining, antigen detection using EIA and rapid assays and immunotyping of isolates can be performed if facilities are available.[37]

The recommended regimen is azithromycin 1 gm once weekly for 3 weeks or erythromycin base 500 mg orally 4 times a day for 21 days.[35]

11.2.7 Chancroid in Pregnancy

Chancroid is caused by a nonmotile, non-spore forming Gram-negative bacterium, *Hemophilus ducreyi*.

Usually multiple ulcers are documented. They are non-indurated, tender, deep, with irregular and undermined edges and bleed on touch. In pregnancy, ulcers are more vascular and larger in size. Painful inguinal lymphadenopathy usually appears within 7–14 days of ulceration. No adverse pregnancy outcomes have been reported.[38,39]

It should be treated with azithromycin 1 gm single dose, inj. ceftriaxone 250 mg intramuscularly in single dose or erythromycin base 500 mg three times a day for 7 days.[35]

11.3 VIRAL STDs

11.3.1 Herpes Simplex in Pregnancy

Herpes genitalis is caused by *Herpes simplex virus* 1 and 2 (HSV 1 and 2), double-stranded DNA viruses of the Herpes viridae family. With the recent rise in viral STDs, the incidence of herpes has increased in the last decade. It has been estimated that the prevalence of herpes in pregnancy is about 2–3%.[40]

11.3.1.1   Clinical Features

Herpes genitalis can present as primary genital herpes, first episode non-primary genital herpes and recurrent genital herpes. Primary genital herpes may initially be associated with the eruption of erythematous macules and papules, which subsequently vesiculate and lead to formation of multiple painful, non-vascular, superficial, coalescing ulcers with erythematous, irregular margins and serous and non-indurated base. External dysuria; vaginal discharge; dyspareunia; and bilateral, tender lymphadenopathy usually accompany them. Systemic symptoms like fever, headache and malaise may be present. Various complications include disseminated herpes, encephalitis, aseptic meningitis, hepatitis, cervicitis, pneumonitis, PID and neonatal herpes. First episode non-primary genital herpes occurs in patients who are already seropositive for either HSV1 or 2 and are then exposed to the other strain. Due to structural similarities between the antigens, the antibodies already present try to neutralise this virus, and thus the episode is less severe than the primary episode.[41] Recurrences are commoner with HSV-2. In 4/5th of the women with recently acquired herpes infection in pregnancy, about 2–4 symptomatic recurrences may occur. Asymptomatic viral shedding is usually brief but more in primary infection.

One of the dreaded complications of herpes in pregnancy is neonatal herpes. Up to 30–50% of pregnant females acquiring the infection near term transmit the infection to their neonate. On the contrary, there is <1% chance of transmission if infection was acquired prenatally or during early pregnancy. All women with no history of genital herpes should be asked to abstain from sexual intercourse in third trimester and also oro-genital contact if a history of orolabial herpes is absent.[42]

11.3.1.2   Neonatal Herpes Infection

Intrauterine HSV infection accounts for approximately 5% of HSV infections in neonates and leads to congenital herpes infection. It may result in stillbirth and abortion. If the fetus survives, it may develop neonatal herpes, which can be clinically classified into disease localised to the skin, eye and/or mouth; encephalitis with or without skin, eye and/or mouth involvement; and disseminated HSV which manifests as severe multi-organ dysfunction. Skin involvement can be in form of vesicles and scarring; ocular lesions may present as chorioretinitis, microphthalmia and cataract; neurologic damage may manifest in the form of intracranial calcifications, microcephaly, encephalomalacia, seizures and growth retardation. In 85–90% of neonatal HSV infections, HSV is acquired at the time of delivery and 5–10% is caused by early postnatal viral acquisition. Thus it is acutely important to elicit the history of genital herpes in all pregnant and intra-partum females, as even caesarean section doesn't eliminate the risk of transmission; it lowers it significantly in mothers suffering a clinical episode, prodrome or asymptomatic shedding.[43]

11.3.1.3   Diagnosis

Herpes genitalis can be diagnosed using viral detection or antibody detection methods. Viral detection can be done by cytological tests (POC), viral culture, viral antigen detection and molecular tests. A Tzanck smear may show multinucleate giant cells but is not useful for diagnosis.[44] Viral culture is considered the gold standard. Its specificity is almost 100% but not widely available. Immunofluorescence detects infected cells from genital ulcers with a specificity of >95%. NAAT, like Aptima HSV 1 and 2, has the highest sensitivity.[45] Serology can be done in pregnant females not giving history of genital herpes but has an infected partner. It can also diagnose infection in absence of genital lesions. HerpeSelect ELISA is an FDA-approved serological test with a sensitivity and specificity of 96–100%.[46]

11.3.1.4   Management

Acyclovir 400 mg orally thrice a day for 7–10 days or valacyclovir 1 gm orally twice a day for 7–10 days is recommended.[35] Acyclovir is the preferred regimen during pregnancy.[13] It can be safely administered to all women orally or parenterally depending on severity of infection. Women with active lesions or symptoms of prodrome should be delivered by caesarean section to reduce neonatal transmission.[35] Use of instruments or invasive fetal monitors should be avoided during labour.

Women with a history of active lesions at term and with absence of antibody response should be offered delivery by caesarean section, especially before rupture of membranes. Suppressive therapy from the 36th week of gestation in women with a history of recurrent genital herpes with the acyclovir regime has been recommended.[47]

11.3.2   GENITAL WARTS

Genital warts are caused by human papillomavirus (HPV), mainly type 6 and 11. HPV is a non-enveloped, double stranded DNA virus belonging to the Papoviridae family. Prevalence ranges from 5.5%–65% depending upon various factors like age of the mother, gestational age and geography. In a study, it was found that the prevalence of genital warts in pregnancy was higher than in non-pregnant state (16.82% vs 12.25%).[48]

11.3.2.1   Clinical Features

Anogenital warts are predominantly present over the vulva or peri-anal area with internal extension, cervix and adjacent extra-mucosal areas. Urethral meatus involvement is less common in females compared to males. These warts may have irregular and finger-like projections and are called acuminate warts. These are usually mucosal. Those with macular, flat and barely palpable papules are called flat warts. The third variant, the papular variety, is seen on the extra-mucosal aspect of genitalia.[49] In pregnancy, lesions are florid, and they increase in size, sometimes obstructing the introitus (Figure 11.3). These lesions rapidly diminish in size and number postpartum due to loss of vascularity and restoration of immunity. However, women with HPV infection have reported adverse pregnancy outcomes like miscarriage, IUGR, pregnancy-induced hypertensive disorders (PIHD), preterm birth, low birth weight, premature rupture of membranes (PROM) and fetal death.[50] Another notable finding is that of juvenile onset recurrent respiratory papillomatosis, characterised by exophytic papillomatosis in the respiratory tract of neonates and children born to mothers with HPV. It is usually due to HPV 6 and 11 and presents as stridor and hoarseness. This is very rare, and it is inconclusive if

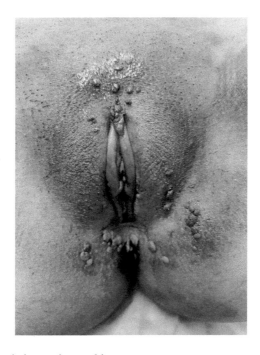

FIGURE 11.3   Multiple genital warts in a multipara.

caesarean delivery prevents this complication.[51] Genital warts in neonates due to perinatal transmission are rare. There are no specific screening recommendations for these in pregnancy.[5]

11.3.2.2 Diagnosis

Genital warts are mainly diagnosed clinically. Doubtful lesions can be subjected to histology, which shows the presence of hyperkeratosis, papillomatosis and koilocytosis.[52] The acetowhite staining technique may be used to diagnose flat or macular warts. Pap smear can be combined with the hybrid capture HPV DNA test 2 (HC2), which is FDA approved to detect HPV.[53] PCR can also be performed if facilities are available.

11.3.2.3 Management

Recommended therapeutic modalities include trichloroacetic acid (TCA) or bichloroacetic acid (BCA) 80–90% solution or cryotherapy with liquid nitrogen or surgical excision by tangential scissor excision, curettage, laser, tangential shave excision or electrosurgery.[13,54] Podophyllin should not be used. Caesarean delivery is indicated only if the pelvic outlet is obstructed or if vaginal delivery will lead to excessive bleeding.[54] The HPV vaccine is not recommended during pregnancy.

11.3.3 *MOLLUSCUM CONTAGIOSUM*

Molluscum is caused by the *Molluscum contagiosum* virus (MCV), belonging to the Molluscipox family. Of the four genotypes, MCV 1 and 2 are encountered most commonly.[55]

11.3.3.1 Clinical Features

It is characterised by the presence of single or multiple clustered or discrete skin-coloured to pink-coloured, firm, round, shiny and umbilicated papules of size about 2–5 mm (Figure 11.4). In pregnancy, due to relative immunosuppression, lesions may be larger (giant molluscum) and more numerous (>100) and resolve slowly. Eczematous plaques may develop around 1–2 lesions, called molluscum dermatitis.[56] The beginning of the end (BOTE) phenomenon refers to development of inflammation around a lesion due to immune response and reflects imminent self-resolution of the lesion.[57]

Congenital molluscum may develop in neonates born via infected birth canal. In such cases, lesions are usually present over the scalp and may be present at birth or may appear by the second or third month of life, given the incubation period of MCV.[58]

11.3.3.2 Diagnosis

It is mainly clinical diagnosis. However, it can be subjected to dermoscopy, which shows multilobular, white to yellowish, amorphous structureless areas with central umbilication and a peripheral

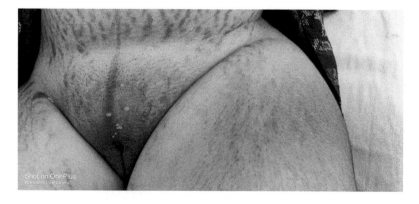

FIGURE 11.4 Multiple genital molluscum contagiosum lesions in a pregnant female.

crown of vessels.[59] Histology reveals lobular proliferation of the affected epidermis with the presence of eosinophilic intracytoplasmic inclusion bodies, called Henderson–Patterson bodies.[60]

11.3.3.3 Management

Mechanical removal (evisceration) of the lesions followed by chemical cautery with 30% TCA, tape stripping, curettage, diathermy and cryosurgery can be performed.[56]

11.3.4 HEPATITIS VIRUS

Hepatitis B virus (HBV) and hepatitis C virus (HCV) are sexually transmitted viruses. While cutaneous manifestations are not predominant, sexually transmitted viral hepatitis warrants mention because unvaccinated neonates have >95% risk of developing chronic hepatitis B (CHB) when infected due to mother-to-child transmission (MTCT), and there have been reports of preterm births and IUGR. All pregnant women should be screened at the first prenatal visit for HBV and HCV. Sera should be tested for HBsAg, HCV, anti-HBsAg and anti-HCV.[61] In the third trimester, all those who were not screened prenatally or who engage in behaviours that put them at high risk for infection and those with signs or symptoms of hepatitis at the time of admission to the hospital for delivery should be tested.[5]

Treatment is symptomatic. When exposed to a person with active HBV infection, pregnant patients should receive both vaccinations as well as hepatitis B immunoglobulin (HBIG). If exposure is with a person with chronic HBV, only vaccination is deemed necessary. Babies born to carrier women must receive a vaccine and HBIG within 12 hours of birth. Mothers with high viremia in the third trimester (HBVDNA levels > 6 log10 copies/mL) should receive oral antivirals to reduce the risk of transmission in the neonate. Three oral nucleos(t)ide analogs considered safe in pregnancy are lamivudine, telbivudine and tenofovir disoproxil fumarate (TDF). TDF is preferred due to a better resistance profile and safety.[62]

11.3.5 CYTOMEGALOVIRUS

Cytomegalovirus (CMV), a double-stranded DNA virus, is acquired most commonly via direct contact with an infected person through saliva, urine or body fluids. In pregnancy, contact with infected young children in the family is the commonest source of infection. The pregnant woman herself is usually asymptomatic, but there is a 40% chance of transmission of the infection to the fetus, causing congenital CMV infection. Other adverse outcomes include stillbirth and preterm delivery. About 1–10% newborns infected with virus exhibit signs and symptoms of the infection in the form of hearing loss, vision problems (including chrioretinitis and blindness), hepatosplenomegaly, LBW, microcephaly and neurological disturbances. Extramedullary erythropoiesis can present as blueberry muffin syndrome.

It can be diagnosed with the help of ultrasonography (placentomegaly, microcephaly, IUGR) and amniocentesis. PCR of body fluids like saliva and urine can be performed in newborns with suspected infection, apart from serological markers for congenital infection. Treatment of the mother with valacyclovir and ganciclovir can reduce the risk of transmission.[63]

11.4 FUNGAL AND PROTOZOAL STDs

11.4.1 VULVOVAGINAL CANDIDIASIS

Vulvovaginal candidiasis (VVC) may or may not be sexually transmitted. *Candida albicans* (*C. albicans*) is the commonest species.

VVC in pregnancy can be attributed to decreased cell-mediated immunity, increased oestrogen levels and increased vaginal mucosal glycogen production. Increased oestrogen facilitates adherence of yeast to vaginal mucosal epithelial cells. Clinically, VVC is characterised by scanty to moderate, clumped, cheesy, adherent plaques of thick curdy white discharge (Figure 11.5), along with

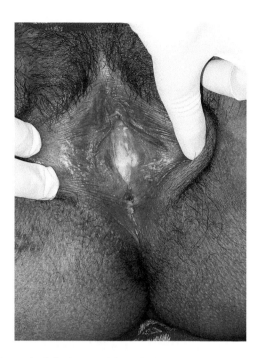

FIGURE 11.5   Curdy white vaginal discharge with genital wart at posterior fourchette.

vaginal and vulval erythema and excoriations. Associated complaints like vulvar itching, external dysuria and dyspareunia are usually present. Cervicitis is usually not seen. Perianal involvement, satellite micropustules around labia majora and post-thrush vestibulitis may be present.[64]

Congenital candidiasis presents at birth or within a few hours of birth in the form of extensive erythematous maculopapular, progressing vesicopustules on erythematous bases over the next 1–3 days. The distribution is predominantly on the head, trunk and extremities Palmoplantar pustules are considered a hallmark of the disease, and mucosae and the napkin area are spared. Onychomycosis and paronychia may rarely be limited to nails. Aspiration of infected amniotic fluid may lead to severe gastrointestinal and respiratory tract involvement that may eventually lead to candidal septicemia.[65]

A 10% KOH mount is the POC test.[66] A culture for VVC is performed if clinical features are suggestive of VVC, but either no organism can be visualised on microscopy or in patients in whom either the infecting organism is suspected to be resistant to azoles or is a non-albicans species.[31] Molecular tests like Aptima CV/TV and BD MAX can be used if facility is available.[67]

Pregnant females should be treated only with topical azoles. Topical formulations in short course, that is, regimens for 1–3 days, are effective for uncomplicated VVC. Clotrimazole 1% cream 5 grams intravaginally for 7 days, miconazole 2% cream 5 grams intravaginally for 7 days or tioconazole 6.5% ointment 5 grams intravaginally in a single application can be given. Clotrimazole vaginal pessaries 100 mg intravaginally once a day for 7 days or 500 mg intravaginally once can be used in place or in combination with topical clotrimazole. Severe VVC, that is, the presence of extensive vulvar erythema, oedema fissures and excoriations, and recurrent cases can be treated with extended topical treatment for 7–14 days.[13,31]

11.4.2   Trichomoniasis

It is caused by *Trichomonas vaginalis,* which is a flagellated protozoan parasite that survives in strictly anaerobic environments but in a wide range of pH values (3.5–8).[68]

11.4.2.1 Clinical Features

It is characterised by profuse, frothy, greenish yellow discharge, along with vulval and vaginal erythema, intense itching and external dysuria. Patients may also complain of irregular bleeding or post-coital bleeding and pelvic pain. However, a significant proportion of women may be asymptomatic. Speculum examination may show strawberry cervix with punctate haemorrhagic points.[68]

Trichomoniasis in pregnancy has been associated with pelvic inflammatory disease and adverse pregnancy outcomes like premature rupture of membranes, preterm delivery and low birth weight baby. Vertical transmission can result in genitourinary and respiratory tract infection in the newborn.[69]

11.4.2.2 Diagnosis

While screening in asymptomatic patients for trichomoniasis is not recommended, patients co-infected with HIV should be screened in the first trimester to reduce vertical transmission of HIV.[5,31]

Wet mount is the POC test for trichomoniasis with sensitivity of about 60–70%. Culture on Diamond's media was considered the gold standard with sensitivity of up to 95% and specificity of >95%. However, culture has now been replaced by NAAT.[70] One of the most common PCR-based tests, the Aptima *T. vaginalis* assay has sensitivity and specificity of 95–100%. It is FDA approved.[71] Other available NAATs include Amplicore, Xpert TV and NuSwab VG. The BD MAX test also detects candida and bacterial vaginosis. It is FDA approved for the same. Rapid antigen hybridisation assays are useful mainly for vaginal swabs. AFFIRM VP III involves DNA hybridisation and gives results in 45 minutes with sensitivity and specificity of about 95%.[72] The OSOM Trichomonas rapid test uses immunochromatographic technology and gives result in 10 minutes with sensitivity of 82–95% and specificity of 97–100%.[73]

11.4.2.3 Management

Metronidazole can be safely used in pregnancy. Recommended regimens include metronidazole 400 mg twice a day for 7 days or metronidazole 2 grams orally in a single dose.[13,31] Tinidazole should avoided in pregnancy.

Table 11.2 summarises the pharmacological agents that are indicated and contraindicated in pregnancy, and Table 11.3 summarises management of select STDs if presentation is at term.

TABLE 11.2

Drugs to Be Given and Drugs to Be Avoided

	Drugs to Be Given	Drugs to Be Avoided
Syphilis	Inj. Benzathine Penicillin G 2.4 million IU I.M. Erythromycin 500 mg orally four times a day for 15 days (penicillin allergy	Doxycycline, fluoroquinolones
Gonorrhoea	Inj. ceftriaxone 500 mg IM single dose/cefixime 400 mg single dose/spectinomycin 2 gm single dose	Fluoroquinolones, tetracycline, aminoglycosides
Chlamydia	Azithromycin 1 gm single dose	Fluoroquinolones, tetracycline, aminoglycosides
Bacterial vaginosis	Metronidazole 500 mg twice daily for 7 days.	Tinidazole
Herpes simplex	Acyclovir 400 mg orally thrice a day for 7–10 days/ valacyclovir 1 gm orally twice a day for 7–10 days	Famciclovir
Viral warts	Cryotherapy/chemical cautery/excision/radiofrequency ablation	Imiquimod, podophyllin, interferons, 5-fluorouracil
Molluscum contagiosum	Extirpation, tape stripping	Imiquimod, podophyllin, interferons, 5-fluorouracil
Vulvovaginal candidiasis	Clotrimazole 1% cream 5 gram intravaginally for 7 days	Fluconazole
Trichomoniasis	Metronidazole 2 gm single dose	Tinidazole

TABLE 11.3

Management When Presentation Is at Term

Syphilis	Treat mother with Inj. Benzathine Penicillin G 2.4 million IU I.M. If VDRL/RPR reactive; monitor neonate for congenital syphilis.
Gonorrhoea	Treat mother; erythromycin 0.5% opthalmic ointment to be used for both eyes to prevent ophthalmia neonatorum
Herpes simplex	Treat mother, Deliver by caesarean section if active lesions or prodrome, monitor neonate
Viral warts	Deliver vaginally if no obstruction of introitus with warts, explain about risk of juvenile laryngeal papillomatosis

11.5   CONCLUSION

STDs in pregnancy pose a significant public health problem worldwide. Therefore, it is imperative that proper screening, diagnosis and treatment be carried out by ensuring adequate antenatal care, especially in resource-poor countries. Proper counselling at every antenatal visit can help not only bringing down the incidence of these infections in the pregnant females but also prevent mother-to-child transmission, thereby improving fetal wellbeing.

REFERENCES

1. WHO. *Data on Syphilis* [internet], accessed 10/08/2023, available at: www.who.int/data/gho/data/themes/topics/data-on-syphilis.
2. Malhotra S. Sexually transmitted infections and pregnancy. In: Gupta S, Kumar B, eds. *Sexually Transmitted Infections*. 2nd edition. New Delhi. Elsevier; 2012: 1081–1094.
3. French P, Gupta S, Kumar B. Infectious syphilis. In: Gupta S, Kumar B, eds. *Sexually Transmitted Infections*. 2nd edition. New Delhi. Elsevier; 2012: 429–457.
4. Shafii T, Radolf JD, Sanchez PJ, et al., eds. Congenital syphilis. In: Holmes KK, Sparling PF, Stamm WE, et al., eds. *Sexually Transmitted Diseases*. 4th edition. New York. McGraw-Hill; 2007: 1577–1612.
5. CDC. *STDs During Pregnancy—CDC Detailed Fact Sheet*, 2023 [internet], available at: www.cdc.gov/std/pregnancy/stdfact-pregnancy-detailed.htm.
6. Ratnam S. The laboratory diagnosis of syphilis. *Can J Infect Dis Med Microbiol*. 2005;16(1):45–51.
7. Quatresooz P, Piérard GE. Skin homing of *Treponema pallidum* in early syphilis: An immunohistochemical study. *Appl Immunohistochem Mol Morphol*. 2009;17(1):47–50.
8. Shields M, Guy RJ, Jeoffreys NJ, et al. A longitudinal evaluation of *Treponema pallidum* PCR testing in early syphilis. *BMC Infect Dis*. 2012;12:353.
9. Tuddenham S, Katz SS, Ghanem KG. Syphilis laboratory guidelines: Performance characteristics of nontreponemal antibody tests. *Clin Infect Dis*. 2020;71(Supplement_1):S21–S42.
10. Henao-Martínez AF, Johnson SC. Diagnostic tests for syphilis: New tests and new algorithms. *Neurol Clin Pract*. 2014;4(2):114–122.
11. WHO. *Dual HIV/Syphilis Rapid Diagnostic Tests* [internet], accessed 10/08/2023, available at: www.who.int/teams/global-hiv-hepatitis-and-stis-programmes/stis/testing-diagnostics/dual-hiv-syphilis-rapid-diagnostic-tests.
12. Workowsky KA, Bachmann LH, Chan PA, et al. Syphilis. *MMWR Recomm Rep*. 2021;70(4):39–56.
13. National AIDS Control Organization, Ministry of Health and Family Welfare Government of India. *National Guidelines on Prevention, Management and Control of Reproductive Tract Infections and Sexually Transmitted Infections*. New Delhi, India; 2014.
14. Vaezzadeh K, Sepidarkish M, Mollalo A, et al. Global prevalence of Neisseria gonorrhoeae infection in pregnant women: A systematic review and meta-analysis. *Clin Microbiol Infect*. 2023;29(1):22–31.
15. Tjahyadi D, Ropii B, Tjandraprawira KD, et al. Female urogenital chlamydia: Epidemiology, chlamydia on pregnancy, current diagnosis, and treatment. *Ann Med Surg (Lond)*. 2022;75:103448.
16. Reekie J, Donovan B, Guy R, et al. Chlamydia and reproductive health outcome investigators; chlamydia and reproductive health outcome investigators. Risk of pelvic inflammatory disease in relation to

chlamydia and gonorrhea testing, repeat testing, and positivity: A population-based cohort study. *Clin Infect Dis.* 2018;66(3):437–443.

17. Reddy BSN, Khandpur S, Sethi S, et al. Gonococcal infections. In: Gupta S, Kumar B, eds. *Sexually Transmitted Infections.* 2nd edition. New Delhi: Elsevier; 2012: 473–493.
18. Steedman N. *Chlamydia trachomatis* infections. In: Gupta S, Kumar B, eds. *Sexually Transmitted Infections.* 2nd edition. New Delhi: Elsevier; 2012: 494–505.
19. Papp JR, Schachter J, Gaydos CA, et al. Recommendations for the laboratory-based detection of *Chlamydia trachomatis* and *Neisseria gonorrhoeae*—2014. *MMWR. Recomm Rep.* 2014;63:1.
20. Knox J, Tabrizi SN, Miller P, et al. Evaluation of self-collected samples in contrast to practitioner-collected samples for detection of *Chlamydia trachomatis, Neisseria gonorrhoeae,* and *Trichomonas vaginalis* by polymerase chain reaction among women living in remote areas. *Sex Transm Infect.* 2002;29(11): 647–654.
21. Gaydos CA, Van Der Pol B, Jett-Goheen M, et al. Performance of the Cepheid CT/NG Xpert rapid PCR test for detection of *Chlamydia trachomatis* and *Neisseria gonorrhoeae. J Clin Microbiol.* 2013;51(6):1666–1672.
22. US Food and Drug Administration. *510(k) Substantial Equivalence Determination Decision Summary: Binx Health io CT/NG Assay.*
23. St. Cyr S, Barbee L, Workowski KA, et al. Update to CDC's treatment guidelines for gonococcal infection, 2020. *MMWR Morb Mortal Wkly Rep.* 2020;69:1911–1916.
24. Hay P, Chandeying V. Bacterial vaginosis. In: Gupta S, Kumar B, eds. *Sexually Transmitted Infections.* 2nd edition. New Delhi: Elsevier; 2012: 542–556.
25. Amsel R, Totten PA, Spiegel CA, et al. Nonspecific vaginitis: Diagnostic criteria and microbial and epidemiologic associations. *Am J Med.* 1983;74(1):14–22.
26. Nugent RP, Krohn MA, Hillier SL. Reliability of diagnosing bacterial vaginosis is improved by a standardized method of gram stain interpretation. *J Clin Microbiol.* 1991;29(2):297–301.
27. Money D. The laboratory diagnosis of bacterial vaginosis. *Can J Infect Dis Med Microbiol.* 2005; 16(2):77–79.
28. Bradshaw CS, Morton AN, Garland SM, et al. Evaluation of a point-of-care test, BVBlue, and clinical and laboratory criteria for diagnosis of bacterial vaginosis. *J Clin Microbiol.* 2005;43(3):1304–1308.
29. Briselden AM, Hillier SL. Evaluation of affirm VP microbial identification test for *Gardnerella vaginalis* and *Trichomonas vaginalis. J Clin Microbiol.* 1994;32(1):148–152.
30. Schwebke JR, Taylor SN, Ackerman R, et al. Clinical validation of the Aptima *Bacterial Vaginosis* and Aptima *Candida/Trichomonas* vaginitis assays: Results from a prospective multicenter clinical study. *J Clin Microbiol.* 2020;58(2):e01643–19.
31. Workowsky KA, Bachmann LH, Chan PA, et al. Diseases characterized by vulvovaginal itching, burning, irritation, odor, or discharge. *MMWR Recomm Rep.* 2021;70(4):82–94.
32. Velho PE, Souza EM, Belda Jr W. Donovanosis. *Braz J Infect Dis.* 2008;12(6):521–525.
33. O'Farrell N. Donovanosis (granuloma inguinale) in pregnancy. *Int J STD AIDS.* 1991;2(6):447–448.
34. Richens J. Donovanosis (granuloma inguinale). *Sex Transm Infect.* 2006;82(Suppl 4):21–22.
35. Workowsky KA, Bachmann LH, Chan PA, et al. Diseases characterized by genital, anal or perianal ulcers. *MMWR Recomm Rep.* 2021;70(4):29–41.
36. Mabey D, Peeling RW. Lymphogranuloma venereum. *Sex Transm Infect.* 2002;78:90.
37. Ceovic R, Gulin SJ. Lymphogranuloma venereum: Diagnostic and treatment challenges. *Infect Drug Resist.* 2015;8:39–47.
38. Lewis DA. Chancroid: Clinical manifestations, diagnosis, and management. *Sex Transm Infect.* 2003;79(1):68–71.
39. Donders GG. Treatment of sexually transmitted bacterial diseases in pregnant women. *Drugs.* 2000;59(3):477–485.
40. Hammad WAB, Konje JC. Herpes simplex virus infection in pregnancy—An update. *Eur J Obstet Gynecol Reprod Biol.* 2021;259:38–45.
41. Sauerbrei A. Herpes genitalis: Diagnosis, treatment and prevention. *Geburtshilfe Frauenheilkd.* 2016;76(12):1310–1317.
42. Straface G, Selmin A, Zanardo V, et al. Herpes simplex virus infection in pregnancy. *Infect Dis Obstet Gynecol.* 2012:385697.
43. Kimberlin DW. Neonatal herpes simplex infection. *Clin Microbiol Rev.* 2004(1):1–13.
44. Yaeen A, Ahmad QM, Farhana A, et al. Diagnostic value of Tzanck smear in various erosive, vesicular, and bullous skin lesions. *Indian Dermatol Online J.* 2015;6(6):381–386.

45. Sam SS, Caliendo AM, Ingersoll J, et al. Performance evaluation of the Aptima HSV-1 and 2 assay for the detection of HSV in cutaneous and mucocutaneous lesion specimens. *J Clin Virol.* 2018;99(100):1–4.
46. Al-Shobaili H, Hassanein KM, Mostafa MS et al. Evaluation of the HerpeSelect express rapid test in the detection of *Herpes simplex virus* type 2 antibodies in patients with genital ulcer disease. *J Clin Lab Anal.* 2015;29(1):43–46.
47. Foley E, Clarke E, Beckett VA, et al., *Management of Genital Herpes in Pregnancy, RCOG Guidelines*, London; 2014 [internet], available at: www.rcog.org.uk/guidance/browse-all-guidance/other-guidelines-and-reports/management-of-genital-herpes-in-pregnancy/
48. Condrat CE, Filip L, Gherghe M, et al. Maternal HPV infection: Effects on pregnancy outcome. *Viruses.* 2021;13(12):2455.
49. Yanofsky VR, Patel RV, Goldenberg G. Genital warts: A comprehensive review. *J Clin Aesthet Dermatol.* 2012;5(6):25–36.
50. Chilaka VN, Navti OB, Al Beloushi M, et al. Human papillomavirus (HPV) in pregnancy—An update. *Eur J Obstet Gynecol Reprod Biol.* 2021;264:340–348.
51. Lépine C, Voron T, Berrebi D, et al. Juvenile-onset recurrent respiratory papillomatosis aggressiveness: In situ study of the level of transcription of HPV E6 and E7. *Cancers (Basel).* 2020;12(10):2836.
52. Vyas NS, Pierce Campbell CM, Mathew R, et al. Role of histological findings and pathologic diagnosis for detection of human papillomavirus infection in men. *J Med Virol.* 2015;87(10):1777–1787.
53. Kulmala SM, Syrjänen S, Shabalova I, et al. Human papillomavirus testing with the hybrid capture 2 assay and PCR as screening tools. *J Clin Microbiol.* 2004;42(6):2470–2475.
54. Workowsky KA, Bachmann LH, Chan PA, et al. Human papillomavirus infections. *MMWR Recomm Rep.* 2021;70(4):102–115.
55. Zorec TM, Kutnjak D, Hošnjak L, et al. New insights into the evolutionary and genomic landscape of molluscum contagiosum virus (MCV) based on Nine MCV1 and Six MCV2 complete genome sequences. *Viruses.* 2018;10.
56. Meza-Romero R, Navarrete-Dechent C, Downey C. Molluscum contagiosum: An update and review of new perspectives in etiology, diagnosis, and treatment. *Clin Cosmet Investig Dermatol.* 2019;12:373–381.
57. Butala N, Siegfried E, Weissler A. Molluscum BOTE sign: A predictor of imminent resolution. *Pediatrics.* 2013;131(5):e1650–e1653.
58. Neri I, Liberati G, Virdi A, et al. Congenital molluscum contagiosum. *Paediatr Child Health.* 2017;22(5):241–242.
59. Ianhez M, Cestari Sda C, Enokihara MY, et al. Dermoscopic patterns of molluscum contagiosum: A study of 211 lesions confirmed by histopathology. *An Bras Dermatol.* 2011;86(1):74–79.
60. van der Wouden JC, Menke J, Gajadin S, et al. Interventions for cutaneous molluscum contagiosum. *Cochrane Database Syst Rev.* 2017;5:CD004767.
61. Chilaka VN, Konje JC. Viral hepatitis in pregnancy. *Eur J Obstet Gynecol Reprod Biol.* 2021;256:287–296.
62. Joshi SS, Coffin CS. Hepatitis B and pregnancy: Virologic and immunologic characteristics. *Hepatol Commun.* 2020;4(2):157–171.
63. Chiopris G, Veronese P, Cusenza F, et al Congenital cytomegalovirus infection: Update on diagnosis and treatment. *Microorganisms.* 2020;8(10):1516.
64. Say JP. Genital candida infections. In: Gupta S, Kumar B, eds. *Sexually Transmitted Infections.* 2nd edition. New Delhi: Elsevier; 2012: 591–601.
65. Aruna C, Seetharam K. Congenital candidiasis. *Indian Dermatol Online J.* 2014;5(Suppl 1):S44–S47.
66. Ponka D, Baddar F. Microscopic potassium hydroxide preparation. *Can Fam Physician.* 2014;60(1):57.
67. Gaydos CA, Beqaj S, Schwebke JR, et al. Clinical validation of a test for the diagnosis of vaginitis. *Obstet Gynecol.* 2017;130(1):181–189.
68. Kissinger P. Trichomonas vaginalis: A review of epidemiologic, clinical and treatment issues. *BMC Infect Dis.* 2015;15:307.
69. Van Gerwen OT, Craig-Kuhn MC, Jones AT, et al. Trichomoniasis and adverse birth outcomes: A systematic review and meta-analysis. *BJOG.* 2021;128(12):1907–1915.
70. Krieger JN, Tam MR, Stevens CE, et al. Diagnosis of trichomoniasis: Comparison of conventional wet-mount examination with cytologic studies, cultures, and monoclonal antibody staining of direct specimens. *JAMA.* 1988;259(8):1223–1227.
71. Chapin K, Andrea S. APTIMA® *Trichomonas vaginalis*, a transcription-mediated amplification assay for detection of *Trichomonas vaginalis* in urogenital specimens. *Expert Rev. Mol. Diagn.* 2011;11(7):679–688.

72. Andrea SB, Chapin KC. Comparison of Aptima *Trichomonas vaginalis* transcription-mediated amplification assay and BD affirm VPIII for detection of T. vaginalis in symptomatic women: Performance parameters and epidemiological implications. *J Clin Microbiol.* 2011;49(3):866–869.
73. Gaydos CA, Klausner JD, Pai NP, et al. Rapid and point-of-care tests for the diagnosis of *Trichomonas vaginalis* in women and men. *Sex Transm Infect.* 2017;93(S4):S31–S35.

12 Striae Gravidarum and Their Management

Rajat Kandhari and Noor S

12.1   DEFINITION

Striae gravidarum (SG) are one of the most common connective tissue changes seen during pregnancy. These linear atrophic scars, or "stretch marks", are irregular in shape, purple/red/violaceous in colour, wrinkled, and slightly depressed, gradually changing to a silvery-white colour and typically occurring at the sixth to seventh month of gestation. They tend to occur in areas of maximum stretch. SG can cause emotional and psychological distress for many women. Research on risk factors, prevention, and management of SG has often been inconclusive.[1]

12.2   INTRODUCTION

Striae gravidarum is considered one of the most common connective tissue changes during pregnancy. They affect all racial groups[2], and the rate of occurrence ranges between 52 and 90% of women with varying ethnicities.[3–7] Striae become obvious during the third trimester,[8] are commonly seen in primigravida,[9] and have a considerable psychological impact, leading to a decreased quality of life.[10] Literature on risk factors, prevention, and management of this condition is limited or provides conflicting results.[11] Stretch marks are divided into striae atrophicae (thinned skin), striae gravidarum (following pregnancy), striae distensae (stretched skin), striae rubrae (red), striae albae (white), striae nigrae (black), and striae caeruleae (dark blue).[12]

12.3   HISTORY

Pregnancy-related stretch marks have always been a matter of stress to women.

As early as 16 BC, women were self-aborting their pregnancies to avoid stretch marks.[13] Treatment options for stretch marks recorded by ancient Egyptians included numerous preparations; Soranus and Pliny the Elder in the 1st century AD endorsed unripe olive oil and sea salt, respectively.[14] One of the most often recommended treatments included frankincense.[15] Various other topical preparations and surgical methods have been tried.

12.4   CLINICAL FEATURES

The appearance of SG varies from flat, pink-to-red bands (striae rubrae or immature striae) (Figure 12.1) that become raised, longer, wider, and violet-red initially; then over a period, the marks fade and become lighter in colour (striae alba or mature striae) (Figure 12.2), parallel to skin tension lines as scar-like, wrinkled, white, and atrophic marks.[9,16,17] SG can at times be associated with itching, burning, and discomfort. Up to 90% of SG appear in primigravidas.[11] The onset of SG in 43% of women has been reported prior to 24 weeks of gestation, though it is typically seen in the second and third trimester.[11] Both mature and immature striae are well appreciated in cases of multigravida (Figure 12.3).

DOI: 10.1201/9781003449690-12

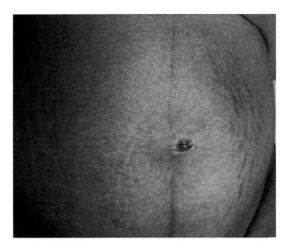

FIGURE.12.1   Striae rubrae seen in primigravida.

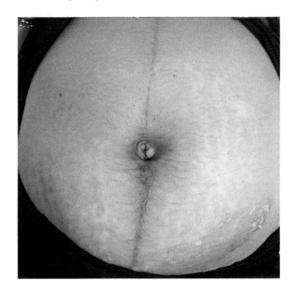

FIGURE.12.2   Striae albae.

12.5   ETIOPATHOGENESIS

According to many investigators, in addition to genetic predisposition,[18] a combination of distension and adrenocortical activity leads to the formation of SG.[19–22] Therefore, etiopathogenesis involves genetic factors[23], hormonal factors,[11,24–26] and increased mechanical stress on connective tissue [6,17,26,27] or a combination of all three. An exact cause of striae gravidarum remains ambiguous.[5]

In a comparative study of an obese population with and without striae, increased excretion of corticosteroids was found in the ones with striae.[28] These studies are further supported by reports of striae development in Cushing's syndrome and in patients treated with systemic and topical corticosteroids.[29]

Tissue stretch—Studies have demonstrated an inconsistent association of SG with maternal weight gain and abdominal, hip girth stretch;[4] it still remains as contentious trigger.

Hormonal factors—When compared with non-pregnant healthy skin, twice as many oestrogen receptors and elevated androgen and glucocorticoid receptors have been observed in SG.[24]

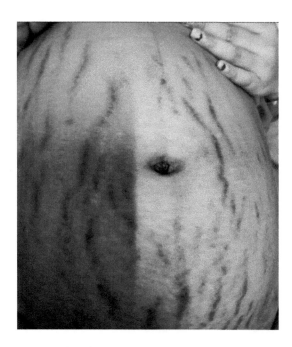

FIGURE.12.3   Striae rubrae and striae albae seen in multigravida.

Pregnancy's distinct hormonal milieu is thought to influence connective tissue that is susceptible to SG when stretched. Ultimately, abnormalities in elastic fibers,[30–32] collagen fibrils,[30,33] and other extracellular membrane components[17] form the pathogenesis of SG.[34] To support this, a study with a comparison between an obese population with and without striae was conducted, in which increased excretion of corticosteroids was seen in the ones with striae.[28] These studies are further supported by reports of striae development in Cushing's syndrome and in patients treated with systemic corticosteroids.[29] Development of atrophic inguinal striae after the prolonged use of a topical steroid cream for intertrigo is also been reported.[35,36]

Several studies support the opinion that they are probably influenced more by increased adrenocortical activity than by increased abdominal circumference,[22] wherein Poidevin[20] in his study found a relationship with increased adrenocortical activity but no correlation with increased abdominal girth.

Priming Stage—In 1974, Liu[18] proposed a series of events that take place during pregnancy leading to the formation of stretch marks. During the first stage, priming of the skin takes place due to hormones that increase during pregnancy, relaxin and oestrogen. These hormones cause an increase in the production of collagen and sulphate-free mucopolysaccharides (MPS), leading to water absorption. This process relaxes the interfibrous cohesive forces causing cleavage or fraying of the collagen fibres, which then easily separate. It appears that "priming" of the dermis is thereby necessary for the formation of striae. However, Shuster[33] believed that stretch with intradermal tears of collagen is the sole factor, without the need of the "priming" for SG formation.

Watson et al.,[17] in an immunohistochemical study of early erythematous striae, demonstrated looser dermal matrix, increased levels of glycosaminoglycans (GAGS), reduced levels of fibrillin and elastic fibres, and alterations in the orientation of elastin and fibrillin in the dermis, suggesting that changes in the skin elements necessary for tensile strength and elasticity, fibrillin, elastin, and collagen, are suspected in the development of striae gravidarum.[37]

In the very early stage of SD, lesional and perilesional clinically uninvolved skin demonstrates sequential changes of elastolysis accompanied by mast cell degranulation, which appears first, followed by an influx of activated macrophages that envelop fragmented elastic fibres, showing the critical roles of elastic fibres, mast cells, and macrophages in the process of SD formation in the initial stages.[31]

It should be noted that the cutaneous changes of pruritic urticarial papules and plaques of pregnancy (PUPPP) are typically localised to abdominal striae in its onset. This suggests that striae damage of the skin leads to a possible exposure of antigenic foci, with secondary inflammatory reactions.[38,39]

Striae associated with pregnancy gradually fade postpartum to pale atrophic lines, but they do not disappear completely.[21,40,41]

The presence of striae also helps in prediction of intraabdominal adhesions. These intraabdominal adhesions are associated with an increase in complications during caesarean section because of recurrent caesarean sections. The diagnostic values of depressed scar, severe striae gravidarum (Figure 12.3), and negative sliding sign were evaluated for predicting intraabdominal adhesions of caesarean candidates in some studies. In the absence of a depressed scar and severe striae gravidarum, there is a 90% chance of no adhesions.[42,43]

12.6   HISTOPATHOLOGY

The histopathological features of striae rubrae on skin biopsy include lack of mast cells, elastolysis, structural changes in collagen bundles, prominent fibroblasts, dermal oedema, perivascular lymphocytes, and reduced fibrillin microfibrils.[44]

Striae albae resemble scar tissue. Epidermal atrophy, loss of skin appendages, and densely packed collagen bundles parallel to the skin surface are observed.[45]

Histologically, in corticosteroid-induced striae, weakening and rupture of dermal elastic fibres are seen as twisted strands at the periphery of the lesions and are absent in the centre of the streaks. Collagen fibres stain weakly and are disposed discretely rather than in interwoven bundles in the dermis.[29]

12.7   RISK FACTORS

Risk factors associated with the development of striae gravidarum have been identified.[4,6] Two of the commonly identified ones are higher weight gain during pregnancy/pre-pregnancy[4,5,7] and higher birth weight babies.[2,4,6,46,47] Other risk factors include young maternal age, family history of SG,[6,7,11,48–50] and personal history of striae.[11] Pre-pregnancy weight or maternal age was not found as a risk factor in studies conducted.[11,51] It was also demonstrated that increased risk of SG was found in women with striae on the breasts; on the other hand, decreased risk of SG was seen in women with striae on the thighs.[11] A study by Chang et al.[11] found a higher prevalence of SG in non-white women.

With regard to socioeconomic status, multiple studies showed that unemployment, receiving state medical assistance, and lower education level were also associated with SG.[1]

Also, factors like expecting a male baby, increased alcohol intake, decreased water intake, and low blood vitamin C levels were also found to be more common among those women with SG in some studies. Limited studies also comment that diabetes and increased serum glucose levels could play a part in the pathogenesis of SG, but not enough data regarding this was found.[1]

12.8   PREVENTION

The highest-quality evidence available on the prevention of striae gravidarum is from a Cochrane Review[52] which assessed the effects of topical preparations on the prevention of stretch marks in pregnancy. Nearly six trials with 800 women were included in this review, which concluded that there was no statistically significant average difference in the groups that developed striae gravidarum despite using topical preparations with active ingredients compared to the group that received a placebo or no treatment. In a survey of 753 pregnant women[53] 78.2% of respondents specified that they used a product to prevent or reduce the development of SG during their current pregnancy, and over 36.5% had used two or more products. There was also no statistically significant average mean difference in the severity of striae gravidarum.

There are many products available which can be used during pregnancy to prevent[54] or treat[55] striae gravidarum.[5,47,53,56,57] While striae appear to be distressing for the patient, unfortunately, therapy remains unsatisfactory.[38,58] Preventative treatments have not proven useful.

Centella asiatica is a medicinal herb containing pentacyclic triterpene derivatives,[59,60] which is thought to increase the production of collagen and elastic fibers.[61] Creams that contain *Centella asiatica* extract are well known and popular for the prevention and reduction of SG.[61,62] A study by Mallol et al. in 1991 demonstrated that creams containing *Centella asiatica* extract, α-tocopherol, and collagen–elastin hydrolysates when applied daily from gestational week 12 until delivery significantly reduced the incidence of SG compared with placebo group. The same was also validated by Garcia Hernandez et al., including that the severity of previous striae significantly increased in the patient group treated with placebo, but this change was not witnessed in the patient group treated with *Centella* cream.[61]

De Buman et al. and Wierrani et al. found that two proprietary creams that contain hyaluronic acid combined with various vitamins and fatty acids were shown to significantly lower the incidence of SG.[63,64] Hyaluronic acid was found to be the active ingredient in both creams, known to increase the resistance to mechanical forces and oppose atrophy through stimulation of fibroblast activity and collagen production.[65,10] The creams in these studies were applied through massage during the second trimester, which poses the question of whether the creams were truly beneficial or the results reflected were the benefits of massage alone.

Other applications containing almond oil, olive oil, or cocoa butter consistently failed to significantly lower the incidence of SG.[66] On the other hand, two studies found that when olive/almond oil was applied with a massage daily, it resulted in a lower incidence of SG development. However, these results could be the benefits of massage alone.[19,67] Contrary to this, Poidevin reported that not only did nightly rubbing of olive oil fail as a prophylactic, but it actually appeared to predispose to the development of striae.[20] There is controversy as to the effectiveness of olive oil and massage, which requires further validation.[19,20]

It should be noted that the application of vitamin E or other oils, in addition to not being proven to work, may also lead to contact dermatitis. Another suggested treatment contains tocopherol, essential fatty acids, panthenol, hyaluronic acid, elastin, and menthol. None of these products are widely available, and the safety of using *Centella asiatica* during pregnancy and the components responsible for their effectiveness has not been fully elucidated.[67] One report describes personal successful experience in preventing striae gravidarum in all pregnant patients with a combination of zinc, ascorbic acid, pyridoxal, and flaxseed oil; however, no large study was conducted to test this observation.[68]

12.9 MANAGEMENT

Though several studies have been conducted on topical and laser treatments for nongestational striae distensae, only a limited number of studies are available on treatment of striae gravidarum. Treatments include topical treatment, lasers, light therapies, microneedling, and others. In order to achieve good results, these treatments should be initiated during the early stages of SG rather than when striae have matured and permanent changes have occurred.

12.9.1 TOPICAL MEDICATIONS

Tretinoin is one of the commonest drugs used in striae treatment. It is known to increase elastin content in the papillary and reticular dermis of the lesions. Limited effectiveness in postpartum treatment of striae distensae has been reported.[69] A 0.1% tretinoin cream used in an open-label study showed a decrease in the severity of striae gravidarum after 3 months of application.[70] Ash et al., in a study, found that tretinoin 0.05% and 0.1% creams used on a daily basis in patients with SG for 3 to 7 months consistently resulted in overall global improvement, up to 47%.[71] Also, a double-blinded placebo-controlled trial of 0.025% tretinoin cream was conducted where this formulation was applied for 7 months to striae gravidarum, and it failed to demonstrate significant improvements over the placebo.[72] Another study with tretinoin cream, along with a combination of 20% glycolic acid and 10% ascorbic acid, showed improvement in SG. Rangel et al. reported decreased mean length and width up to 20% and 23%, respectively, of lesions,[70] while Pribanich et al. demonstrated the minimum effective concentration of tretinoin cream to be 0.05% for striae management.[72] Twenty percent glycolic acid combined with either 10% ascorbic acid or 0.05% tretinoin improved the appearance of SG, although there was no statistically significant difference between the two combinations.[71]

12.9.2 LASER TREATMENTS

For striae with no gestational origin, both fractional and non-fractional lasers have been studied. Among fractional lasers, both non-ablative erbium (Er):glass, erbium fibre, and ablative carbon dioxide (CO_2) lasers have been used.

At 3 months post-treatment, a statistically significant clinical improvement in SG with 1540-nm non-ablative fractional laser was seen that ranged from 1% to 24%.[73]An average of 50–75% improvement in lesions after 2 to 6 sessions with nonablative Er:glass treatments was also reported by Bak et al., De Angelis et al., and Tretti Clementoni and Lavangno,[74–76] which was supported by histologic studies where an increase in elastic fibres and collagen production was appreciated. This laser was generally safe, and treatments were well tolerated by patients. Most recent studies have shown that patients with SG of different types (rubra/alba) benefit from treatment with non-ablating fractional laser (NAFL), experiencing minimal transient side effects. Hence, it can be considered a safe and partially effective treatment option for stretch marks of patients with SG.[77]

Although Cho et al. reported inconsistent results in their studies,[78] a 50–75% improvement was demonstrated, especially in striae alba, with ablative CO_2 lasers in a study by Lee et al.[79] Ablative lasers like CO_2 lasers are more painful, may have longer down time than non-ablative lasers, and may lead to post inflammatory pigmentation. The use of tretinoin between laser sessions may help.

Different non-fractional laser modalities like excimer, pulsed dye, neodymium-doped yttrium aluminium garnet (Nd:YAG), copper bromide, and diode have been studied in the treatment of SD of patients of nongestational origin. Pulsed dye lasers are used to treat erythema in cases of striae rubra2 while having limited benefits in striae alba. [80,81]

The 308-nm excimer laser, on the other hand, is a modality utilised to induce pigmentation in cases of mature hypopigmented striae (i.e., striae alba). Repigmentation was achieved, with up to a 75% increase in pigmentation; however, results are generally temporary, and pigmentation of the normal surrounding skin is an unfavourable consequence.[82] In a small study that used a copper bromide laser, 13 out of 15 women experienced a complete resolution or modest improvement of striae for up to 2 years.[83] In dark-skinned individuals, a diode laser was used to treat SD, where this laser was ineffective and 64% of patients developed undesirable hyperpigmentation.[84] A long-pulsed Nd:YAG laser demonstrated excellent improvement of up to 70% or more, despite being specifically indicated for immature striae rubrae.[85]

12.9.3 LIGHT TREATMENTS

Light therapy modalities such as intense pulsed light (IPL), ultraviolet (UV) light, and infrared light have been employed for the treatment of non-gestational SD. IPL seems to result in moderate improvement of striae,[86] but persistent erythema and post-inflammatory hyperpigmentation were found to be common complications of this treatment. UV light, especially broadband (i.e., a combination of UV-B and UV-A), has shown consistent repigmentation of striae alba. However, the results are not promising and maintenance treatment is required.[87] Four treatment sessions with infrared light at 800 to 1800 nm resulted in 25–50% improvement in striae alba. Long-term studies with larger sample sizes are lacking to confirm these results.[88] When IPL was combined with erbium fractional laser, it was found to improve the atrophy of SG, lighten the colour, and increase the elasticity and thickness of the skin, with a high treatment safety and remarkable clinical results.[89]

12.9.4 OTHER MODALITIES

Modalities such as microdermabrasion and microneedling have been found to be effective treatments in nongestational striae in various studies. Microdermabrasion involves application and subsequent vacuuming of abrasive substances (like aluminium oxide) to the treated area. Microdermabrasion has been especially effective for striae rubrae.[90] In a comparative study, although microdermabrasion with sonophoresis improved striae, needling therapy that causes controlled skin injury with the goal of producing new collagen and elastin in the papillary dermis was found to yield an even greater, statistically significant improvement in SG compared to microdermabrasion.[91]

In the recent past, non-ablative and fractional microneedle radiofrequency (MNRF) devices have been used for tightening of the skin with significant efficacy and safety profile. RF uses a coupling method to generate high energy fluences that deliver energy to the dermis and subcutaneous tissue without damaging the epidermis. The skin's impedance reacts with this electric energy and converts it into thermal energy, which in turn stimulates fibroblasts with contraction and denaturation of the fibrillar collagen structure. These changes promote neocollagenosis, neoelastogenesis, and changes in the ECM.[92] Bipolar radiofrequency demonstrated clinical and histologic improvements in SD,[93] while tripolar third-generation radiofrequency was found to provide 25% to 75% improvement at 1 week post-final treatment.[94]

Platelet-rich plasma (PRP) is used alone or in combination with microneedling. PRP containing various growth factors and protein, when injected intradermally, acts by augmenting dermal elasticity by stimulation of ECM and inducing synthesis of new collagen.[92]

Carboxytherapy: Depending upon the age of striae, CO_2 gas is injected subcutaneously at the depth of 5–6 mm in striae at weekly intervals for 3–12 sessions. This stimulates blood circulation and increases the release of oxygen by means of oxyhaemoglobin. It also activates the synthesis of collagenase, elastin, and hyaluronic acid by stimulation of fibroblast function.[92]

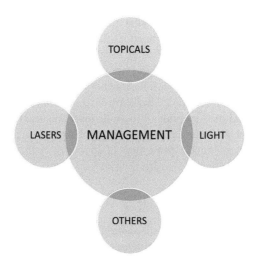

FIGURE 12.4 Management options.

Amongst the aforementioned modalities, a combination of lasers and/or MNRF or bipolar radiofrequency may be utilised to provide superior outcomes. When combining two modalities in the same session, the user must tread cautiously in order to avoid untoward effects such as post-inflammatory pigmentation around the striae. The surrounding areas should always be treated in order to provide a "stretch effect" to make the global appearance of the region smoother.

Oral tretinoin therapy was also suggested as a potential postpartum therapy.[95] Surgical excision of striae with abdominoplasty was also found to give favourable results when there is accompanying redundant abdominal skin.

Other minimally invasive modalities such as monofilament threads, PLLA threads, collagen bioremodellers, galvanopuncture, and pulsed dye laser may be tried to enhance the outcome as adjuvant therapies.

12.10 CONCLUSION

SG is a common, disfiguring, and distressing change found in many women postpartum. While the risk factors are well studied, there are no proven preventive measures. It is important to counsel and reassure the pregnant woman regarding the use of lubrication and massage during pregnancy as possible preventive measures, on the nature of SG, and that while the discoloration will probably become less noticeable, the lesions may persist. Various therapies have been used to improve the global appearance of SG where fractional lasers and topical medications yielded variable outcomes.

REFERENCES

1. Farahnik B, Park K, Kroumpouzos G, et al. Striae gravidarum: Risk factors, prevention, and management. *Int J Womens Dermatol.* 2016;3(2):77–85.
2. Buchanan K, Fletcher HM, Reid M. Prevention of striae gravidarum with cocoa butter cream. *Int J Gynaecol Obstet.* 2010;108(1):65–68.
3. Muzaffar F, Hussain I, Haroon TS. Physiologic skin changes during pregnancy: A study of 140 cases. *Int J Dermatol.* 1998;37(6):429–431.
4. Atwal GSS, Manku LK, Griffiths CEM, et al. Striae gravidarum in primiparae. *Br J Dermatol.* 2006;55(5):965–969.
5. Osman H, Rubeiz N, Tamim H, et al. Risk factors for the development of striae gravidarum. *Am J Obstet Gynecol.* 2007;196(1):62.e61–65.
6. Ghasemi A, Gorouhi F, Rashighi-Firoozabadi M, et al. Striae Gravidarum: Associated factors. *J Eur Acad Dermatol Venereol.* 2007;21(6):743–746.
7. Bahrami N, Soleimani MA, Nia HS, et al. Striae gravidarum in Iranian women: Prevalence and associated factors. *Life Sci J.* 2012;9(4):3032–3037.
8. Cunningham FG, Leveno KJ, Bloom SL, et al. *Williams obstetrics.* 23rd ed. New York: McGraw Hill; 2010.
9. Salter SA, Kimball AB. Striae gravidarum. *Clin Dermatol.* 2006;24(2):97–100.
10. Korgavkar K, Wang F. Stretch marks during pregnancy: A review of topical prevention. *Br J Dermatol.* 2015;172:606–615.
11. Chang AL, Agredano YZ, Kimball AB. Risk factors associated with striae gravidarum. *J Am Acad Dermatol.* 2004;51:881–885.
12. Oakley AM, Patel BC. Stretch marks. 2023 Apr 3. In: *StatPearls* [Internet]. Treasure Island, FL: StatPearls Publishing; 2023.
13. Rayor DJ, Batstone WW. *Latin lyric and elegiac poetry: An anthology of new translations.* New York: Garland; 1995.
14. Owsei T. *Soranus' gynecology.* Baltimore: John Hopkins University Press; 1991.
15. NWI Trading Co Frank-Incense—Frankincense resin and Frankincense Essential Oil; 2016.
16. Sodhi VK, Sausker WF. Dermatoses of pregnancy. *Am Fam Physician.* 1988;37:131–138.
17. Watson RE, Parry EJ, Humphries JD, et al. Fibrillin microfibrils are reduced in skin exhibiting striae distensae. *Br J Dermatol.* 1998;138:931–937.
18. Liu DT. Letter: Striae gravidarum. *Lancet.* 1974;1:625.
19. Davey CM. Factors associated with the occurrence of striae gravidarum. *J Obstet Gynaecol Br Commonw.* 1972;79:1113–1114.

20. Poidevin L. Striae gravidarum. Their relation to adrenal cortical hyperfunction. *Lancet.* 1959;2:436–439.
21. Wade TR, Wade SL, Jones HE. Skin changes and diseases associated with pregnancy. *Obstet Gynecol.* 1978;52:233–242.
22. Wong RC, Ellis CN. Physiologic skin changes in pregnancy. *J Am Acad Dermatol.* 1984;10:929–940.
23. Di Lernia V, Bonci A, Cattania M, et al. Striae distensae (rubrae) in monozygotic twins. *Pediatr Dermatol.* z2001;18:261–262.
24. Cordeiro RC, Zecchin KG, de Moraes AM. Expression of estrogen, androgen, and glucocorticoid receptors in recent striae distensae. *Int J Dermatol.* 2010;49:30–32.
25. Lurie S, Matas Z, Fux A, et al. Association of serum relaxin with striae gravidarum in pregnant women. *Arch Gynecol Obstet.* 2011;283:219–222.
26. Murphy KW, Dunphy B, O'Herlihy C. Increased maternal age protects against striae gravidarum. *J Obstet Gynaecol.* 1992;12:297–300.
27. Fitzpatrick TB, Wolff K. *Fitzpatrick's dermatology in general medicine.* New York: McGraw-Hill Medical; 2008.
28. Simkin B, Arce R. Steroid excretion in obese patients with colored abdominal striae. *N Engl J Med.* 1962;266:1031–1035.
29. McKenzie AW. Skin disorders in pregnancy. *Practitioner.* 1971;206:773–780.
30. Pinkus H, Keech MK, Mehregan AH. Histopathology of striae distensae, with special reference to striae and wound healing in the Marfan syndrome. *J Invest Dermatol.* 1966;46:283–292.
31. Sheu HM, Yu HS, Chang CH. Mast cell degranulation and elastolysis in the early stage of striae distensae. *J Cutan Pathol.* 1991;18:410–416.
32. Tsuji T, Sawabe M. Elastic fibers in striae distensae. *J Cutan Pathol.* 1988;15:215–222.
33. Shuster S. The cause of striae distensae. *Acta Derm Venereol Suppl (Stockh).* 1979;59:161–169.
34. Wang F, Calderone K, Smith NR, et al. Marked disruption and aberrant regulation of elastic fibres in early striae gravidarum. *Br J Dermatol.* 2015;173:1420–1430.
35. Chernosky ME, Knox JM. Atrophic striae after occlusive corticosteroid therapy. *Arch Dermatol.* 1964;90:15–19.
36. Epstein N, Epstein W, Epstein J. Atopic striae in patients with inguinal intertrigo. *Arch Dermatol.* 1963;87:450.
37. Nussbaum R, Benedetto AV. Cosmetic aspects of pregnancy. *Clin Dermatol.* 2006;24:133–141.
38. Elling SV, Powell FC. Physiological changes in the skin during pregnancy. *Clin Dermatol.* 1997;15:35–43.
39. Powell F, Dervan P, Wayte J, et al. Pruritic urticarial papules and plaques of pregnancy (PUPPP): A clinicopathological review of 35 patients. *J Eur Acad Dermatol Venereol.* 1996;6:105–111.
40. Hellreich P. The skin changes of pregnancy. *Cutis.* 1974;13:82–86.
41. Winton GB, Lewis CW. Dermatoses of pregnancy. *J Am Acad Dermatol.* 1982;6:977–998.
42. Mokhtari M, Yaghmaei M, Akbari Jami N, et al. Prediction of intraperitoneal adhesions in repeated cesarean section using sliding sign, striae gravidarum, and cesarean scar. *Med J Islam Repub Iran.* 2022;36:44.
43. Shafti V, Azarboo A, Ghaemi M, et al. E. Prediction of intraperitoneal adhesions in repeated cesarean sections: A systematic review and meta-analysis. *Eur J Obstet Gynecol Reprod Biol.* 2023;287:97–108.
44. Rook A, Wilkinson DS, Ebling FJB, et al., eds. *Textbook of dermatology.* 4th ed. Blackwell Scientific Publications.
45. Al-Himdani S, Ud-Din S, Gilmore S, et al. Striae distensae: A comprehensive review and evidence-based evaluation of prophylaxis and treatment. *Br J Dermatol.* 2014;170(3):527–547.
46. Thomas RGR, Liston WA. Clinical associations of striae gravidarum. *J Obstet Gynaecol.* 2004;24(3):270–271.
47. Lerdpienpitayakul R, Manusirivithaya S, Wiriyasirivaj B, et al. Prevalence and risk factors of Striae Gravidarum in Primiparae. *Thai J Obstet Gynaecol.* 2009;17:70–79.
48. Kasielska-Trojan A, Sobczak M, Antoszewski B. Risk factors of striae gravidarum. *Int J Cosmet Sci.* 2015;37(2):236–240.
49. Durmazlar SPK, Eskioglu F. Striae gravidarum: Associated factors in primiparae. *J Turk Acad Dermatol.* 2009;3(4):93401a.
50. Narin R, Nazik H, Narin MA, et al. Can different geographic conditions affect the formation of striae gravidarum? A multicentric study. *J Obstet Gynaecol Res.* 2015;41(9):1377–1383.
51. Findik RB, Hascelik NK, Akin KO, et al. Striae gravidarum, vitamin C and other related factors. *Int J Vitam Nutr Res.* 2011;81:43–48.
52. Brennan M, Young G, Devane D. Topical preparations for preventing stretch marks in pregnancy. *Cochrane Database Syst Rev.* 2012;11:CD000066.
53. Brennan M, Clarke M, Devane D. The use of anti stretch marks products by women in pregnancy: A descriptive, cross-sectional survey. *BMC Pregnancy Childbirth.* 2016;16:276.

54. Summers B, Lategan M. The effect of a topically-applied cosmetic oil formulation on striae distensae. *S Afr Fam Pract*. 2009;51(4):332–336.
55. Osman H, Usta IM, Rubeiz N, et al. Cocoa butter lotion for prevention of striae gravidarum: A double-blind, randomised and placebo-controlled trial. *Br J Obstet Gynaecol*. 2008;115(9):1138–1142.
56. Madlon-Kay DJ. Striae gravidarum. Folklore and fact. *Arch Fam Med*. 1993;2(5):507–511.
57. Yamaguchi K, Suganuma N, Ohashi K. Prevention of striae gravidarum and quality of life among pregnant Japanese women. *Midwifery*. 2014;30(6):595–599.
58. Muallem MM, Rubeiz NG. Physiological and biological skin changes in pregnancy. *Clin Dermatol*. 2006;24:80–83.
59. Brinkhaus B, Lindner M, Schuppan D, et al. Chemical, pharmacological and clinical profile of the East Asian medical plant Centella asiatica. *Phytomedicine*. 2000;7:427–448.
60. Young GL, Jewell D. Creams for preventing stretch marks in pregnancy. *Cochrane Data-base Syst Rev*. 2000;CD000066.
61. García Hernández JÁ, Madera González D, Padilla Castillo M, et al. Use of a specific anti-stretch mark cream for preventing or reducing the severity of striae gravidarum. Randomized, double-blind, controlled trial. *Int J Cosmet Sci*. 2013;35:233–237.
62. Mallol J, Belda MA, Costa D, et al. Prophylaxis of Striae gravidarum with a topical formulation. A double-blind trial. *Int J Cosmet Sci*. 1991;13:51–57.
63. de Buman M, Walther M, de Weck R. Effectiveness of alphastria cream in the prevention of pregnancy stretch marks (striae distensae). Results of a double-blind study. *Gynakol Rundsch*. 1987;27:79–84.
64. Wierrani F, Kozak W, Schramm W, et al. Attempt of preventive treatment of striae gravidarum using preventive massage ointment administration. *Wien Klin Wochenschr*. 1992;104:42–44.
65. Elsaie ML, Baumann LS, Elsaaiee LT. Striae distensae (stretch marks) and different modalities of therapy: An update. *Dermatol Surg*. 2009;35:563–573.
66. Taşhan S, Kafkaslı A. The effect of bitter almond oil and massaging on striae gravidarum in primiparous women. *J Clin Nursing*. 2012;21:1570–1576.
67. Ernst E. Herbal medicinal products during pregnancy: Are they safe? *BJOG*. 2002;109:227–235.
68. Levin WM. Striae gravidarum: Folklore and fact. *Arch Fam Med*. 1995;4:98.
69. Elson ML Treatment of striae distensae with topical tretinoin. *J Dermatol Surg Oncol*. 1990;16:267–270.
70. Rangel O, Arias I, Garcia E, et al. Topical tretinoin 0.1% for pregnancy-related abdominal striae: An open-label, multicenter, prospective study. *Adv Ther*. 2001;18:181–186.
71. Ash K, Lord J, Zukowski M, et al. Comparison of topical therapy for striae alba (20% glycolic acid/0.05% tretinoin versus 20% glycolic acid/10% L-ascorbic acid). *Dermatol Surg*. 1998;24:849–856.
72. Pribanich S, Simpson FG, Held B, et al. Low-dose tretinoin does not improve striae distensae: A double-blind, placebo-controlled study. *Cutis*. 1994;54:121–124.
73. Malekzad F, Shakoei S, Ayatollahi A, et al. The safety and efficacy of the 1540nm non-ablative fractional XD probe of star lux 500 device in the treatment of striae alba: Before-after study. *J Lasers Med Sci*. 2014;5:194–198.
74. Bak H, Kim BJ, Lee WJ, et al. Treatment of striae distensae with fractional photothermolysis. *Dermatol Surg*. 2009;35:1215–1220.
75. de Angelis F, Kolesnikova L, Renato F, et al. Fractional nonablative 1540-nm laser treatment of striae distensae in Fitzpatrick skin types II to IV: Clinical and histological results. *Aesthet Surg J*. 2011;31:411–419.
76. Tretti Clementoni M, Lavagno R. A novel 1565 nm non-ablative fractional device for stretch marks: A preliminary report. *J Cosmet Laser Ther*. 2015;17:148–155.
77. Nourmohammadpour P, Ehsani AH, Hatami P, et al. Striae gravidarum treatment: Evaluating non-ablating fractional laser (NAFL) efficacy and safety. *J Cosmet Laser Ther*. 2023;12:1–5.
78. Cho SB, Lee SJ, Lee JE, et al. Treatment of striae alba using the 10,600-nm carbon dioxide fractional laser. *J Cosmet Laser Ther*. 2010;12:118–119.
79. Lee SE, Kim JH, Lee SJ, et al. Treatment of striae distensae using an ablative 10,600-nm carbon dioxide fractional laser: A retrospective review of 27 participants. *Dermatol Surg*. 2010;36:1683–1690.
80. McDaniel DH, Ash K, Zukowski M. Treatment of stretch marks with the 585-nm flashlamp-pumped pulsed dye laser. *Dermatol Surg*. 1996;22:332–337.
81. Aldahan AS, Shah VV, Mlacker S, et al. Laser and light treatments for striae distensae: A comprehensive review of the literature. *Am J Clin Dermatol*. 2016;17:239–256.
82. Goldberg DJ, Sarradet D, Hussain M. 308-nm Excimer laser treatment of mature hypopigmented striae. *Dermatol Surg*. 2003;29:596–598. discussion 598–599.
83. Longo L, Postiglione MG, Marangoni O, et al Two-year follow-up results of copper bromide laser treatment of striae. *J Clin Laser Med Surg*. 2003;21:157–160.

84. Tay YK, Kwok C, Tan E. Non-ablative 1,450-nm diode laser treatment of striae distensae. *Lasers Surg Med*. 2006;38:196–199.

85. Goldman A, Rossato F, Prati C. Stretch marks: Treatment using the 1,064-nm Nd:YAG laser. *Dermatol Surg*. 2008;34:686–691. discussion 691–692.

86. Al-Dhalimi MA, Abo Nasyria AA. A comparative study of the effectiveness of intense pulsed light wavelengths (650 nm vs 590 nm) in the treatment of striae distensae. *J Cosmet Laser Ther*. 2013;15:120–125.

87. Sadick NS, Magro C, Hoenig A. Prospective clinical and histological study to evaluate the efficacy and safety of a targeted high-intensity narrow band UVB/UVA1 therapy for striae alba. *J Cosmet Laser Ther*. 2007;9:79–83.

88. Trelles MA, Levy JL, Ghersetich I. Effects achieved on stretch marks by a nonfractional broadband infrared light system treatment. *Aesthetic Plast Surg*. 2008;32:523–530.

89. Wang Y, Song Y. Efficacy of combined treatment with intense pulsed light and erbium fractional laser in striae gravidarum. *Clin Cosmet Investig Dermatol*. 2022;15:2817–2824.

90. Abdel-Latif AM, Elbendary A. Treatment of striae distensae with microdermabrasion: A clinical and molecular study. *J Egypt Wom Dermatol Soc*. 2008;5:24–30.

91. Nassar A, Ghomey S, El Gohary Y, et al. Treatment of striae distensae with needling therapy versus microdermabrasion with sonophoresis. *J Cosmet Laser Ther*. 2016;18:330–334.

92. Lokhande AJ, Mysore V. Striae distensae treatment review and update. *Indian Dermatol Online J*. 2019;10(4):380–395.

93. Montesi G, Calvieri S, Balzani A, et al. Bipolar radiofrequency in the treatment of dermatologic imperfections: Clinicopathological and immunohistochemical aspects. *J Drugs Dermatol*. 2007;6:890–896.

94. Manuskiatti W, Boonthaweeyuwat E, Varothai S. Treatment of striae distensae with a TriPollar radiofrequency device: A pilot study. *J Dermatolog Treat*. 2009;20:359–364.

95. Tunzi M, Gray GR. Common skin conditions during pregnancy. *Am Fam Physician*. 2007;75:211–218.

13 Keloids during Pregnancy

Anuradha Kakkanatt Babu and Anncilla Jose

13.1 INTRODUCTION

Cutaneous wound healing is a complex process which follows an injury that helps to restore the integrity of skin. Keloids and hypertrophic scars result from excess formation of fibrous tissue during wound healing. Keloids extend beyond the margins of the original wound, whereas hypertrophic scars are confined to it.

The term keloid is derived from the Greek word 'chele', meaning crab, since the lateral outgrowth of fibrous tissue onto the normal skin resembles claw of a crab, and 'oid', meaning 'like' (Figure 13.1).[1]

Keloids occur spontaneously or at sites of trauma. They usually occur at sites of acne, folliculitis, burns, varicella, vaccination sites, or surgical wounds. Spontaneous formation of keloids in the absence of any injury is rare. During pregnancy, hormonal changes can influence pre-existing scars, and also termination of pregnancy can result in episiotomy or C-section scars.

13.2 EPIDEMIOLOGY

Keloids can occur at any age, more commonly during the first and second decades of life. Genetic and environmental factors play a role in the development of keloids.[2] Some individuals are predisposed to develop keloids. Both men and women are equally susceptible to the formation of keloids. A slightly higher incidence of keloids is reported in females because skin piercings (ear) are done more by them, and they also seek more treatment due to cosmetic disfigurement compared to males.

The incidence of keloids is variable with racial differences. It is reported more in people with skin of colour than whites, more in Blacks and Asians compared to Caucasians, as they are genetically predisposed to produce more collagen during wound healing.[3,4] The tendency to develop keloids runs in families.[5] Keloids with a familial tendency tend to present early and occurs at multiple sites with greater severity.

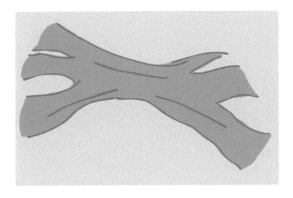

FIGURE 13.1 Keloid resembling claw of a crab.

DOI: 10.1201/9781003449690-13

13.3 RISK FACTORS FOR KELOIDS

Local mechanical stimulus contributes to the development and progression of keloids. Keloid-prone areas include the anterior aspect of chest, shoulders, and other sites with skin tension or wounds closed under tension. Skin tension and friction on the areas can influence the shape of keloids as well, for example, a butterfly-shaped keloid on the front of the chest (Figure 13.2A) and a dumbbell-shaped keloid on the scapular area (Figure 13.2B).[6]

During pregnancy and puberty, due to the interplay of hormonal factors in wound healing, appearance, reoccurrence, or increase in size of keloids are reported.[7]

Patients with Rubinstein–Taybi syndrome, Ehlers–Danlos syndrome, Lowe syndrome, and the novel X-linked syndrome are found to have increased risk of developing keloids.[8]

13.4 PATHOPHYSIOLOGY

A cutaneous wound results from any kind of trauma that disrupts the anatomical integrity of skin. Wounds limited to the epidermis of the skin heal without any scar formation.

Scars result from any injury to the deep dermis as a result of the complex wound healing process that includes the phases of inflammation, proliferation, and remodelling (Figure 13.3).[9] The inflammatory phase involves inflammation as well as haemostasis. Haemostasis is attained by vasoconstriction and formation of a fibrin clot. Fibrin clots also act as a scaffolding for platelets and inflammatory cells. Vasodilatation that follows the immediate vasoconstrictive response results in erythema and oedema at the wound site.

During the phase of inflammation, cells (neutrophils and macrophages) that produce proinflammatory growth factors and cytokines are recruited. This inflammatory cascade clears the injured tissue and invading microorganisms.[10]

The phase of proliferation is characterised by the formation of granulation tissue and restoration of the vascular network. Fibroblasts and endothelial cells are the major cells that contribute to this

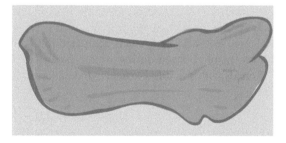

FIGURE 13.2A   Butterfly-shaped keloid commonly seen on anterior aspect of chest.

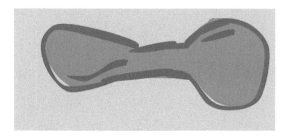

FIGURE 13.2B   Dumbbell-shaped keloid commonly seen on scapular area.

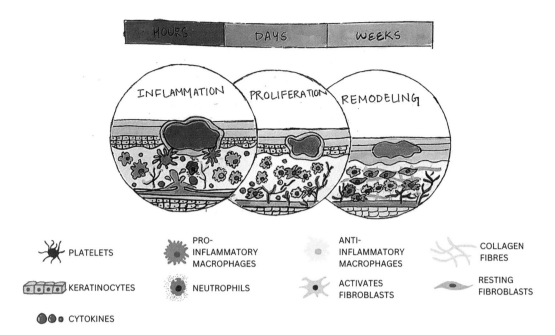

FIGURE 13.3 Phases of inflammation and the major cellular and extracellular components involved.

proliferative phase. As the cells proliferate, a hypoxic stimulus that evokes angiogenic response is produced. Cytokines, interleukins, and growth factors (TGF-beta, VEGF, PDGF) have a major role in this phase. Meanwhile epithelisation starts from the edge of the wound under the influence of inflammatory cytokines and growth factors.

The remodelling phase follows the proliferative phase. Any imbalance between synthesis and degradation of tissues can result in abnormal scar formation. During remodelling, formation of granulation tissue stops and maturation of the scar begins. Type I collagen replaces type III and thus strengthens the scar. Matrix metallo proteinases (MMPs) have a major role in the remodelling phase. The cells remaining in the scar undergo apoptosis, and angiogenic responses diminish, resulting in the contraction of the scar.

Any imbalance or abnormality in wound healing, like excess collagen formation or turnover or excess accumulation of extracellular matrix, leads to the formation of keloids and hypertrophic scars.

The aetiopathogenesis of keloids is poorly understood; hence several hypotheses have been put forward to explain the formation of keloids. Hypotheses in keloid formation:[11]

1. Sebum autoimmune hypothesis
2. Hypoxia hypothesis
3. Tension hypothesis
4. Stiffness gap hypothesis
5. Hormonal hypothesis

The sebum autoimmune hypothesis states that sebum that gets into the dermis through trauma acts as an antigen that triggers keloid formation. Points favouring this hypothesis are that keloids are more seen in seborrheic areas, not reported in the volar skin where sebaceous glands are absent, and seen after onset of puberty when the sebaceous glands are active.

Hypoxia in abnormal scars stimulates excess formation of collagen. Hypoxia inducible factor-1 is found more in keloids, which provide an environment for keloidal keratinocytes to become fibroblasts. Histopathological examination of keloids shows that blood vessels are narrower due to obliteration by myofibroblast and endothelial cells.[12] This also provides a hypoxic microenvironment.

Tension in wounds can result in the formation of keloids.[13] Mechanical forces are an important trigger in keloid development in predisposed individuals. Skin incisions made parallel to skin tension lines rarely result in abnormal scars.

The stiffness gap hypothesis illustrates the mechanism of the progression of keloids: ECM stiffness (the dominant ECM ingredients in keloids are collagen type I) and cell stiffness (predominant cells in keloids are dermal fibroblasts) is not well balanced in keloids, with ECM stiffness increasingly higher than cell stiffness, and such a continuously enlarged stiffness gap potentiates cellular changes towards keloid progression.[14]

The hormonal theory is supported by the facts that keloids are seen after the onset of puberty and exacerbated during pregnancy (Figure 13.4) and rarely occur after menopause. Male hormone-related sebum overproduction, acne lesions in polycystic ovarian syndrome patients, and prolonged cutaneous inflammation stimulated by androgens may also contribute to keloid pathogenesis.[15]

Abnormal production of various growth factors and cytokines like interleukin-6, -17, and TGF-β1 and -β2 and aberrant expression of its receptors are seen in keloidal fibroblasts.

During pregnancy, the placenta is a source of oestrogens, which have a definite role in the growth of keloids.[16] It has been hypothesised that Activin-A (a dimeric protein and a member of the transforming growth factor-beta superfamily) that regulates various aspects of cell growth and differentiation as well as keloid development is produced by stromal endometrial cells during pregnancy.[17]

13.5   CLINICAL FEATURES

Keloids present as firm asymptomatic or pruritic or painful nodules or swellings, more commonly on the chest, shoulders, earlobes, and upper back. Patients seek treatment mostly because of cosmetic disfigurement. Previously treated keloids are also shown to be reactivated during pregnancy.[18] Kim et al. report a case where a patient had activation of a quiescent scar at times of two pregnancies.[19] There is one report with herpes zoster during pregnancy resulting in keloids with no prior keloidal tendency.[17] The differences between keloid and hypertrophic scars are illustrated in Table 13.1.

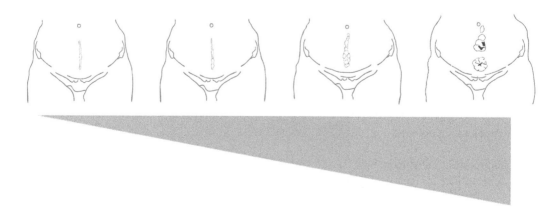

FIGURE 13.4   Change in size of keloid during pregnancy with expansion of abdomen.

TABLE 13.1

Differences between Hypertrophic Scars and Keloids

	Keloids	Hypertrophic Scars
Clinical Features		
Frequency of occurrence	Rare	Common
Prior history of trauma or any cutaneous inflammation	Not always	Always present
Time of onset	May appear spontaneously May not appear for months after surgery or trauma	Occur soon after surgery or trauma
Confined to area of original tissue damage	No	Yes
Common sites	Earlobes, chest, shoulders	Any sites, more across joints and flexor surfaces
Familial predisposition	Yes	No
Skin types	More in pigmented skin	Any
Regression	No	Frequent
Histopathology		
Keloidal collagen	Present	Absent
Arrangement of collagen	Haphazard or whorled	Parallel
Ratio of collagen I/III ratio	Highest	Higher compared to normal tissue
Myofibroblasts and alpha smooth muscle actin	+	++
Response to Treatment		
Recurrence after surgical excision	Yes	Less chance

13.6 HISTOPATHOLOGY OF KELOIDS AND HYPERTROPHIC SCARS

Well-formed keloidal collagen is the histologic hallmark of keloids. Histopathologically, a keloid is characterised by the presence of whorls and nodules of thick, hyalinised collagen bundles (keloidal collagen) with a tongue-like advancing edge and a prominent fascia-like band with mucinous ground substance. But little or no keloidal collagen is found in hypertrophic scars.[20] On the other hand, the presence of α-SMA-positive myofibroblasts and dermal nodules is more in favour of hypertrophic scars.[21]

13.7 KELOIDS AND C-SECTION SCARS

Women with keloids on the caesarean scar have increased adhesions between the uterus and the bladder and between the uterus and the abdominal wall.[22] The chances for developing keloids can be reduced to some extent by careful surgical techniques. Wound closure with absorbable subcuticular sutures provides better cosmetic results than surgical staples.[23]

Transverse incisions on skin are better compared to vertical, as there is a decreased chance of the development of hypertrophic scars, keloids, and incisional hernia and hence improved cosmetic results (Figure 13.5A and 13.5B).[24] The risk of wound disruption and secondary bacterial infections, which are risk factors for keloids, are also lower for transverse incisions.

Measures for preventing secondary infections at the surgical site should be taken, as it is a risk factor for keloids. Silicone gel sheets kept on wound sites can prevent occurrence of keloids and hypertrophic scars. Removal of abnormal scars of previous C-sections at the time of a C-section is found to be promising.[25] Emergency C-sections are also reported to be a risk factor for the recurrence of keloids and hypertrophic scars.

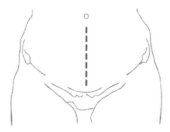

FIGURE 13.5A   Vertical incision on skin for C-section.

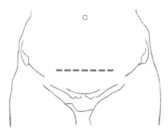

FIGURE 13.5B   Transverse incision on skin for C-section.

13.8   TREATMENT OPTIONS

There is no single treatment modality that gives a complete cure for keloids. A history of a tendency towards keloids should be elicited, and preventive measures can be taken. Surgical excision can remove the existing abnormal scar, but there is a 45–100% chance of recurrence.[26] Conservative management can be done during pregnancy, like pressure therapy, silicone sheeting, and scar massage. Keloids with pruritus can be treated with topical steroids. Intralesional steroids are better avoided, but a single injection may be given in cases of severe pruritus or to reduce size. Limited studies on intralesional injections during pregnancy have shown no adverse effects on mother or baby.[27,28] Cryotherapy can be safely administered during pregnancy.

Patients with keloids after a first C-section can be treated during a second delivery C-section with complete excision.[29]

Active interventions can be undertaken once pregnancy is terminated. Intralesional steroid (triamcinolone acetonide) injections provide a response of 50–100%. Cryotherapy can be used as monotherapy and in combination with intralesional steroid therapy. Carbon dioxide lasers can also be used in the management of keloids, alone or in combination with steroids (topical or intralesional).[30] Pulsed dye lasers give promising results for young immature scars, especially in reducing erythema. Apart from steroids, 5-flurouracil, bleomycin, and Interferon-α2b are given as intralesional injections.[31] Botulinum toxin is used to reduce skin tension around wounds and helps to decrease the chance of keloid formation.

REFERENCES

1. Alibert JLM. Quelques recherches sur la cheloide. *Mem Soc Med d'Emul.* 1817;744.
2. Betarbet U, Blalock TW. Keloids: A review of etiology, prevention, and treatment. *J Clin Aesthetic Dermatol.* 2020;13(2):33–43.
3. Louw L. Keloids in rural black South Africans. Part 1: General overview and essential fatty acid hypotheses for keloid formation and prevention. *Prostaglandins Leukot Essent Fatty Acids.* 2000;63(5):237–245.
4. Fujiwara M, Muragaki Y, Ooshima A. Keloid-derived fibroblasts show increased secretion of factors involved in collagen turnover and depend on matrix metalloproteinase for migration. *Br J Dermatol.* 2005;153(2):295–300.

5. Santos-Cortez RLP, Hu Y, Sun F, et al. Identification of ASAH1 as a susceptibility gene for familial keloids. *Eur J Hum Genet EJHG*. 2017;25(10):1155–1161.
6. Ogawa R, Okai K, Tokumura F, et al. The relationship between skin stretching/contraction and pathologic scarring: The important role of mechanical forces in keloid generation. *Wound Repair Regen Off Publ Wound Heal Soc Eur Tissue Repair Soc*. 2012;20(2):149–157.
7. Ibrahim NE, Shaharan S, Dheansa B. Adverse effects of pregnancy on keloids and hypertrophic scars. *Cureus*. 2020;12(12):e12154.
8. Huang C, Wu Z, Du Y, Ogawa R. The epidemiology of keloids. In: Téot L, Mustoe TA, Middelkoop E, Gauglitz GG, editors. *Textbook on Scar Management: State of the Art Management and Emerging Technologies*. Cham: Springer International Publishing; 2020: 29–35.
9. *Wound Healing—StatPearls—NCBI Bookshelf* [Internet]. [cited 2023 Jun 27]. Available from: www.ncbi.nlm.nih.gov/books/NBK535406/
10. Ulrich MMW. Fetal wound healing. In: *Textbook on Scar Management: State of the Art Management and Emerging Technologies*. Internet: Springer; 2020.
11. Venkataram M. *ACS (I) Textbook of Cutaneous & Aesthetic Surgery*, 2nd ed. New Delhi: Jaypee Brothers; 2017.
12. Steinbrech DS, Mehrara BJ, Chau D, et al. Hypoxia upregulates VEGF production in keloid fibroblasts. *Ann Plast Surg*. 1999;42(5):514–519.
13. Ogawa R. Keloid and hypertrophic scarring may result from a mechanoreceptor or mechanosensitive nociceptor disorder. *Med Hypotheses*. 2008;71(4):493–500.
14. Huang C, Liu L, You Z, et al. Keloid progression: A stiffness gap hypothesis. *Int Wound J*. 2016;14(5): 764–771.
15. Yang Y, Chen Z, Wu X, et al. Androgen-related disorders and hormone therapy for patients with keloids. *Chin J Plast Reconstr Surg*. 2022;4(1):44–48.
16. Moustafa MF, Abdel-Fattah MA, Abdel-Fattah DC. Presumptive evidence of the effect of pregnancy estrogens on keloid growth. Case report. *Plast Reconstr Surg*. 1975;56(4):450–453.
17. Verma SB, Wollina U. Herpes zoster in pregnancy leading to keloids and post herpetic neuralgia: A double whammy? *Indian Dermatol Online J*. 2013;4(2):158–159.
18. Park TH, Chang CH. Keloid recurrence in pregnancy. *Aesthetic Plast Surg*. 2012;36(5):1271–1272.
19. Kim HD, Hwang SM, Lim KR, et al. Recurrent auricular keloids during pregnancy. *Arch Plast Surg*. 2013;40(1):70–72.
20. Lee JYY, Yang CC, Chao SC, Wong TW. Histopathological differential diagnosis of keloid and hypertrophic scar. *Am J Dermatopathol*. 2004;26(5):379–384.
21. Limandjaja GC, Niessen FB, Scheper RJ, Gibbs S. Hypertrophic scars and keloids: Overview of the evidence and practical guide for differentiating between these abnormal scars. *Exp Dermatol*. 2021;30(1):146–161.
22. Tulandi T, Al-Sannan B, Akbar G, et al. Prospective study of intraabdominal adhesions among women of different races with or without keloids. *Am J Obstet Gynecol*. 2011;204(2):132.e1–132.e4.
23. Alderdice F, McKenna D, Dornan J. Techniques and materials for skin closure in caesarean section. *Cochrane Database Syst Rev*. 2003;2:CD003577.
24. Maaløe N, Aabakke AJM, Secher NJ. Midline versus transverse incision for cesarean delivery in low-income countries. *Int J Gynecol Obstet*. 2014;125(1):1–2
25. Bağlı İ, Ogawa R, Bakır S, et al. Predictors of the recurrence of surgically removed previous caesarean skin scars at caesarean section: A retrospective cohort study. *Scars Burns Heal*. 2021;7:20595131211023388.
26. Mustoe TA, Cooter RD, Gold MH, et al. International clinical recommendations on scar management. *Plast Reconstr Surg*. 2002;110(2):560–571.
27. Toktas O, Toprak N. Treatment results of intralesional steroid injection and topical steroid administration in pregnant women with idiopathic granulomatous mastitis. *Eur J Breast Health*. 2021;17(3):283–287.
28. Filippini C, Saran S, Chari B. Musculoskeletal steroid injections in pregnancy: A review. *Skeletal Radiol*. 2023;52(8):1465–1473.
29. Kim J, Lee SH. Therapeutic results and safety of postoperative radiotherapy for keloid after repeated Cesarean section in immediate postpartum period. *Radiat Oncol J*. 2012;30(2):49–52.
30. Tawaranurak N, Pliensiri P, Tawaranurak K. Combination of fractional carbon dioxide laser and topical triamcinolone vs intralesional triamcinolone for keloid treatment: A randomised clinical trial. *Int Wound J*. 2022;19(7):1729–1735.
31. Gauglitz GG. Management of keloids and hypertrophic scars: Current and emerging options. *Clin Cosmet Investig Dermatol*. 2013;6:103–114.

14 Safety of Dermatological Drugs in Pregnancy and in Lactation

Sara D Ragi, Emily Garelick, Mark W Hocevar,
Julia Cheng and Jenny E Murase

14.1 INTRODUCTION

Pharmacologic therapies play an essential role in human health, but it is important that the unique circumstances of each individual patient be considered when prescribing medications. Studies have shown that about 59% of pregnant women are prescribed a drug or recommended to use an over-the-counter supplement (1). However, pregnancy may affect the pharmacokinetics of certain medications, and drugs that reach the fetus have the potential to cause teratogenic effects (1). It can be challenging to determine the safety of drug use during pregnancy, as randomised-controlled studies would risk harm to the fetus. Most testing is done on animals, but the results do not always translate to humans.

The FDA has pregnancy category ratings based on animal and human studies that provide recommendations on the safety of various dermatologic medications during pregnancy. The categories are A, B, C, D, and X. Category A includes drugs for which controlled studies show no increased risk of fetal abnormalities (1). Category B includes drugs that have no evidence of risk in humans for which no adequate human studies have been performed and for which animal studies are negative. Category C includes drugs where risk cannot be ruled out because human studies are lacking, and animal studies are either positive for fetal risks or lacking as well, although the benefits may outweigh the risks of use. Category D includes drugs with evidence of adverse effects based on adverse reaction data; however, the benefits may outweigh the risks of use if no safer alternatives are available. Category X drugs are contraindicated in pregnancy, with the risks of medication clearly outweighing the benefits due to the evidence of risk based on human or animal studies and/or adverse reaction data. Category N drugs were not classified (1). In 2015, the FDA discontinued use of these pregnancy categories and implemented the Pregnancy and Lactation Label Ruling (PLLR) as a replacement, providing more detailed information regarding safety considerations and increasing the complexity of safety medication counselling in pregnancy (2). In this review, we provide the previous pregnancy category references for informational purposes.

It is important for dermatologists to explain both the benefits of treatment and the risk of potential effects on the developing fetus when counselling patients regarding the safety of medications in pregnancy and lactation (3). Similar considerations arise regarding drug safety during lactation and breastfeeding. The effect that a drug has during pregnancy may not always reflect its effects on nursing infants. Here, we provide a guide for physicians and other healthcare providers on the use and safety of various dermatologic drugs during pregnancy and lactation.

14.2 TOPICAL THERAPIES FOR ACNE AND HAIR LOSS

Topical formulations of azelaic acid, benzoyl peroxide, salicylic acid, adapalene, tretinoin, and tazarotene are commonly used in the treatment of acne vulgaris.

DOI: 10.1201/9781003449690-14

14.2.1 AZELAIC ACID

Azelaic acid [former Pregnancy Category B] does not have any well-controlled studies showing the outcome of this medication in women who are pregnant and lacks adverse effects on fertility in animals. Studies demonstrated embryotoxicity in rats given 2500 mg/kg/day, rabbits given 150 mg/kg/day, and monkeys given 500 mg/kg/day. These doses were also found to be toxic maternally, and they ranged from 19 to 162 times the recommended human dose based on body surface area. These studies showed that there were no teratogenic effects in any of these animals, but there were slight postnatal developmental disturbances. This medication has not been tested dermally in animals or humans for effects on pregnant patients and their offspring, but topical application only results in only 4% systemic absorption (4).

When using equilibrium dialysis to test human milk in lactating mothers, it was found that azelaic acid can be passed into maternal milk. Use on limited body surface areas such as the face would be unlikely to result in any significant systemic absorption or maternal milk levels (4). It can be concluded that azelaic acid can be used in pregnant and lactating patients.

14.2.2 BENZOYL PEROXIDE

Benzoyl peroxide [former Pregnancy Category C] is about 5% absorbed systemically. It has a fast renal clearance, which decreases the risk of congenital malformations, making it safe during pregnancy (5). Benzoyl peroxide is quickly converted to benzoic acid, which is a food derivative, in the skin. Given the low level of systemic absorption when applied to limited body surface areas, it is considered safe to use while breastfeeding (6). If directly applied to the nipple, benzoyl peroxide should be washed before breastfeeding (7).

14.2.3 SALICYLIC ACID

Salicylic acid [former Pregnancy Category C] has limited testing in pregnant women. Animal studies have found malformations in rat embryos from systemic salicylic acid use during pregnancy. There is limited absorption when applied to small body surface areas, and it is thought to be safe in pregnancy (5). It is unlikely that salicylic acid would be absorbed into breast milk, so it is safe to use for lactating mothers (8).

14.2.4 ADAPALENE

Adapalene [former Pregnancy Category C] became an over-the-counter (OTC) medication in the United States in 2016. During the switch of adapalene to OTC, the safety of adapalene during pregnancy was studied. Adapalene has a large and reassuring margin of safety (MOS). Studies demonstrate that there is no teratogenic risk. Therefore, adapalene 0.1% gel is a safe and effective medication for the treatment of acne, as there is no prescription needed and there is no risk of harm to the fetus (9).

There is minimal systemic absorption when used on small body surface areas, and it is unlikely to pass into women's breast milk, so it is considered safe during lactation (10).

14.2.5 TRETINOIN

Tretinoin [former Pregnancy Category C] at commonly used strengths and body surface area results in minimal systemic absorption. There have been a few cases reported of congenital malformations after use of topical tretinoin, but there is no definitive pattern of teratogenicity with specific association. Reports have shown that topical tretinoin used in Wistar rats at doses that are greater than ten times the maximum recommended dose can cause teratogenic effects. Topical tretinoin is fetotoxic in rabbits at ten times the maximum recommended dose. Oral tretinoin has been reported as teratogenic in animal studies, including growth retardation and lower neonatal survival in doses that are 19 times the maximum recommended dose. It has specifically been noted as fetotoxic at 24 times the maximum recommended dose (11). Tretinoin is considered a viable option in pregnancy if benefits outweigh the risks.

It is unlikely that tretinoin is excreted in human milk when applied to limited body surface area, so it is considered safe in lactation (11).

14.2.6 TAZAROTENE

Tazarotene [former Pregnancy Category X] is used for acne and psoriasis. This drug is known to be teratogenic, but the specific amount of exposure that causes this effect is unknown (12). Therefore, this drug is contraindicated in pregnant patients.

Animal studies with lactating rats showed topical tazarotene was passed to the mother's milk after only a single use. This has not been tested on humans, but it is not recommended that patients use this drug while nursing if the medication is used on large body surface areas resulting in potential systemic absorption (12).

14.2.7 MINOXIDIL

Minoxidil [former Pregnancy Category C] is used for alopecia both topically and orally (11). Although there is one case report in the literature of a child born to a mother with congenital defects who was using topical minoxidil throughout pregnancy, it is unclear if this is directly related to the use of topical minoxidil as a single case report given the low systemic absorption when using topical minoxidil on a limited body surface area (13). However, it is generally recommended to avoid all cosmetic topical therapy in pregnancy, including topical minoxidil.

It is expected that topical minoxidil should not cause an issue when breast-feeding. however, it is recommended that maternal use be avoided when breastfeeding and in preterm or neonatal infants. One study reported an infant developing facial hypertrichosis while the nursing mother was using 5% minoxidil topically twice daily. Therefore, caution should be taken with topical use of this drug while nursing, but it is not contraindicated (14, 15).

14.3 SYSTEMIC MEDICATIONS FOR ACNE AND HAIR LOSS

Spironolactone and isotretinoin are oral acne medications commonly used by patients with severe acne.

14.3.1 SPIRONOLACTONE

Spironolactone [former Pregnancy Category C] can potentially affect sex differentiation during embryogenesis. Animal studies with rats showed that pregnant rats with spironolactone exposure had feminisation of their male fetuses. It has also been reported that both the mother and offspring can have heart failure, hypertension, and cirrhosis with use of the drug during pregnancy (16). The potential adverse fetal effects are a risk during pregnancy, so it is recommended that this drug be avoided, particularly in the first trimester of pregnancy.

There is no specific data reporting whether spironolactone has any effect on milk production, and no adverse effects have been reported with breastfeeding (16). Spironolactone is thought to be compatible with breastfeeding.

14.3.2 ISOTRETINOIN

Isotretinoin [former Pregnancy Category X] is an oral medication that is highly contraindicated during pregnancy. It is teratogenic, causing severe birth defects, miscarriages, premature births, and fetal deaths. This drug should never be taken while pregnant, and extreme caution must be taken to prevent pregnancy while in use. Patients are not allowed to breastfeed while taking isotretinoin and must wait one month after stopping isotretinoin to begin breastfeeding (17, 18).

Oral formulas of finasteride and minoxidil are used by patients suffering from hair loss.

14.3.3 FINASTERIDE (ORAL)

Finasteride [former Pregnancy Category X] cannot be used during pregnancy. It is an inhibitor of Type II 5-alpha-reductase inhibitor, blocking the conversion of testosterone to 5-alpha-dihydrotestosterone (DHT). Animal studies showed that with the lack of DHT from finasteride, male rat offspring had abnormal development of external genitalia. However, this is highly unlikely to occur due to the extremely low levels of finasteride in semen and the very low likelihood that these low levels would enter the maternal blood circulation through exposure in vaginal intercourse. It is recommended to avoid finasteride during nursing, as it is not known whether it can transfer to human milk and cause developmental effects in offspring (19).

14.3.4 MINOXIDIL (ORAL)

Minoxidil [former Pregnancy Category C] is not recommended in pregnancy. Oral administration has been shown to increase fetal absorption in rabbits; however, this was at five times the recommended dose. Even though animal studies did not show any teratogenic effects even with maternally toxic doses, studies with patients using oral minoxidil resulted in minoxidil-induced fetal toxicity or fetal minoxidil syndrome. This results in newborns with congenital heart defects, neurodevelopmental abnormalities, limb malformations, and more (14).

Oral minoxidil has been shown to transfer to breast milk, where milk levels paralleled serum levels. One study showed no abnormal side effects in infants with mothers breastfeeding while orally taking this drug, but there are limited data. Generally, it is best to advise avoidance of cosmetic therapy in pregnancy and lactation (15).

14.4 ANAESTHETICS

14.4.1 LIDOCAINE AND EPINEPHRINE

Lidocaine [former Pregnancy Category B] is safe to use during pregnancy (21). Breastfeeding while using lidocaine is not known to cause any problems for a nursing baby. Lidocaine can transfer into breast milk, but it is not absorbed well by the feeding infant (20). While lidocaine is used as an anaesthetic in dermatologic procedures, it is a vasodilator, which means that there can be substantial bleeding if used on its own. It is commonly combined with epinephrine, which is a vasoconstrictor, to help reduce the amount of bleeding (21, 22). Given that epinephrine is used in very small amounts to cause localised vasoconstriction for medical procedures, and given that catecholamines are inactivated at the level of the placenta, it is recommended that patients who are pregnant or breastfeeding only use lidocaine with epinephrine for small surgical procedures in dermatology (23, 24).

14.5 TOPICAL ANTIBIOTICS

Topical antibiotics, including bacitracin and mupirocin, are commonly used in patients who have skin injuries or need post-operative treatment to a wound.

14.5.1 BACITRACIN

The topical antibiotic bacitracin [former Pregnancy Category C] is safe to use during pregnancy. There is no evidence showing that there could be increased risk of harm to fetal development. This medication is also safe to use while breastfeeding because it has minimal absorption into the skin and therefore minimal risk to the nursing baby (25).

14.5.2 MUPIROCIN

The topical antibiotic mupirocin [former Pregnancy Category B] is safe to use during pregnancy and lactation. There are no human studies, but animal studies in rats and rabbits with mupirocin that was subcutaneously administered at 43 times the highest recommended human dose showed no harm to the fetus (26, 27).

14.6 SYSTEMIC ANTIBIOTICS

Systemic antibiotics are commonly prescribed by dermatologists in patients suffering from bacterial infections affecting the skin. This includes cephalosporins, clindamycin, metronidazole, penicillin, trimethoprim-sulfamethoxazole, dapsone, ciprofloxacin, and doxycycline.

14.6.1 CEPHALOSPORINS

Cephalosporins are known to be safe to use during pregnancy. A case study of the teratogenic potential of cephalosporin use during pregnancy concluded that there are no detectable teratogenic risks (28). Studies of lactation have shown that cephalosporins can be present in low levels in milk if used while nursing, but adverse effects in infants are rare. Some results have shown that infants can have some rare gastrointestinal upset, but cephalosporins may not be the direct cause (29).

14.6.2 CLINDAMYCIN

Clindamycin [former Pregnancy Category B] is an antibiotic that can be used both topically and orally and has not resulted in congenital abnormalities with systemic use during pregnancy. Clindamycin has been reported to transfer to breast milk, so it should be used to treat a complicated skin infection only when medically indicated (30).

14.6.3 METRONIDAZOLE

Studies of metronidazole [former Pregnancy Category C] have not demonstrated increased risk of preterm delivery, congenital anomalies, or other adverse effects on the fetus in more than 5000 women who have used this drug during pregnancy. One study reported an increased risk of cleft lip, but there was no confirmation of these findings (31).

This drug is transferred to human milk proportional to maternal serum levels. Animal studies with mice and rats showed a potential risk for tumorigenicity, so there is a risk to nursing while taking this medication. A physician and mother must consider how important the use of this drug is and whether it should be discontinued. There is also the option to pump and discard milk until 24 hours after use of metronidazole (31).

14.6.4 PENICILLIN

Penicillin V can be taken orally, and penicillin G can be administered by injection. Penicillins [former Pregnancy Category B] are safe to use during pregnancy. Animal studies have not shown any adverse effects on the fetus, and none have been reported in humans (32). Of note, it has been shown that a higher dose might be necessary during pregnancy due to higher rates of elimination of penicillin in pregnant patients (33). It has also been reported that penicillins are transferred to human milk, so nursing mothers should use only when medically indicated (32).

14.6.5   TRIMETHOPRIM-SULFAMETHOXAZOLE

Trimethoprim-sulfamethoxazole [former Pregnancy Category C] has been shown to produce teratogenic effects in rat studies when taken orally. This drug affects folic acid metabolism, which can harm fetal development and has resulted in cleft palates in offspring without maternal folic acid supplementation. Animal studies with rabbits reported an increase in the loss of the fetus while taking this drug. Regarding third trimester risk, this drug does pass through the placenta, and it also is excreted in milk, predisposing to an increase in bilirubin levels and a predisposition for kernicterus in newborns and neonates, so it should be used only when medically indicated in the third trimester or when nursing a baby during the first 3 months of life (34).

14.6.6   DAPSONE

Dapsone [former Pregnancy Category C] must be used with caution in pregnancy because there are not enough data to determine the risk. Animal studies have demonstrated embryonical effects when administered at 250 times the recommended maximum human dose. In animal studies with administration 400 times the maximum recommended dose for humans, there was an increase in stillbirths and decreased weight (35). Dapsone is contraindicated in the third trimester due to the increased risk of hyperbilirubinemia and kernicterus in newborns.

Oral administration in lactation does transfer to breast milk, leading to a risk of haemolytic anaemia and hyperbilirubinemia in infants with glucose-6-phosphate dehydrogenase (G6PD) deficiency. Therefore, systemic administration is not recommended when nursing during the first 3 months of life (35).

14.6.7   CIPROFLOXACIN

Ciprofloxacin [former Pregnancy Category C] is not recommended for use during pregnancy unless medically indicated. Published data concluded that teratogenic effects are unlikely if taken while pregnant. Additional studies did not find any changes in birth weight, increase in prematurity, or spontaneous abortions. (36).

It is known that ciprofloxacin is excreted in milk, so it is not recommended that mothers use this drug while nursing unless clinically indicated. There has been a report of a breastfeeding newborn developing colitis who was exposed to ciprofloxacin through maternal use (36).

14.6.8   DOXYCYCLINE

Doxycycline [former Pregnancy Category D] is contraindicated during pregnancy. Doxycycline is part of the tetracycline class of drugs, and if used during the second and third trimesters of pregnancy, it can lead to discoloration of teeth. Animal studies have shown that there is potential for embryotoxicity, causing a slowing of skeletal development if this drug is taken early in the pregnancy. Tetracyclines are also excreted in human milk, but the amount that is transferred is unknown. It is recommended that the use of doxycycline be avoided in nursing mothers if taken for a period that is greater than 2 weeks. However, there is typically minimal absorption by the nursing infant because tetracyclines, like doxycycline, bind to milk calcium (37).

14.7   TOPICAL ANTIFUNGALS

Topical antifungals are commonly used to treat fungal infections of the skin. Three widely prescribed antifungal medications are clotrimazole, nystatin, and ciclopirox.

14.7.1 CLOTRIMAZOLE

Clotrimazole [former Pregnancy Category B] is considered safe for use during pregnancy. Multiple studies have shown no adverse effects or associations with congenital defects (38, 39). When applied dermally or intravaginally, there is minimal absorption; therefore, only topical is recommended (40). Animal studies have also not shown any adverse effects. Therefore, clotrimazole is the topical antifungal of choice during pregnancy (39). It is also compatible with breastfeeding and has no adverse effects on fertility in animal studies (41).

14.7.2 NYSTATIN

Nystatin [former Pregnancy Category C topically and A vaginally] has not been associated with congenital malformations (42–44). Similar to clotrimazole, in pregnant individuals, nystatin has minimal absorption when applied dermally or vaginally. It is considered safe during pregnancy and is a topical antifungal commonly used for candida infections (40). Limited safety data are available regarding its use during breastfeeding; however, due to its minimal absorption, it is considered safe to use during breastfeeding (41).

14.7.3 CICLOPIROX

Ciclopirox [former Pregnancy Class B] is absorbed 1.3% with topical application, and there are no reports of congenital abnormalities associated with its use (45). Animal studies have also not shown any teratogenic effects. It is likely safe for use during pregnancy (45). The excretion of ciclopirox into breast milk is thought to be negligible (45). Therefore, it is likely compatible with breastfeeding. Similar to the other antifungals mentioned, ciclopirox has no adverse effects on fertility in animal studies.

14.8 SYSTEMIC ANTIFUNGALS

Systemic antifungals are commonly used to treat fungal infection in all populations, including pregnant individuals.

14.8.1 TERBINAFINE

Terbinafine [former Pregnancy Class B] is a commonly used systemic antifungal medication. Studies have shown no increased risk of major malformations or spontaneous abortions associated with its topical or oral use (46). Animal studies have also indicated no teratogenicity or embryofetal toxicity. When applied topically, less than 5% of terbinafine is systemically absorbed (47). Limited use of terbinafine during pregnancy is likely safe if medically necessary (48). Treatment of onychomycosis can be postponed until after pregnancy is completed. Terbinafine is excreted in low amounts in breast milk, and it is thought to be compatible with breastfeeding (85).

14.8.2 GRISEOFULVIN

Due to potential risks, griseofulvin [former Pregnancy Category B] is an antifungal medication that warrants careful consideration during pregnancy and breastfeeding. It has been associated with reports of adverse effects, including conjoined twins and fetal abnormalities, mainly when used during the first trimester of pregnancy (49). Animal studies have demonstrated teratogenic and embryotoxic properties at higher doses, and the medication is known to cross the placenta (50). As a result, griseofulvin is contraindicated in pregnancy, and women of child-bearing potential must use effective contraception while taking the drug (51). Limited safety data are available regarding its use during breastfeeding, and due to concerns about tumorigenicity, griseofulvin is not recommended unless medically necessary (51).

14.8.3 FLUCONAZOLE

Fluconazole [former Pregnancy Category C] is a medication commonly used for yeast and fungal infections and poses specific considerations during pregnancy and breastfeeding. Although there are no well-controlled studies in pregnant women, reports have linked first-trimester exposure to congenital anomalies, including cleft palate, craniofacial and bone abnormalities, and cardiovascular defects (52). While no specific patterns have been identified, more extensive studies have reported spontaneous abortions and congenital disabilities. Animal studies have shown teratogenic and embryotoxic effects (53). As a result, fluconazole is generally contraindicated during pregnancy except when treating severe or potentially life-threatening fungal infections. Limited use in low doses and short-term treatment for vaginal candidiasis during the first trimester was not shown to increase congenital defects, but first-trimester exposure should prompt fetal ultrasound assessment between 18 and 20 weeks gestation (54). Fluconazole is excreted in breast milk and is thought to be compatible with breastfeeding (55). It is often prescribed during breastfeeding, as the dose to the infant is estimated to be lower than what would be administered directly for treatment of infection.

14.8.4 KETOCONAZOLE

Ketoconazole [former Pregnancy Category C], a medication used to treat fungal infections, requires careful consideration during pregnancy and breastfeeding due to limited data and potential risks. While no well-controlled studies have been conducted in pregnant women, there have been reports of adverse effects associated with first-trimester exposure to ketoconazole, including cardiovascular, skeletal, craniofacial, and neural defects in infants (56). However, a large study did not observe significant congenital disabilities with oral ketoconazole use in the first trimester (57). Animal studies have shown teratogenic and embryotoxic effects, such as syndactyly and oligodactyly, at high doses (58). As a result, it is generally advised to avoid ketoconazole during pregnancy, although limited use after the first trimester at low doses may be considered safe. Fetal ultrasound assessment at 18–20 weeks gestation is recommended for women exposed to ketoconazole in the first trimester (59). Ketoconazole is excreted in breast milk, but it is likely compatible with breastfeeding, as no adverse effects have been reported (59).

14.8.5 ITRACONAZOLE

Itraconazole [former Pregnancy Category B], a medication used to treat fungal infections, warrants careful consideration during pregnancy and breastfeeding due to limited data and potential risks. Animal studies have demonstrated teratogenic and embryotoxic effects at doses exceeding the recommended human dose, resulting in skeletal defects in rats, encephaloceles, and macroglossia in mice (60). Although post-marketing reports have suggested a potential association with congenital abnormalities, a causal relationship with itraconazole has not been firmly established (61). Published studies involving short courses of itraconazole during the first trimester have not shown an increased rate of significant congenital disabilities; however, there were methodological limitations, such as short exposure durations or lack of therapy duration data (62). Despite the lack of well-controlled studies, itraconazole is generally contraindicated during pregnancy. At low doses, limited use after the first trimester may be regarded as safe, accompanied by fetal ultrasound assessment following first-trimester exposure. Itraconazole is excreted in breast milk, and although no adverse effects have been reported, its use is not recommended during breastfeeding.

14.9   TOPICAL IMMUNOMODULATORS

There are a variety of topical creams that are immunomodulators used for patients with different dermatologic conditions.

14.9.1   CALCIPOTRIENE

Calcipotriene [former Pregnancy Category C] is considered safe to use topically due to a low amount of systemic absorption (63). Animal studies of teratogenicity were done using an oral route and showed that there was a potential for an increase in forelimb phalanges, increase in pubic bones, and incomplete ossification of bone in rabbit offspring at high doses when administered systemically. In rat offspring, there was an increase in skeletal abnormalities as well. There are no well-controlled studies done in humans (64).

Topical calcipotriene is thought to be compatible with breastfeeding given the low chance of systemic absorption when administered topically in the mother (64).

14.9.2   CORTICOSTEROIDS

Topical corticosteroids [former Pregnancy Category C] are generally considered safe to use during pregnancy (65). Topical corticosteroids are the only medication with a formal review in the Cochrane database to document the safety in pregnancy. There has been no increased risk of congenital malformations, such as the increased risk of oral cleft palate with systemic cortisone exposure in the first trimester, but there was the potential for increase in low birth weight if more than 300 grams of a high-potency topical corticosteroid was dispensed throughout the course of the pregnancy (65).

It is most likely safe to use during breastfeeding. Only class one corticosteroids (the most potent, such as clobetasol) should not be applied to the nipple area. Systemically administered corticosteroids are transferred into the breast milk and can cause growth suppression, interference with endogenous corticosteroid production, and more. Therefore, caution must be taken if taking long-term corticosteroids orally while nursing (66, 67).

14.9.3   TACROLIMUS

Tacrolimus ointment [former Pregnancy Category C] has <5% bioavailability and has not been specifically associated with any fetal anomalies. Teratogenic effects in animal studies have only been reported with systemic use. Therefore, the topical formulation is considered safe to use during pregnancy by providers if the benefits outweigh the potential risks (68, 69). Nursing mothers should not use tacrolimus topically on the nipple because oral consumption by the infant could be significant (68, 69).

14.9.4   CRISABOROLE

Crisaborole is a topical medication used for mild to moderate atopic dermatitis. There are not enough data to determine whether this drug can cause major birth defects, loss of babies, or other adverse events in development; therefore, it should be used with caution in pregnant women. Animal studies have shown that there are no adverse developmental effects when two to three times the normal dose of crisaborole is orally administered to rats and rabbits. Also, it is unknown if crisaborole is excreted in human milk. It is known that the drug is systemically absorbed, so caution should be taken in nursing mothers using the medication on large body surface areas (70).

14.10 SYSTEMIC IMMUNOMODULATORS

Systemic immunomodulators can be used to treat certain dermatologic conditions in pregnant women for conditions such as atopic dermatitis, psoriasis, and blistering diseases.

14.10.1 INTRAVENOUS IMMUNOGLOBULIN

Intravenous immunoglobulin (IVIG) is FDA approved to treat a variety of dermatologic conditions such as autoimmune bullous disease and toxic epidermal necrolysis. IVIG is also used outside of dermatology during pregnancy for a variety of conditions, including autoimmune thrombocytopenia, fetal haemolytic disease, gestational alloimmune liver disease, or antiphospholipid syndrome. It is only recommended that intravenous immunoglobulin be used for conditions for which the benefits of controlling the underlying dermatologic condition outweigh the risks of no therapy (71, 72). Given that this does potentially increase the risk of headaches, renal failure, and hypertension, pregnant women do need to be monitored given that these potential side effects mimic pre-eclampsia. Studies with nursing mothers have shown that IVIG is well tolerated in pregnant women, and there are no serious adverse events when breastfeeding while using intravenous immunoglobulin (73). Additionally, there are studies being performed to see if the use of IVIG can help to improve pregnancy outcomes in women with recent histories of pregnancy loss (74). Protein immunoglobulins are known to transfer into the milk, but there have not been significant adverse effects noted (7). Therefore, this treatment is compatible with both pregnancy and breastfeeding.

14.10.2 HYDROXYCHLOROQUINE

Hydroxychloroquine is a drug that is used for patients suffering from various forms of connective tissue disease such as lupus and dermatomyositis as well as arthritis (75). This drug is known to be safe for use during pregnancy if it is within an appropriate therapeutic dose range. Hydroxychloroquine can be used at dose ≤ 400mg/day during pregnancy and is considered the first-line treatment for inflammatory or rheumatologic diseases that require systemic treatment (74). There are data that suggest that this drug can cross the placenta, but there have not been any concerns of toxicity to the developing neonate (74). It is often important to use this drug because the underlying connective tissue disease, if left untreated, can cause premature birth and growth problems (75).

Hydroxychloroquine can be excreted in breast milk in small amounts but is considered compatible with breastfeeding (75). It is recommended that patients using this drug during breastfeeding take their baby for regular checkups to monitor for haemolysis and jaundice, specifically for premature infants or neonates who are younger than 1 month (7).

14.10.3 PREDNISONE

Prednisone is an oral corticosteroid that can be used for skin conditions such as atopic dermatitis or autoimmune blistering diseases to suppress inflammation and immune responses. Prednisone should not significantly increase the risk of a fetus being born with a birth defect, especially when prescribed at low levels (10–15 mg/day) (74). However, if prednisone is prescribed at higher doses, there is a greater risk of birth defects, so a detailed fetal ultrasound is indicated. Epidemiologic studies indicated a threefold increased risk of orofacial clefts 4 weeks before conception to 12 weeks after conception. There is also a risk of preterm delivery or low birth weight when taking prednisone while pregnant, so it is important to determine the benefits versus the potential fetal risks of using systemic corticosteroids during the early and late stages of pregnancy (74, 76).

The use of prednisone during breastfeeding is usually safe because there are low amounts transferred into the breast milk, and they are similar to naturally produced hormones. This means that there are unlikely to be harmful effects on the infant that is nursing. Percentages of transfer range from 0.35–0.53% of prednisone from the maternal dose into the infant's circulation and 0.09–0.18% of its active metabolite, prednisolone, from the maternal dose into the infant's circulation. Studies have shown that there is a peak of prednisone in breast milk at 1 to 2 hours after administration of the medication. This serum level significantly decreases 4 hours after taking the medication, so it is recommended that patients wait 4 hours before pumping breast milk or nursing. High doses of prednisone can cause temporary reduction in milk supply, so it is best to prescribe low doses if possible. There should be no need for pumping and dumping (7, 76).

14.10.4　Azathioprine

Azathioprine is an immunomodulatory drug that can be used for bullous, autoimmune diseases, intractable pruritus, photodermatoses, psoriasis, atopic dermatitis, and more (77, 78). This drug is safe for use during pregnancy when it is given at a dose that is ≤2 mg/kg. This low dose is needed to limit the risk of infantile leukopenia and thrombocytopenia. It is important for patients to have monthly complete blood counts to ensure there is no risk of toxicity (74). At higher doses, there been a risk of increased prematurity rate, but it is difficult to determine if this is directly related to use of the medication or other comorbidities. It has not been associated with a specific pattern of congenital malformation outside of a possible increased risk of atrial or ventricular septal defects (77–79).

Azathioprine can be transferred into breast milk in small amounts, so there is a risk of neutropenia or immunosuppression. The 1988 WHO's report "Drugs and Human Lactation" recommended that patients avoid breastfeeding while taking azathioprine. However, more recent North American and European guidelines believe that this medication is most likely safe for use during breastfeeding. It is recommended that patients wait 4 hours after taking the medication to feed their babies to avoid peak levels of ingestion and absorption into the baby's bloodstream. Also, infant blood counts should be checked periodically to check for toxicity (7).

14.10.5　Mycophenolate Mofetil

Mycophenolate mofetil [former Pregnancy Category D] is used to treat autoimmune conditions, including atopic dermatitis, autoimmune blistering diseases, forms of vasculitis, erythema multiforme, and connective tissue disease such as lupus nephritis. Studies with patients exposed to this drug during pregnancy have shown associations with miscarriages and malformations including orofacial clefts, congenital heart defects, and more. It is recommended that the use of mycophenolate mofetil be stopped 6 weeks before conception and during pregnancy. The patient should not attempt conception until 4 weeks after discontinuation of the medication and should not use oral contraception alone, since this medication has been shown to compromise the efficacy of the birth control pill. This drug is also excreted in breast milk, so it is contraindicated in nursing mothers (80).

14.10.6　Rituximab

Rituximab [former Pregnancy Category C] is an anti-CD20 monoclonal antibody that is used for off-label dermatologic conditions, including chronic graft-versus-host disease and pemphigus vulgaris (81). Animal studies performed in monkeys did not show any teratogenic effects, but B-cell lymphoid tissue was decreased in the fetus. These B-cell counts then returned to normal levels within 6 months after birth (82). Women should be counselled to avoid pregnancy for at least 12 months after rituximab exposure.

Rituximab can be minimally excreted into the breast milk and absorbed through the baby's gastrointestinal tract, but it is unlikely due to its high molecular weight. However, there is the risk of it affecting the infant's development of the gastrointestinal tract, so it should be avoided while breastfeeding (7).

14.10.7 OMALIZUMAB

Omalizumab is indicated for use in patients with chronic idiopathic urticaria who have not received any relief from over 3 months of layered antihistamine treatment. This drug is considered safe in pregnancy (74). Animal studies of monkeys were done with ten times the maximum recommended human dose, and there was no result of fetal harm (83).

There is minimal transfer of omalizumab into the breast milk because of its low molecular weight. Additionally, studies demonstrated that there were no adverse effects on infant health or development after breastfeeding from a mother using omalizumab. Using this drug while breast-feeding is considered safe (7).

14.10.8 DUPILUMAB

Dupilumab is used for severe atopic dermatitis that has not resolved with topical therapy. Preclinical studies showed that weekly exposure to dupilumab during pregnancy did not cause any maternal–fetal complications, infantile immunosuppression, or other fetal complications. Additionally, seven case reports of dupilumab use during pregnancy did not show any adverse pregnancy outcomes, congenital malformations, or fetal death. All pregnancies resulted in live births, and one of them was premature (74). Animal studies where monkeys were given subcutaneous doses of the drug did not result in adverse developmental effects with doses ten times the maximum recommended dose (84). Overall, there are currently no safety signals regarding dupilumab's use in pregnancy.

Dupilumab is a large protein that is degraded by proteolytic enzymes and avid in the gut of the infant. This means that there is insignificant infant exposure to this drug if the mother needs to take it while breastfeeding. No adverse effects were reported in any case report or series. However, during the first 3 postpartum days, there are large wide gaps in breast alveolar harbour cells that allow for the passage of immunoglobulins. This means that there may be minimal transfer during this short postpartum period in infants who are preterm and have an immature gastrointestinal tract. Current studies are being performed, and the results of the pregnancy and lactation registries regarding dupilumab and breastfeeding are expected in 2027 (7).

14.11 JANUS KINASE INHIBITORS

Topical ruxolitinib and oral abrocitinib, baricitinib, tofacitinib, and updacitinib are Janus kinase inhibitors (JAK) inhibitors that are approved for a variety of inflammatory skin and hair disorders. There are no definitive clinical studies that monitor their use in pregnant patients, but there are pre-clinical studies showing that in utero exposure to JAK inhibitors can cause decreased fetal weight and survival and teratogenicity, including cardiovascular and skeletal malformations. For this rea-son, JAK inhibitors should still be avoided during pregnancy and discontinued for 2–6 weeks before conception. Smaller cohort studies did not show any pregnancy complications with JAK inhibitor usage, but larger cohort studies are ongoing and will be able to determine exposure risk more defini-tively in the future (74).

None of these drugs have safety data available regarding use during breastfeeding. Animal stud-ies show that there is a high level of transfer into breast milk, specifically amounts that parallel maternal serum levels. It is recommended that the use of JAK inhibitors be discontinued 2 weeks before breastfeeding begins to avoid potential infant toxicity (7).

14.11.1 RUXOLITINIB

Ruxolitinib [formerly Pregnancy Category C] is a topical JAK inhibitor that is for inflammatory skin and hair disorders. Even though there are no definitive clinical studies that monitor their use in pregnant patients, preclinical studies resulted in lower fetal weight, survival, cardiovascular, and skeletal malformations. Ruxolitinib should be avoided during pregnancy and discontinued for 2–6 weeks before conception as of now with the current clinical results (74, 85, 86).

Breastfeeding while taking ruxolitinib is not considered safe due to the potential for severe adverse reactions in nursing infants. The limited safety data available predict a high amount of transfer into breast milk, so the decision should be made to either discontinue nursing or discontinue the drug, considering its significance to the mother (7).

14.11.2 ABROCITINIB

Current data suggest that abrocitinib, an oral JAK inhibitor, is not safe for use during pregnancy. Animal studies showed potential fetal risks when abrocitinib was administered to pregnant rats and rabbits at doses higher than the recommended human dose (87, 88). The risk of fetal survival and developmental issues is a risk with JAK inhibitors, so it is recommended that patients avoid use of this drug during pregnancy. There are also limited data regarding breastfeeding, but current data show that the high risk of transfer into the mother's milk makes breastfeeding a huge risk. This means that abrocitinib should be avoided as well for at least 2 weeks before nursing begins (7, 74).

14.11.3 BARICITINIB

Baricitinib, a medication used to treat alopecia areata, presents considerations regarding its use during pregnancy and breastfeeding. The available data suggest that the use of baricitinib during pregnancy should be carefully evaluated, as the potential benefits need to be weighed against the possible risks to the fetus. Limited human data are available, and JAK inhibitors affect cell adhesion and embryonic development, putting patients at risk for reduced fetal birth weight and teratogenic effects (74, 89, 90).

It is important to note that baricitinib has been detected in rat milk, but its presence and potential impact on human milk are unknown (91). However, caution is advised for breastfeeding mothers, and alternative agents may be preferred, particularly when breastfeeding newborn or preterm infants. Use of baricitinib is ultimately contraindicated in pregnancy and should be avoided for up to 4 days after use in breastfeeding and lactation (7, 74).

14.11.4 TOFACITINIB

Tofacitinib, a medication used to treat certain inflammatory conditions, presents limited information regarding its use in pregnancy and breastfeeding. In animal studies, teratogenic effects have been observed at exposures significantly higher than the standard human dosage (92, 93). As a drug inhibiting the JAK pathway, patients who take this during pregnancy are putting their fetus at risk for reduced birth weight and teratogenic effects (74). Regarding breastfeeding, the manufacturer and expert recommendations advise discontinuing breastfeeding while using tofacitinib and for 18 hours after the last dose (94). There are limited human research data available, but it is currently recommended to avoid using tofacitinib during pregnancy and breastfeeding.

14.11.5 UPADACITINIB

Upadacitinib, a medication used to treat certain inflammatory conditions, has shown potential for fetal harm in animal studies when administered at exposures equal to or greater than the maximum recommended human dose (95, 96). These studies have indicated an increased risk of skeletal and cardiovascular malformations and decreased fetal body weights due to inhibition of the JAK pathway. No controlled data are available on the use of upadacitinib in human pregnancy, but current data show that upadacitinib is contraindicated in pregnancy. As for breastfeeding, there are limited data available, but JAK inhibitors have the risk of high amounts transferring into breast milk. Therefore, it is recommended that patients do not use this drug while breastfeeding (7).

14.12 PSORIASIS THERAPIES

Some important drugs that are used for patients suffering with psoriasis include certolizumab, etanercept, adalimumab, cyclosporine, apremilast, methotrexate, secukinumab, ustekinumab, ixekizumab, and guselkumab.

14.12.1 CERTOLIZUMAB

Certolizumab, an anti-tumour necrosis factor (TNF) biologic therapy, is safe during pregnancy given that it is an Fc-free pegylated antibody that cannot attach to the neonatal Fc receptor for IgG and therefore does not cross the placenta (97, 98). Certolizumab is the biologic of choice in pregnancy for patients suffering from psoriasis (74). This drug is known to be of large size, preventing it from passing significantly into breast milk. The limited data available show that it is not well absorbed when swallowed as breast milk, further decreasing its chances of affecting a baby (97, 98). This makes certolizumab compatible for use during pregnancy and breastfeeding.

14.12.2 ETANERCEPT

Etanercept, also an anti-TNF biologic therapy, crosses the placenta through simple diffusion as a fusion protein, so cord blood levels range from 4–8% of maternal dose in the newborn. The majority of published studies show that this drug does not increase the rate of miscarriage of birth defects in the fetuses of pregnant mothers taking this drug. This drug is also a large protein that does not transfer well into breast milk, so it is most likely safe for nursing mothers (99). Current data suggest that etanercept is compatible with pregnancy and breastfeeding (7, 74).

14.12.3 ADALIMUMAB

Adalimumab, an anti-TNF biologic, is not known to increase the chance of miscarriages or birth defects. Cord blood levels are approximately 160% of maternal levels given that there is an increase in the transfer of the medication across the placenta late in the third trimester. Due to the possibility of immunosuppression in the fetus, live vaccines, particularly the BCG vaccine, should be avoided in the first 6 months of life. Breastfeeding is also thought to be safe while taking this drug because of the low levels that travel into the milk. There are very few reported cases of newborns that were exposed to adalimumab through breast milk, but those who were did not show any negative symptoms (100). This drug is compatible with both pregnancy and breastfeeding.

14.12.4 CYCLOSPORINE

Cyclosporine is a drug that can be used during pregnancy if determined to be medically necessary by the treating physician. There are always risks in using drugs during pregnancy, and careful thought should be put into making this decision. The data that exist for this drug are primarily from the transplant literature and registry data. This medication should be used with caution in doses greater than 8 mg/kg/day due to higher rates of prematurity, intrauterine growth restriction, and the need for caesarean delivery. Additionally, there is an increased risk of maternal complications, including hypertension and pre-eclampsia (74). Many cases include women who have pre-existing maternal comorbidities because this drug is commonly used for organ transplant rejection prevention and more. This means that it is difficult to determine if any premature births or developmental problems to the fetus were due to this drug or another medical condition of the carrying mother (101).

This drug has not commonly been detected in the blood of feeding infants. However, detection is possible, so nursing mothers must take caution and only use this drug if necessary while breastfeeding. If breastfed, infants should be frequently monitored to make sure there is no concern of toxicity (102).

14.12.5 APREMILAST

Apremilast is an oral medication for moderate to severe psoriasis and psoriatic arthritis. This drug must be used with caution during pregnancy because it has not been well studied. It is unknown whether this drug will increase the risk of birth defects of miscarriages, given that animal studies did show an increased risk of spontaneous abortions at higher doses of apremilast (103).

It is not recommended that patients breastfeed while using this medication unless the benefits outweigh possible risks. The drug is small enough that it can transfer into breast milk, so it is recommended that patients avoid using apremilast while breastfeeding (7, 103).

14.12.6 METHOTREXATE

Methotrexate should be avoided in pregnancy because it can induce abortions, stop the growth of cells, and interfere with folic acid metabolism, which is essential during pregnancy. It is recommended that parents wait 3 to 6 months after stopping this drug before fertilisation if possible. This drug increases the risk of miscarriage and birth defects, including limb, bone, and face malformations. It can also lead to delayed development and intellectual issues later in the life of the affected fetus (104). This drug is also known to pass into breast milk in small amounts and cause toxic tissue accumulation, so it is recommended to avoid this drug while nursing. Mothers must wait 1 week after taking a dose of methotrexate before breastfeeding again (104).

14.12.7 SECUKINUMAB

An embryo-fetal development study using secukinumab, an interleukin-17A inhibitor, was done on monkeys with 30 times the maximum recommended human dose and resulted in no adverse effects on the development of the infant. A retrospective study with 292 women exposed to secukinumab during pregnancy had rates of spontaneous abortion, congenital malformations, and preterm deliveries comparable to the general population. However, 50% of pregnant women in this study did not follow up and therefore had "unknown" outcomes (105, 106). Therefore, secukinumab does not have as much data as several agents in the TNF-alpha biologic class, so it should be used when benefits outweigh the risks

There are also limited data on the effect that this drug has on human milk and ingestion in the fetus (107). Current data show that there is low excretion of secukinumab into breast milk, so it is most likely compatible (7).

14.12.8 USTEKINUMAB

Limited data exist for the chance of miscarriage or birth defects with use of ustekinumab, an interleukin-12/23 inhibitor. Animal studies have shown that there is no increased chance of birth defects. In cases where the TNF-alpha agents are not feasible, ustekinumab has the second most reassuring safety data in pregnancy and lactation (74). Data show that the protein in ustekinumab is large, meaning that very little can transfer into the milk. It is also not absorbed very well, so there is only a very small chance that any would get into the baby's bloodstream when feeding. This drug is most likely compatible during pregnancy and breastfeeding (108).

14.12.9 Ixekizumab

Ixekizumab, an interleukin-17A inhibitor, also has more limited data during pregnancy. In an embryo fetal study done in pregnant monkeys, researchers injected 19 times the maximum recommended human dose and found no adverse effect on fetal development. Therefore, ixekizumab can be used with caution during pregnancy if clinically indicated and other agents that have more reassuring safety data are not available. There are limited data involving nursing mothers. An animal study with monkeys showed some detection of the drug in monkey's milk (109). Data shows that the excretion into breast milk is limited, and this drug is most likely compatible in nursing mothers (74).

14.12.10 Guselkumab

Guselkumab, a monoclonal IgG1 antibody that inhibits interleukin-23A, did not have any adverse pregnancy outcomes or immunological effects in babies. Seven documented cases of exposure to guselkumab during the first trimester of pregnancy resulted in all live full-term births with no complications or teratogenicity. Data show that there is low risk of guselkumab having negative effects on the fetus during pregnancy, but given that safety data are more limited, it should be used when other agents with more safety data are not feasible (74).

There are limited data on the effects that this drug can have on a breastfeeding child, but the large antibody makes it unlikely to be passed into breast milk and absorbed into the baby's bloodstream. It is expected that there is low excretion into breast milk, and it is likely compatible with breastfeeding (74, 110).

14.13 ANTIPRURITIC THERAPIES

When contemplating the administration of medications to alleviate pruritus during pregnancy, healthcare professionals must exercise caution, thoroughly assess potential side effects, and engage in informed discussions with patients to make prudent decisions regarding their safety and effectiveness.

14.13.1 Diphenhydramine

Diphenhydramine [former Pregnancy Category B], an antihistamine commonly used as an antipruritic and sleep aid, requires careful consideration during pregnancy and breastfeeding. While one study has suggested an increased risk for cleft palate, other extensive studies have found no associations with teratogenicity (111–113). Diphenhydramine is considered safe during pregnancy and is often recommended as a first-line antihistamine, with first-generation antihistamines preferred over second generation. However, its use near delivery should be avoided due to its sedating effects on the child. It is excreted in breast milk, and while short-term drowsiness and irritability have been reported in breastfed infants, no other adverse effects have been found (114). It is likely compatible with breastfeeding, but monitoring the infant for sedation is recommended.

14.13.2 Cetirizine

Cetirizine [former Pregnancy Category B], a non-sedating antihistamine commonly used for allergy relief, is generally considered safe during pregnancy and breastfeeding. While more well-controlled studies on pregnant women need to be undertaken, there have been no associations with teratogenicity in existing studies, and animal studies have not shown any teratogenic effects (115–117). It is a first-line antihistamine drug, and there is low risk of harm to the baby if used during pregnancy. It is minimally excreted in breast milk, but it is considered compatible with breastfeeding, and second-generation antihistamines like cetirizine are generally preferred over first generation due to less sedating effects (118). While further research is needed, the available evidence suggests that cetirizine does not pose significant risks to pregnancy or breastfeeding.

14.13.3 LORATADINE

Loratadine [former Pregnancy Category B], a widely used non-sedating antihistamine for allergy relief, is generally considered safe during pregnancy and breastfeeding. Extensive studies with over 5000 exposed pregnancies have not shown an increased risk of congenital disabilities (119, 120). However, one study suggested a potential association with hypospadias that was not supported by other studies. Animal studies have not demonstrated teratogenic effects (121, 122). Loratadine is recommended as the first choice among non-sedating antihistamines during pregnancy, with first-generation antihistamines preferred over second-generation ones. It is minimally excreted in breast milk but compatible with breastfeeding and has less risk of sedation (123). Loratadine is considered a safe choice for allergy relief during pregnancy and breastfeeding.

14.13.4 HYDROXYZINE

Hydroxyzine, an antihistamine commonly prescribed for various conditions such as anxiety and allergies, requires careful consideration during pregnancy and breastfeeding due to its associated risks. In pregnancy, exposure to hydroxyzine may lead to hypotension, myoclonus, movement disorders, hypoxia, central nervous system depression, and urinary retention (124). Hydroxyzine crosses the placenta, raising concerns about potential adverse effects on the developing fetus, especially in the first trimester (125). This drug should be used with caution during pregnancy and only if the benefits are determined to outweigh the risks. While data on the drug concentration in breast milk are limited, the excretion of its metabolite cetirizine has been reported, and seizures have been observed in breastfed infants at high doses of hydroxyzine (150 mg daily) (126). The risk of seizures as well as sedation and drowsiness suggest that hydroxyzine should be used with caution in breastfeeding mothers.

14.14 ANTIVIRAL MEDICATIONS

14.14.1 ACYCLOVIR

Acyclovir [former Pregnancy Category B], a widely prescribed antiviral medication utilised for treating herpes simplex virus (HSV) and varicella-zoster virus infections, is generally regarded as safe and effective during pregnancy. Extensive studies have been conducted to evaluate the potential risks associated with acyclovir use, particularly in the first trimester, and have found no significant increase in the occurrence of major congenital disabilities (127, 128). These findings reassure pregnant individuals requiring treatment for viral infections and support the utilisation of acyclovir as the first-choice antiviral therapy for managing herpes infections during pregnancy (129). Animal studies have further corroborated the safety profile of acyclovir, as teratogenic effects have not been observed (130).

Regarding breastfeeding, a low concentration of acyclovir is excreted in breast milk after oral administration. The topical application of acyclovir away from the breast is considered to pose a negligible risk to breastfed infants, and no adverse effects have been reported. As such, acyclovir is generally compatible with breastfeeding, as the amount in breast milk is only about 1% of a typical infant dosage (131). Overall, acyclovir is considered a safe and valuable treatment option for managing HSV and varicella-zoster virus infections during pregnancy and breastfeeding.

14.15 LICE AND SCABIES MEDICATIONS

14.15.1 PERMETHRIN

Permethrin, a topical medication widely used to treat scabies and lice, is considered safe and effective during pregnancy. Extensive studies have demonstrated the absence of adverse effects associated with its use, and animal studies have provided reassurance by not showing any detrimental impacts on fetal development (132–134). With its topical application, permethrin is minimally absorbed and rapidly metabolised to inactive metabolites, further supporting its safety profile during pregnancy.

Permethrin is recommended as the first-line treatment for scabies during pregnancy and the second-line treatment for lice. Its compatibility with breastfeeding is attributed to its safe application directly on infants' skin and the rapid metabolism of inactive compounds (135). Permethrin is widely regarded as a safe and effective treatment option for scabies and lice during pregnancy and breastfeeding.

14.15.2 IVERMECTIN

The safety of ivermectin during pregnancy remains uncertain due to the lack of well-controlled studies in pregnant women. While no adverse effects have been reported with its use, at high cumulative doses, animal studies have shown teratogenic and embryo-fetal toxic effects at higher doses, including cleft palate, carpal flexure, decreased fetal weight, and behavioural development abnormalities (136–138). Despite these findings, ivermectin is recommended as a treatment option for scabies if topical therapies are ineffective, highlighting the importance of carefully considering its use in pregnancy on a case-by-case basis. This drug should generally be avoided during pregnancy unless there is a compelling indication for its use. Regarding breastfeeding, ivermectin is poorly excreted into breast milk after oral administration. Although neonatal toxicity has been observed in animal studies, it is believed to be related to poorly developed blood–brain barriers in rats. If topical therapies for scabies are ineffective, ivermectin can be considered compatible with breastfeeding, as the amounts ingested by breastfed infants are small and unlikely to cause adverse effects in infants over 7 days of age (139). Nonetheless, the limited data warrant caution and generally avoiding use during pregnancy but show compatibility with breastfeeding.

14.16 WART TREATMENTS

14.16.1 IMIQUIMOD

Imiquimod [former Pregnancy Category C] is an immune response modifier that is utilised in the treatment of warts but which should be used with caution during pregnancy. Limited human data available on the effects of imiquimod in pregnancy suggest that there is a low risk, but it should still be avoided during pregnancy. Animal studies conducted on rats and rabbits that were administered 98 times the maximum recommended human dose did not show any fetal toxicity or teratogenicity. It is also unknown whether imiquimod is transferred to breast milk, and there a no human data available. It is most likely compatible with use while breastfeeding, but only if deemed to be necessary (140).

14.17 CONCLUSION

The use of medications during pregnancy and breastfeeding necessitates careful consideration, weighing the available information and individual circumstances. Each medication should be prescribed individually, tailored to the specific needs and risks of the pregnant or breastfeeding individual. It is crucial to balance addressing the health condition effectively and ensuring the safety of both the mother and the developing or breastfed infant. Nonetheless, further research is needed to expand our understanding and ensure the utmost safety in these populations. By continuing to investigate the effects of medications during pregnancy and breastfeeding, healthcare professionals can make informed decisions and provide safe and effective care to pregnant and breastfeeding individuals.

REFERENCES

1. Sachdeva P, Patel BG, Patel BK. Drug use in pregnancy; a point to ponder! *Indian J Pharm Sci*, 2009;71(1):1–7.
2. Blattner CM, Danesh M, Safaee M, et al. Understanding the new FDA pregnancy and lactation labeling rules. *Int J Women's Dermatol*. 2016;2(1):5–7.
3. Dathe K, Schaefer C. The use of medication in pregnancy. *Dtsch Arztebl Int*. 2019;116(46):783–790.
4. Finacea (azelaic acid) gel label. *Food and Drug Administration*; 2010, available at www.accessdata.fda.gov/drugsatfda_docs/label/2010/021470s005lbl.pdf.

5. Chien AL, Qi J, Rainer B, et al. Treatment of acne in pregnancy. *J Am Board Family Med.* 2016;29(2):254–263.
6. Adapalene and benzoyl peroxide [package insert]. *Hawthorne.* New York: Taro Pharmaceuticals, Inc.; 2020.
7. Butler DC, Heller MM, Murase JE. Safety of dermatologic medications in pregnancy and lactation: Part II. Lactation. *J Am Acad Dermatol.* 2014;70(3):417e411–410; quiz 427.
8. *Drugs and Lactation Database (LactMed®)* [Internet]. Bethesda, MD: National Institute of Child Health and Human Development; 2006. Salicylic Acid [updated 2021 Jun 21], available at www.ncbi.nlm.nih.gov/books/NBK500675.
9. Weiss J, Mallavalli S, Meckfessel M et al. Safe use of adapalene 0.1 % gel in a non-prescription environment. *J Drugs Dermatol.* 2021;20(12):1330–1335.
10. Differin (adapalene) gel label. *Food and Drug Administration*; 2012, available at www.accessdata.fda.gov/drugsatfda_docs/label/2012/021753s004lbl.pdf.
11. Retin-A Micro (tretinoin) Gel microsphere 0.1%, 0.08% and 0.04% for topical use. *Food and Drug Administration*; 2014, available at www.accessdata.fda.gov/drugsatfda_docs/label/2014/020475s021lbl.pdf.
12. *Tazorac—Food and Drug Administration*; 2011, available at www.accessdata.fda.gov/drugsatfda_docs/label/2011/020600s008lbl.pdf.
13. Smorlesi C, Caldarella A, Caramelli L, et al. Topically applied minoxidil may cause fetal malformation: A case report. *Birth Defects Res A Clin Mol Teratol.* 2003;67(12):997–1001.
14. U.S. Department of Health and Human Services. *Fetal Minoxidil Syndrome—About the Disease.* Genetic and Rare Diseases Information Center; 2023, available at https://rarediseases.info.nih.gov/diseases/2308/fetal-minoxidil-syndrome.
15. Drugs and Lactation Database (LactMed®) [Internet]. Bethesda, MD: National Institute of Child Health and Human Development; 2006. Minoxidil [updated 2022], available at www.ncbi.nlm.nih.gov/books/NBK501032/
16. ALDACTONE® (spironolactone) tablets for oral use. *Food and Drug Administration*; 2018, available at www.accessdata.fda.gov/drugsatfda_docs/label/2018/012151s075lbl.pdf.
17. Center for Drug Evaluation and Research. *Isotretinoin Capsule Information.* U.S. Food and Drug Administration; 2021, available at www.fda.gov/drugs/postmarket-drug-safety-information-patients-and-providers/isotretinoin-capsule-information#:~:text=Isotretinoin%20is%20a%20potentially%20dangerous,births%2C%20and%20death%20in%20babies.
18. Accutane (isotretinoin) capsules label. *Food and Drug Administration*; 2002, available at www.accessdata.fda.gov/drugsatfda_docs/label/2002/18662s051lbl.pdf.
19. PROPECIA (finasteride) tablets for oral use. *Food and Drug Administration*; 2021, available at www.accessdata.fda.gov/drugsatfda_docs/label/2021/020788s028lbl.pdf.
20. Chiaravalloti A, Jinna S. Dermatologic surgical considerations in the pregnant female. *J Am Acad Dermatol.* 2019;81(4):AB191.
21. Mother to Baby, Fact Sheets [Internet]. Brentwood, TN: Organization of Teratology Information Specialists (OTIS); 1994. Lidocaine; 2021, available at www.ncbi.nlm.nih.gov/books/NBK582791/
22. Kim H, Hwang K, Yun SM, et al. Usage of epinephrine mixed with lidocaine in plastic surgery. *J Craniofacial Surg.* 2020;31(3):791–793.
23. Goldberg D, Maloney M. Dermatologic surgery and cosmetic procedures during pregnancy and the postpartum period. *Dermatol Ther.* 2103;26(4):321–330.
24. Lee JM, Shin TJ. Use of local anesthetics for dental treatment during pregnancy; safety for parturient. *J Dental Anesthesia Pain Med.* 2017;17(2):81–90.
25. Nguyen R, Khanna NR, Safadi AO, et al. Bacitracin topical [updated 2022]. In: *StatPearls* [Internet]. Treasure Island, FL: StatPearls Publishing; 2023, available at www.ncbi.nlm.nih.gov/books/NBK536993/
26. BACTROBAN Ointment (mupirocin ointment, 2%). *Food and Drug Administration*; 2015, available at www.accessdata.fda.gov/drugsatfda_docs/label/2015/050591s030lbl.pdf.
27. *Drugs and Lactation Database (LactMed®)* [Internet]. Bethesda, MD: National Institute of Child Health and Human Development; 2006. Mupirocin [updated 2018 Oct 31], available at www.ncbi.nlm.nih.gov/books/NBK501429/
28. Czeizel AE, Rockenbauer M, Sørensen HT, et al. Use of cephalosporins during pregnancy and in the presence of congenital abnormalities: A population-based, case-control study. *Am J Obstet Gynecol.* 2001;184(6):1289–1296.
29. *Drugs and Lactation Database (LactMed®)* [Internet]. Bethesda, MD: National Institute of Child Health and Human Development; 2006. Cephalexin [updated 2021], available at www.ncbi.nlm.nih.gov/books/NBK501487/

30. CLEOCIN HCL (clindamycin hydrochloride) capsules, USP. *Food and Drug Administration*; n.d., available at www.accessdata.fda.gov/drugsatfda_docs/label/2014/050162s092s093lbl.pdf.
31. Metronidazole Tablets. *Food and Drug Administration*; 2020, available at www.accessdata.fda.gov/drugsatfda_docs/label/2020/018845s014,018930s013lbl.pdf.
32. Penicillin G Potassium. *Food and Drug Administration*; 2016, available at www.accessdata.fda.gov/drugsatfda_docs/label/2016/050638s019lbl.pdf.
33. Heikkilä AM, Erkkola RU. The need for adjustment of dosage regimen of penicillin V during pregnancy. *Obstet Gynecol*. 1993;81(6):919–921.
34. BACTRIM Sulfamethoxazole and trimethoprim DS (double strength) tablets and tablets USP. *Food and Drug Administration*; 2010, available at www.accessdata.fda.gov/drugsatfda_docs/label/2010/017377s067lbl.pdf.
35. ACZONE Gel, 5% safely and effectively. *Food and Drug Administration*; 2018, available at www.accessdata.fda.gov/drugsatfda_docs/label/2018/021794s016lbl.pdf.
36. CIPRO (ciprofloxacin hydrochloride) tablet, for oral use. *Food and Drug Administration*; 2016, available at www.accessdata.fda.gov/drugsatfda_docs/label/2016/019537s086lbl.pdf.
37. DORYX (doxycycline hayclate) Delayed-release tablets. *Food and Drug Administration*; 2008, available at www.accessdata.fda.gov/drugsatfda_docs/label/2008/050795s005lbl.pdf.
38. Czeizel AE, Tóth M, Rockenbauer M. No teratogenic effect after clotrimazole therapy during pregnancy. *Epidemiology*. 1999;10(4):437–440.
39. Khatter NJ, Khan MAB. Clotrimazole [updated 2022]. In: *StatPearls* [Internet]. Treasure Island, FL: StatPearls Publishing; 2023, available at www.ncbi.nlm.nih.gov/books/NBK560643/
40. van Schalkwyk J, Yudin MH. Infectious disease committee. Vulvovaginitis: Screening for and management of trichomoniasis, vulvovaginal candidiasis, and bacterial vaginosis. *J Obstet Gynaecol Can*. 2015;37(3):266–274.
41. Spencer JP, Gonzalez LS, Barnhart DJ. Medications in the breast-feeding mother. *Am Fam Physician*. 2001;64(1):119–126.
42. Czeizel AE, Kazy Z, Puhó E. A population-based case-control teratological study of oral nystatin treatment during pregnancy. *Scand J Infect Dis*. 2003;35(11–12):830–835.
43. King CT, Rogers PD, Cleary JD, et al. Antifungal therapy during pregnancy. *Clin Infect Dis*. 1998;27(5):1151–1160.
44. *Drugs and Lactation Database (LactMed®)* [Internet]. Bethesda, MD: National Institute of Child Health and Human Development; 2006. Nystatin [updated 2021], available at www.ncbi.nlm.nih.gov/books/NBK501241/
45. *Drugs and Lactation Database (LactMed®)* [Internet]. Bethesda, MD: National Institute of Child Health and Human Development; 2006. Ciclopirox [updated 2018], available at www.ncbi.nlm.nih.gov/books/NBK501434/
46. Andersson NW, Thomsen SF, Andersen JT. Evaluation of association between oral and topical terbinafine use in pregnancy and risk of major malformations and spontaneous abortion. *JAMA Dermatol*. 2020;156(4):375–383.
47. Andersson NW, Thomsen SF, Andersen JT. Evaluation of association between oral and topical terbinafine use in pregnancy and risk of major malformations and spontaneous abortion. *JAMA Dermatol*. 2020;156(4):375–383.
48. Maxfield L, Preuss CV, Bermudez R. Terbinafine [updated 2023 May 29]. In: *StatPearls* [Internet]. Treasure Island, FL: StatPearls Publishing; 2023, available at www.ncbi.nlm.nih.gov/books/NBK545218/
49. Czeizel AE, Métneki J, Kazy Z, et al. A population-based case-control study of oral griseofulvin treatment during pregnancy. *Acta Obstet Gynecol Scand*. 2004;83(9):827–831.
50. Klein MF, Beall JR. Griseofulvin: A teratogenic study. *Science*. 1972;175(4029):1483–1484.
51. Olson JM, Troxell T. Griseofulvin. In: *StatPearls* [Internet]. Treasure Island, FL: StatPearls Publishing; 2023, available at www.ncbi.nlm.nih.gov/books/NBK537323/
52. Mølgaard-Nielsen D, Pasternak B, Hviid A. Use of oral fluconazole during pregnancy and the risk of birth defects. *N Engl J Med*. 2013;369(9):830–839.
53. Pursley TJ, Blomquist IK, Abraham J, et al. Fluconazole-induced congenital anomalies in three infants. *Clin Infect Dis*. 1996;22(2):336–340.
54. Bérard A, Sheehy O, Zhao JP, et al. Associations between low- and high-dose oral fluconazole and pregnancy outcomes: 3 nested case-control studies. *CMAJ*. 2019;191(7):E179–E187.
55. *Drugs and Lactation Database (LactMed®)* [Internet]. Bethesda, MD: National Institute of Child Health and Human Development; 2006. Fluconazole; 2018.

56. Moudgal VV, Sobel JD. Antifungal drugs in pregnancy: A review. *Expert Opin Drug Saf.* 2003;2(5): 475–483.

57. Kazy Z, Puhó E, Czeizel AE. Population-based case-control study of oral ketoconazole treatment for birth outcomes. *Congenit Anom (Kyoto).* 2005;45(1):5–8.

58. Van Cauteren H, Lampo A, Vandenberghe J, et al. Safety aspects of oral antifungal agents. *Br J Clin Pract Suppl.* 1990;71:47–49.

59. Koh YP, Tian EA, Oon HH. New changes in pregnancy and lactation labelling: Review of dermatologic drugs. *Int J Womens Dermatol.* 2019;5(4):216–226.

60. El-Shershaby AF, Imam A, Helmy M, et al. In utero exposure to itraconazole during different gestational periods of rats. *Toxicol Mech Methods.* 2014;24(1):50–59.

61. De Santis M, Di Gianantonio E, Cesari E, et al. First-trimester itraconazole exposure and pregnancy outcome: A prospective cohort study of women contacting teratology information services in Italy. *Drug Saf.* 2009;32(3):239–244.

62. Liu D, Zhang C, Wu L, et al. Fetal outcomes after maternal exposure to oral antifungal agents during pregnancy: A systematic review and meta-analysis. *Int J Gynaecol Obstet.* 2020;148(1):6–13.

63. NHS. *Pregnancy, Breastfeeding and Fertility While Using Calcipotriol.* NHS Choices; 2022, available at www.nhs.uk/medicines/calcipotriol/pregnancy-breastfeeding-and-fertility-while-using-calcipotriol/#:~:text=Calcipotriol%20 and%20pregnancy,if%20used%20in%20this%20way.

64. DOVONEX (calcipiotriene) Cream, 0.005%. *Food and Drug Administration*; 2015, available at www. accessdata.fda.gov/drugsatfda_docs/label/2015/020273s013,020554s012lbl.pdf.

65. Chi CC, Wang SH, Kirtschig G. Safety of topical corticosteroids in pregnancy. *JAMA Dermatol.* 2016;152(8):934–935.

66. Hydrocortisone Butyrae Cream, 0.1% (Lipophilic). *Food and Drug Administration*; n.d., available at www.accessdata.fda.gov/drugsatfda_docs/label/2013/202145Orig1lbl.pdf.

67. KENALOG Creams Rx only Triamcinolone Acetonide Cream USP. *Food and Drug Administration*; n.d., available at www.accessdata.fda.gov/drugsatfda_docs/label/pre96/011601s036lbl.pdf.

68. PROTOPIC (tacrolimus). *Food and Drug Administration*; 2011, available at www.accessdata.fda.gov/ drugsatfda_docs/label/2011/050777s018lbl.pdf.

69. Weatherhead S, Robson SC, Reynolds NJ. Eczema in pregnancy. *BMJ (Clinical Research).* 2007;335 (7611):152–154.

70. *Eucrisa Indications and Usage (Crisaborole).* EUCRISA Indications and Usage (crisaborole) | Pfizer Medical Information—US; n.d., available at www.pfizermedicalinformation.com/en-us/eucrisa/ indications-usage.

71. Dhar S. Intravenous immunoglobulin in dermatology. *Ind J Dermatol.* 2009;54(1):77–79.

72. D'Mello RJ, Hsu CD, Chaiworapongsa P, et al. Update on the use of intravenous immunoglobulin in pregnancy. *NeoReviews.* 2021;22(1):e7–e24.

73. *Drugs and Lactation Database (LactMed®)* [Internet]. Bethesda, MD: National Institute of Child Health and Human Development; 2006. Immune Globulin [updated 2023], available at www.ncbi.nlm.nih.gov/ books/NBK501437/.

74. Murase JE, Heller MM, Butler DC. Safety of dermatologic medications in pregnancy and lactation: Part I. Pregnancy. *J Am Acad Dermatol.* 2014;70(3):401, e401–414; quiz 415.

75. NHS. *NHS Choices*; 2022, available at www.nhs.uk/medicines/hydroxychloroquine/pregnancy- breastfeeding-and-fertility-while-taking-hydroxychloroquine/#:~:text=You%20can%20safely%20 take%20hydroxychloroquine,you%20and%20your%20baby%20well.

76. *Prednisone/Prednisolone—Mother to Baby | Fact Sheets—NCBI Bookshelf*; 2022, available at www.ncbi. nlm.nih.gov/books/NBK582908/.

77. Chavez-Alvarez S, Herz-Ruelas M, Villarreal-Martinez A, et al. Azathioprine: Its uses in dermatology. *An Bras Dermatol.* 2020;95(6):731–736.

78. Natekar A, Pupco A, Bozzo P, et al. Safety of azathioprine use during pregnancy. *Can Fam Physician.* 2011;57(12):1401–1402.

79. NHS. *Pregnancy, Breastfeeding and Fertility While Taking Azathioprine.* NHS Choices; 2023, available at www.nhs.uk/medicines/azathioprine/pregnancy-breastfeeding-and-fertility-while-taking-azathioprine/#:~: text=Azathioprine%20and%20breastfeeding&text=Azathioprine%20passes%20into%20breast%20 milk,need%20some%20extra%20blood%20tests.

80. Coscia LA, Armenti DP, King RW, et al. Update on the teratogenicity of maternal mycophenolate mofetil. *J Pediatric Genet.* 2015;4(2):42–55.

81. Gleghorn K, Wilson J, Wilkerson M. Rituximab: Uses in dermatology. *Skin Ther Lett.* 2016;21(5):5–7.

82. Rituxan (rituximab) Injection for Intravenous Use. *Food and Drug Administration*; 2010, available at www.accessdata.fda.gov/drugsatfda_docs/label/2010/103705s5311lbl.pdf.

83. XOLAIR® (omalizumab) for Injection, for Subcutaneous Use. *Food and Drug Administration*; 2016, available at www.accessdata.fda.gov/drugsatfda_docs/label/2016/103976s5225lbl.pdf.

84. DUPIXENT® (dupilumab) Injection, for Subcutaneous Use. *Food and Drug Administration*; 2022, available at www.accessdata.fda.gov/drugsatfda_docs/label/2022/761055s040lbl.pdf.

85. Raedler LA. Jakafi (Ruxolitinib): First FDA-approved medication for the treatment of patients with polycythemia vera. *Am Health Drug Benefits*. 2015;8(Spec Feature):75–79.

86. *Jakafi (ruxolitinib) Tablets [Prescribing Information]*. Wilmington, DE: Incyte Corporation; 2014.

87. Iznardo H, Roé E, Serra-Baldrich E, et al. Efficacy and safety of JAK1 inhibitor abrocitinib in atopic dermatitis. *Pharmaceutics*. 2023;15(2):385.

88. Napolitano M, Ruggiero A, Fontanella G, et al. New emergent therapies for atopic dermatitis: A review of safety profile with respect to female fertility, pregnancy, and breastfeeding. *Dermatol Ther*. 2021;34(1):e14475.

89. Costanzo G, Firinu D, Losa F, et al. Baricitinib exposure during pregnancy in rheumatoid arthritis. *Ther Adv Musculoskelet Dis*. 2020;12:1759720X19899296.

90. Peterson EA, Lynton J, Bernard A, et al. Rheumatologic medication use during pregnancy. *Obstet Gynecol*. 2020;135(5):1161–1176.

91. Ahmad A, Zaheer M, Balis FJ. Baricitinib [updated 2022]. In: *StatPearls* [Internet]. Treasure Island, FL: StatPearls Publishing; 2023.

92. Clowse ME, Feldman SR, Isaacs JD, et al. Pregnancy outcomes in the tofacitinib safety databases for rheumatoid arthritis and psoriasis. *Drug Saf*. 2016;39(8):755–762.

93. Götestam Skorpen C, Hoeltzenbein M, Tincani A, et al. The EULAR points to consider for use of antirheumatic drugs before pregnancy, and during pregnancy and lactation. *Ann Rheum Dis*. 2016;75:795–810.

94. Pfizer Inc. *XeljanzPrescribing Information*; 2014, available at http://labeling.pfizer.com/ShowLabeling.aspx?id=959.

95. Upadacitinib for rheumatoid arthritis. *Aust Prescr*. 2020;43(5):178–179.

96. Padda IS, Bhatt R, Parmar M. Upadacitinib [updated 2023]. In: *StatPearls* [Internet]. Treasure Island, FL: StatPearls Publishing; 2023.

97. Mother to Baby, *Fact Sheets* [Internet]. Brentwood, TN: Organization of Teratology Information Specialists (OTIS); 1994. Certolizumab Pegol (Cimzia®) 2022, Available at www.ncbi.nlm.nih.gov/books/NBK582625/.

98. CIMZIA (certolizumab pegol) for injection, for subcutaneous use. *Food and Drug Administration*; 2016, available at www.accessdata.fda.gov/drugsatfda_docs/label/2017/125160s270lbl.pdf.

99. Mother to Baby, *Fact Sheets* [Internet]. Brentwood, TN: Organization of Teratology Information Specialists (OTIS); 1994. Etanercept (Enbrel®) 2021, available at www.ncbi.nlm.nih.gov/books/NBK582693/.

100. Mother to Baby, *Fact Sheets* [Internet]. Brentwood, TN: Organization of Teratology Information Specialists (OTIS); 1994. Adalimumab (Humira®) 2021, Available at www.ncbi.nlm.nih.gov/books/NBK582559/.

101. Paziana K, Del Monaco M, Cardonick E, et al. Ciclosporin use during pregnancy. *Drug Saf*. 2013;36(5):279–294.

102. *Drugs and Lactation Database (LactMed®)* [Internet]. Bethesda, MD: National Institute of Child Health and Human Development; 2006. Cyclosporine [updated 2023], available at www.ncbi.nlm.nih.gov/books/NBK501683/.

103. Mother to Baby, *Fact Sheets* [Internet]. Brentwood, TN: Organization of Teratology Information Specialists (OTIS); 1994. Apremilast (Otezla®) 2022, available at www.ncbi.nlm.nih.gov/books/NBK582579/.

104. Mother to Baby, *Fact Sheets* [Internet]. Brentwood, TN: Organization of Teratology Information Specialists (OTIS); 1994. Methotrexate; 2023, available at www.ncbi.nlm.nih.gov/books/NBK582834/.

105. Warren RB, Reich K, Langley RG, et al. Secukinumab in pregnancy: Outcomes in psoriasis, psoriatic arthritis and ankylosing spondylitis from the global safety database. *Br J Dermatol*. 2018;179(5):1205–1207.

106. Kimball AB, Guenther L, Kalia S, et al. Pregnancy outcomes in women with moderate-to-severe psoriasis from the psoriasis longitudinal assessment and registry (PSOLAR). *JAMA Dermatol*. 2021;157(3):301–306.

107. COSENTYX (secukinumab) Injection, for Subcutaneous Use. *Food and Drug Administration*; 2015, available at www.accessdata.fda.gov/drugsatfda_docs/label/2021/125504s043lbl.pdf.

108. Mother to Baby, *Fact Sheets* [Internet]. Brentwood, TN: Organization of Teratology Information Specialists (OTIS); 1994. Ustekinumab (Stelara®) 2023, available at www.ncbi.nlm.nih.gov/books/NBK583005/.

109. TALTZ (ixekizumab) Injection, for Subcutaneous Use. *Food and Drug Administration*; 2015, available at www.accessdata.fda.gov/drugsatfda_docs/label/2021/125521s014lbl.pdf.

110. Mother to Baby, *Fact Sheets* [Internet]. Brentwood, TN: Organization of Teratology Information Specialists (OTIS); 1994. Guselkumab (Tremfya®) 2021, available at www.ncbi.nlm.nih.gov/books/NBK582737/.

111. Mother to Baby, *Fact Sheets* [Internet]. Brentwood, TN: Organization of Teratology Information Specialists (OTIS); 1994. Diphenhydramine; 2021, available at www.ncbi.nlm.nih.gov/books/NBK582675/

112. Saxén I. Letter: Cleft palate and maternal diphenhydramine intake. *Lancet*. 1974;1(7854):407–408.

113. Schardein JL, Hentz DL, Petrere JA, et al. Teratogenesis studies with diphenhydramine HCl. *Toxicol Appl Pharmacol*. 1971;18(4):971–976.

114. *Drugs and Lactation Database (LactMed®)* [Internet]. Bethesda, MD: National Institute of Child Health and Human Development; 2006. Diphenhydramine [updated 2021], available at www.ncbi.nlm.nih.gov/books/NBK501878/.

115. Golembesky A, Cooney M, Boev R, et al. Safety of cetirizine in pregnancy. *J Obstet Gynaecol*. 2018;38(7):940–945.

116. Weber-Schoendorfer C, Schaefer C. The safety of cetirizine during pregnancy. A prospective observational cohort study. *Reprod Toxicol*. 2008;26(1):19–23.

117. Etwel F, Djokanovic N, Moretti ME, et al. The fetal safety of cetirizine: An observational cohort study and meta-analysis. *J Obstet Gynaecol*. 2014;34(5):392–399.

118. *Drugs and Lactation Database (LactMed®)* [Internet]. Bethesda, MD: National Institute of Child Health and Human Development; 2006. Cetirizine [updated 2022], available at www.ncbi.nlm.nih.gov/books/NBK501509/.

119. Mother to Baby, *Fact Sheets* [Internet]. Brentwood, TN: Organization of Teratology Information Specialists (OTIS); 1994. Loratadine (Claritin®) 2021, available at www.ncbi.nlm.nih.gov/books/NBK582799/.

120. Schwarz EB, Moretti ME, Nayak S, et al. Risk of hypospadias in offspring of women using loratadine during pregnancy: A systematic review and meta-analysis. *Drug Saf*. 2008;31(9):775–788.

121. Pedersen L, Nørgaard M, Rothman KJ, et al. Loratadine during pregnancy and hypospadias. *Epidemiology*. 2008;19(2):359–360.

122. Schwarz EB, Moretti ME, Nayak S, et al. Risk of hypospadias in offspring of women using loratadine during pregnancy: A systematic review and meta-analysis. 2008. In: *Database of Abstracts of Reviews of Effects (DARE): Quality-assessed Reviews* [Internet]. York, UK: Centre for Reviews and Dissemination; 1995, available at www.ncbi.nlm.nih.gov/books/NBK75218/.

123. *Drugs and Lactation Database (LactMed®)* [Internet]. Bethesda, MD: National Institute of Child Health and Human Development; 2006. Loratadine [updated 2018], available at www.ncbi.nlm.nih.gov/books/NBK501009/.

124. Brzezińska-Wcisło L, Zbiciak-Nylec M, Wcisło-Dziadecka D, et al. Pregnancy: A therapeutic dilemma. *Postepy Dermatol Alergol*. 2017;34(5):433–438.

125. Gilboa SM, Ailes EC, Rai RP, Anderson JA, et al. Antihistamines and birth defects: A systematic review of the literature. *Expert Opin Drug Saf*. 2014;13(12):1667–1698.

126. *Drugs and Lactation Database (LactMed®)* [Internet]. Bethesda, MD: National Institute of Child Health and Human Development; 2006. Hydroxyzine; 2021.

127. Haddad J, Messer J, Willard D, et al. Aciclovir et grossesse: Aspects actuels [Acyclovir and pregnancy: Current aspects]. *J Gynecol Obstet Biol Reprod (Paris)*. 1989;18(5):679–683.

128. Ratanajamit C, Vinther Skriver M, Jepsen P, et al. Adverse pregnancy outcome in women exposed to acyclovir during pregnancy: A population-based observational study. *Scand J Infect Dis*. 2003;35(4):255–259.

129. Stone KM, Reiff-Eldridge R, White AD, et al. Pregnancy outcomes following systemic prenatal acyclovir exposure: Conclusions from the international acyclovir pregnancy registry, 1984–1999. *Birth Defects Res A Clin Mol Teratol*. 2004;70(4):201–207.

130. Moore HL Jr, Szczech GM, Rodwell DE, et al. Preclinical toxicology studies with acyclovir: Teratologic, reproductive and neonatal tests. *Fundam Appl Toxicol*. 1983;3(6):560–568.

131. *Drugs and Lactation Database (LactMed®)* [Internet]. Bethesda, MD: National Institute of Child Health and Human Development; 2006. Acyclovir [updated 2018], available at www.ncbi.nlm.nih.gov/books/NBK501195/.

132. Kennedy D, Hurst V, Konradsdottir E, et al. Pregnancy outcome following exposure to permethrin and use of teratogen information. *Am J Perinatol*. 2005;22(2):87–90.

133. Weill A, Bernigaud C, Mokni M, et al. Scabies-infested pregnant women: A critical therapeutic challenge. *PLoS Negl Trop Dis*. 2021;15(1):e0008929.

134. Mytton OT, McGready R, Lee SJ, et al. Safety of benzyl benzoate lotion and permethrin in pregnancy: A retrospective matched cohort study. *BJOG*. 2007;114(5):582–587.
135. *Drugs and Lactation Database (LactMed®)* [Internet]. Bethesda, MD: National Institute of Child Health and Human Development; 2006. Permethrin [updated 2022], available at www.ncbi.nlm.nih.gov/books/ NBK501383/.
136. Nicolas P, Maia MF, Bassat Q, et al. Safety of oral ivermectin during pregnancy: A systematic review and meta-analysis. *Lancet Glob Health*. 2020;8(1):e92–e100.
137. Nicolas P, Maia MF, Bassat Q, et al. Safety of oral ivermectin during pregnancy: A systematic review and meta-analysis. *Lancet Glob Health*. 2020;8(1):e92–e100.
138. Poul JM. Effects of perinatal ivermectin exposure on behavioral development of rats. *Neurotoxicol Teratol*. 1988;10(3):267–272.
139. *Drugs and Lactation Database (LactMed®)* [Internet]. Bethesda, MD: National Institute of Child Health and Human Development; 2006. Ivermectin [updated 2022], available at www.ncbi.nlm.nih.gov/books/ NBK501375/9.
140. ALDARA (imiquimod) Cream, 5%. *Food and Drug Administration*; 2005, available at www.accessdata. fda.gov/drugsatfda_docs/label/2005/020723s018lbl.pdf.

15 Cosmetics and Cosmeceuticals in Pregnancy

Pooja Arora and Soumya Narula

Pregnant women undergo multiple physiological skin changes. Hyperpigmentation is one of the commonest changes seen in pregnant women; hence they are more likely to use cosmetics and other cosmeceutical products during pregnancy.[1] Melasma is the commonest pigmentation experienced during pregnancy. It presents with brownish macules over the cheeks and forehead.[2] Other forms of pigmentation include generalised hyperpigmentation of skin over the areola and linea nigra over the abdomen.

The Drugs and Cosmetics Act, 1940, India, defines a cosmetic as

> any article intended to be rubbed, poured, sprinkled or sprayed on, or introduced into, or otherwise applied to, the human body or any part thereof for cleansing, beautifying, promoting attractiveness, or altering the appearance, and includes any article intended for use as a component of cosmetic.[3]

Cosmeceuticals are products that are said to be somewhere between cosmetics and pharmaceuticals. The term was coined by Dr. Kligman. These products can be purchased without a prescription, and there are no regulations regarding their efficacy and safety profile. These products are not recognised by the United States Food and Drug Administration (US FDA) or the Central Drugs Standard Control Organization (CDSCO) of India.[4]

15.1 KEY ACTIVE INGREDIENTS IN COSMETICS AND COSMECEUTICALS

15.1.1 HYDROQUINONE

It is one the most widely used topical preparations for hyperpigmentation. It inhibits the conversion of dihydroxyphenylalanine to melanin by inhibiting tyrosinase. It is FDA Pregnancy Category C. Animal studies have shown that doses up to 300 mg/kg/day did not have any bearing on pregnancy outcome.[5] Human studies, too, have shown no increase in adverse effects in women who used topical hydroquinone during pregnancy in Senegal.[6] Still, it is advisable to reduce its usage during pregnancy. Hydroquinone is not a component of cosmeceuticals or cosmetics, but it is now available in multiple skin-lightening creams as an over-the-counter (OTC) product, which is alarming. The FDA has issued warning letters to companies that are manufacturing such products.[7]

15.1.2 AZELAIC ACID

It is a dicarboxylic acid which produces depigmentation by inhibition of the tyrosinase enzyme. It has a role in hyperpigmentation such as melasma, acne, and even antiaging properties.[8] It belongs to Pregnancy Category B; thus there has been no risk demonstrated in animal studies, but human studies are lacking. There is minimal systemic absorption through skin, and studies have indicated that it is safe during all trimesters.[9] Thus it can be used in pregnancy in limited amounts and over smaller surface areas. Cosmeceuticals generally contain concentrations up to 10%. Concentrations of 15–20% are available only by prescription.

DOI: 10.1201/9781003449690-15

15.1.3 KOJIC ACID

Kojic acid (5-hydroxy-2-hydroxymethyl-4-pyrone) is a compound derived from organisms such as *Aspergillus, Acetobacter*, and *Penicillium*.[10]

It is available in cosmeceuticals up to a concentration of 2%. It reduces tyrosinase activity by capturing the copper ions which are essential for its functioning and thus reducing melanin synthesis. It also acts as an antioxidant. Multiple animal studies have reported adverse outcomes in pregnant mice, but currently no human data is available. Hence, its safety profile in pregnancy is still dubious, and it is not recommended currently.[11]

15.1.4 SALICYLIC ACID

It is available in numerous OTC products for management of acne. It exerts its action by its keratolytic property. Concentrations ranging from 0.5–2% are approved in OTC products. It is categorised as FDA Pregnancy Category C. There is minimal systemic absorption, and hence it is considered safe in pregnancy. Thus it is advisable to apply minimal quantities without occlusion over smaller surface areas.[9]

15.1.5 RETINOIDS

Retinoids available in cosmeceutical products include retinol, retinaldehyde, retinyl palmitate, and acetate. Their role in hyperpigmentation is through decreasing melanosome transfer and inhibiting matrix metalloproteinase activation. They also enhance the penetration of other active agents by increasing the permeability. Retinol is the most active form and is available in concentrations up to 1%. Retinyl acetate and palmitate are the least effective ones, and retinaldehyde is available in concentrations of 0.05% in antiaging preparations.[10] No data is available regarding these agents available in cosmetics, but data is available on topical tretinoin. The systemic absorption of topical tretinoin is very low. There are a few reported cases of retinoid embropathy after topical tretinoin, use but a recent multivariate analysis reported that the usage of topical tretinoin in first trimester did not reveal any increased risk of malformations compared to the general population.[12] Hence it is still not recommended for use in pregnancy, but accidental exposure does not pose any greater risk to the embryo.

15.1.6 HYALURONIC ACID

It is a glycosaminoglycan which is present in various tissues and fluids in the body. It is available in cosmetic preparations in concentrations ranging from 0.2–1%. It has a beneficial role in skin hydration, as it has the ability to hold moisture (antiaging, particularly high molecular weight hyaluronic acid). This property of hyaluronic acid is also utilised in skin ageing products which incorporate low molecular weight hyaluronic acid. It is available in cosmetic preparations along with other ingredients such as plant extracts, amino acid, peptides, and probiotics and other active agents such as allantoin and lactic acid.[13]

It can be considered safe in pregnancy, as it is found abundantly in the body.

15.1.7 PANTHENOL

It has a role in skin hydration by reducing transepidermal water loss as well as accelerating wound healing; hence, it has a role in post-procedure skin care.[13] It is also considered safe during pregnancy, as it is a normal constituent of skin.

15.1.8 VITAMIN C

It is one of the most popular cosmeceuticals agents for pigmentation. It reduces melanin production by downregulating the tyrosinase enzyme via interaction with copper ions and has an antioxidant role. The most active and stable topical form available is L-ascorbic acid. It is considered safe in pregnancy.[14]

15.1.9 Arbutin

It is a derivative of hydroquinone and reduces melanin synthesis by inhibition of tyrosinase activity and prevents melanocyte maturation. Currently, no animal or human data is available regarding its effects on the reproductive system. Since its systemic absorption is very low and it is less toxic than hydroquinone, it is assumed to be safer in pregnancy.[15]

15.1.10 Nicotinamide

It is a derivative of vitamin B3. It reduces pigmentation by reversible inhibition of melanosome transfer from melanocytes to keratinocytes by action on keratinocyte factors. It is safe in concentrations up to 4%.[16] Since it is a derivative of niacin, that is, vitamin B3, it is considered safe to use in pregnancy. There has been no evidence of teratogenicity in pregnant females taking nicotinamide.[17]

15.1.11 Thiamidol

It is a resorcinyl thiazole derivate and hence a potent inhibitor of the tyrosine enzyme. In a few studies, it has been found to be more efficacious than hydroquinone in treatment of hyperpigmentation.[10] Currently, no data is available regarding its safety during pregnancy.

15.1.12 Alpha-Hydroxy Acids

It is a widely available cosmeceutical for hyperpigmentation and acne. Systemic absorption is dependent upon the vehicle used for the formulation; propylene glycol penetrates more than glycerin-based formulations. Animal studies have found it to be safe in doses up to 250 mg/kg/day, but no human data is available. It is FDA Category B and hence safe to use during pregnancy in concentrations of up to 10% and pH more than 3.5.[15]

15.1.13 Resorcinol

Resorcinol (4-n-butylresorcinol) is a potent inhibitor of melanin synthesis by directly inhibiting tyrosinase activity and its production. It is approved by the FDA as an OTC product for acne in concentrations of 2% along with sulphur.[18] No data is available regarding its safety in pregnancy.

15.1.14 Liquorice Root Extract

Major active agents of liquorice include glabridin and liquiritin. Glabridin inhibits the activity of tyrosinase enzyme, and liquiritin has an effect on melanosomes. It is available in concentrations of 2–4%.[10] Currently, no data is available regarding safety during pregnancy.

15.1.15 Soy

Soy exerts inhibitory effects on melanosome transfer via protease activated receptor 2, which reduces the phagocytosis of melanosomes by keratinocytes and thus reduces melanin transfer.[10] No data is available regarding systemic absorption of topical preparations and its safety during pregnancy.

15.1.16 Lipoic Acid

It is an antioxidant which is found in many antiaging products and has an inhibitory effect on tyrosinase enzyme and decreases the proliferation of melanocytes. The concentration in cosmeceutical products is very low (0.5–1%) and not found to have any toxic effects; hence, it is considered safe for use in pregnancy.[15]

15.1.17 FERULIC ACID

It acts as an antioxidant and acts along with vitamin C as a photoprotective agent. It inhibits the tyrosinase enzyme and reduces proliferation of melanocytes. The recommended cosmeceutical concentration is 0.5–1%. It is found to be safe during pregnancy.[19]

15.1.18 SUNSCREENS

Strict photoprotection remains the mainstay treatment for pigmentary disorders such as melasma.

Physical sunscreens are the most suitable ones for use in pregnancy, as they are not absorbed in circulation. Hence titanium dioxide– and iron oxide–containing sunscreens would be preferable.

Organic UV filters pose a risk due to their dermal absorption. Benzophenone-3 is a commonly used UV filter in chemical sunscreen and has shown adverse outcomes in animal studies done on pregnant mice. There was evidence of intrauterine growth restriction and increased female to male sex ratio.[20] No data is available in humans; hence, it is to be used with caution.

15.2 ADVERSE EFFECTS

Cosmetics may appear to be harmless products, but they can contain a variety of chemical substrates such as parabens, phthalates, phenols, and triclosan. Pregnancy is a crucial time where exposure to such endocrine-disrupting chemicals (EDCs) can have a significant impact on the growing embryo.

There have been reports of the presence of multiple ultraviolet filters and parabens in the umbilical cord blood and thus would be passed on to the growing embryo.[21]

15.2.1 ROUTES OF EXPOSURE OF COSMETICS

The varied routes of exposure to these molecules include direct contact with skin where they cross the barrier to reach circulation, contact with mucous membranes, and inhalation.

15.2.2 ENDOCRINE-DISRUPTING CHEMICALS

EDCs prevent binding of hormones to their receptors and block or activate natural hormone production as well their degradation. Bisphenol A acts mainly through the oestrogen receptors, as it is an oestrogen antagonist.[22] They produce genotoxic effects via modulation of epigenetic processes involving steroid hormones. It might lead to changes in DNA and hence mutation and even death. The epigenetic processes involved include DNA methylation, chromatic modification, and post-translational modification. EDCs have an impact on follicle formation and growth. They can induce apoptosis of ovarian cells, thus leading to infertility, premature ovarian failure, early menopause, and even polycystic ovarian disease.

15.2.3 SHORT-TERM EFFECTS

15.2.3.1 Small for Gestational Age and Preterm Birth

EDCs such as phalates can cross the placental barrier and in turn interfere with growth and development. This can lead to premature births and low birth weight babies. In a study conducted by Li H et al., they evaluated the outcomes in women who used cosmetic products during pregnancy compared to those who didn't. They found that more than 50% of their study participants used some cosmetics during pregnancy and there was an increased risk of the fetus being small for gestational age (SGA) in cosmetic users which increased with increasing frequency of cosmetic use during pregnancy. They postulated that it might be due to the exposure to toxic metals in the cosmetics such as mercury, arsenic, and cadmium that can affect the blood flow and nutrient supply to the fetus.[23]

TABLE 15.1

Topical Cosmetic and Cosmeceutical Ingredients, Their Mechanisms of Action, and Safety in Pregnancy

Topical Agent	Mechanism of Action	Safety in Pregnancy
Azelaic acid	Inhibition of tyrosinase enzyme Role in hyperpigmentation, acne, and antiaging	FDA Category B. Minimal systemic absorption. Safe in all trimesters
Kojic acid	Captures the copper ions essential for tyrosinase functioning	Safety data inadequate and hence not recommended in pregnancy
Hyaluronic acid	Role in skin hydration as it has the ability to hold moisture, antiaging properties	Considered safe in pregnancy
Salicylic acid	Keratolytic action has a role in acne	FDA Category C. Minimal systemic absorption, considered safe in pregnancy
Resorcinol	Inhibits tyrosinase activity and production	No data available
Retinoids	• Decrease melanosome transfer • Inhibit matrix metalloproteinase activation • Enhance the penetration of other active agents	Data is available regarding topical tretinoin, which has low systemic absorption. There are few reported cases of retinoid embryopathy Hence, it is not recommended for use in pregnancy, but accidental exposure does not pose any greater risk to the embryo
Ferulic acid	Inhibits tyrosinase enzyme and reduces proliferation of melanocytes	Safe in pregnancy
Panthenol	Hydration and wound-healing properties	Considered safe, as it is a natural constituent of skin
Vitamin C	Reduces melanin production by interacting with copper ions, antioxidant	Considered safe in pregnancy
Arbutin	Hydroquinone derivative which inhibits tyrosinase	Currently no animal or human data available. Systemic absorption is very low and less toxic than hydroquinone; it is assumed to be safer in pregnancy
Lipoic acid	Inhibitory effect on tyrosinase enzyme and decreases proliferation of melanocytes	Considered safe in pregnancy
Soy	Reduces phagocytosis of melanosomes by keratinocytes and thus reduces melanin transfer	No data available
Liquorice root extract	Inhibitory effect on tyrosinase enzyme	No data available
AHA	Role in hyperpigmentation and acne	FDA Category B, hence safe in pregnancy in concentrations of up to 10% and pH more than 3.5
Nicotinamide	Reversible inhibition of melanosome transfer from melanocytes to keratinocytes	Considered safe in pregnancy
Thiamidol	Resorcinyl thiazole derivative, inhibits tyrosinase enzyme	No data available regarding safety
Hydroquinone	Inhibits tyrosinase	Human studies have shown no increase in adverse effects, but still advisable to reduce use in pregnancy, as it is FDA Category C
Sunscreens	Photoprotective effect from ultra-violet radiation	Physical sunscreens are more suitable Chemical sunscreens to be used with caution

15.2.4 Long-Term Effects

15.2.4.1 Childhood Leukaemia

Exposure to carcinogenic products during pregnancy can affect the hematopoietic system and thus predispose to malignancies such as leukaemias. A case control study reported a greater risk of developing acute lymphoblastic leukaemia before the age of 2 years in children whose mothers used hair dyes and hair-straightening products in the first trimester of pregnancy.[24] Chemicals identified in hair dyes include persulphates, parabens, and phenols, all of which have been associated with haematological malignancies, osteosarcomas, and pulmonary adenocarcinomas.

15.2.4.2 Childhood Intelligence

Exposure to polyhydrocarbons in the prenatal period was associated with increased risk of neurodevelopmental abnormalities in children, which included disorders of attention, motor skills, and abnormal social behaviour. There was also an increased risk of developing depression in adulthood.[25]

15.2.4.3 Eczemas

The urinary concentrations of butyl benzyl phthalate in the prenatal period correlate with increased incidence of early-onset childhood eczemas.[26]

15.2.5 Changes in Usage of Cosmetics during Pregnancy

It was observed in a cross-sectional study that pregnant women consciously made changes in their choice of cosmetics, such as giving up nail polish, nail polish removers, and hair dyes altogether and reducing the frequency of usage of perfumes. Replacement of body lotions and shower gels with ones which harboured fewer chemicals was done. The only product whose frequency of usage increased was body lotions.[27]

15.3 CONCLUSION

There needs to be cautious use of cosmetics and cosmeceuticals during pregnancy. All health care providers who deal with pregnant women, including gynaecologists and dermatologists, need to be aware of the potential risks that are associated with the use of cosmetics and cosmeceuticals. Hence, it is their duty to counsel women to reduce the frequency as well as the quantity of cosmetics and personal care products during pregnancy as much as possible. Among the cosmeceuticals which can be considered safe include those such as azelaic acid, hyaluronic acid, and AHA in limited amounts (see Table 15.1). Products such as nail polish, nail polish removers, hair dyes, and makeup products can be completely eliminated. Those which are essential to maintain hygiene such as body washes and body lotions can be replaced by those which contain the least harmful chemicals.

REFERENCES

1. Erlandson M, Wertz MC, Rosenfeld E. Common skin conditions during pregnancy. *Am Fam Physician* 2023;107(2):152–158.
2. Kroumpouzos G, Cohen LM. Dermatoses of pregnancy. *J Am Acad Dermatol* 2001;45(1):1–22.
3. India Code. *National Informatics Centre*. India, available at www.indiacode.nic.in/handle/123456789/2409? view_type=browse&sam_handle=123456789/1362#:~:text=An%20Act%20to%20regulate%20 the,sale%20of%20drugs%20and%20cosmetics.&text=Notification%3A,dated%20the%2025th%20 August%2C%201941.
4. Pandey A, Jatana GK, Sonthalia S. Cosmeceuticals [Internet]. In: *StatPearls*. StatPearls Publishing; Treasure Island; 2023 [cited 2023 Sep 8], available at www.ncbi.nlm.nih.gov/books/NBK544223/
5. Krasavage WJ, Blacker AM, English JC, Murphy SJ. Hydroquinone: A developmental toxicity study in rats. *Fundam Appl Toxicol Off J Soc Toxicol* 1992;18(3):370–375.
6. Mahé A, Perret JL, Ly F, et al. The cosmetic use of skin-lightening products during pregnancy in Dakar, Senegal: A common and potentially hazardous practice. *Trans R Soc Trop Med Hyg* 2007;101(2):183–187.
7. *FDA Works to Protect Consumers from Potentially Harmful OTC Skin Lightening Products*. FDA [Internet]; 2022 [cited 2023 Sep 8], available at www.fda.gov/drugs/drug-safety-and-availability/ fda-works-protect-consumers-potentially-harmful-otc-skin-lightening-products

8. King S, Campbell J, Rowe R, et al. A systematic review to evaluate the efficacy of azelaic acid in the management of acne, rosacea, melasma and skin aging. *J Cosmet Dermatol* 2023;22:2650–2662 [cited 2023 Aug 29].

9. Murase JE, Heller MM, Butler DC. Safety of dermatologic medications in pregnancy and lactation: Part I. Pregnancy. *J Am Acad Dermatol* 2014;70(3):401.e1–401.e14.

10. Searle T, Al-Niaimi F, Ali FR. The top 10 cosmeceuticals for facial hyperpigmentation. *Dermatol Ther* 2020;33(6):e14095.

11. Burnett CL, Bergfeld WF, Belsito DV, et al. Final report of the safety assessment of Kojic acid as used in cosmetics. *Int J Toxicol* 2010;29(6 Suppl):244S–273S.

12. Panchaud A, Csajka C, Merlob P, et al. Pregnancy outcome following exposure to topical retinoids: A multicenter prospective study. *J Clin Pharmacol* 2012;52(12):1844–1851.

13. Juncan AM, Moisă DG, Santini A, et al. Advantages of hyaluronic acid and its combination with other bioactive ingredients in cosmeceuticals. *Molecules* 2021;26(15):4429.

14. Correia G, Magina S. Efficacy of topical vitamin C in melasma and photoaging: A systematic review. *J Cosmet Dermatol* 2023;22(7):1938–1945.

15. Putra IB, Jusuf NK, Dewi NK. Skin changes and safety profile of topical products during pregnancy. *J Clin Aesthetic Dermatol* 2022;15(2):49–57.

16. Wohlrab J, Kreft D. Niacinamide—Mechanisms of action and its topical use in dermatology. *Skin Pharmacol Physiol* 2014;27(6):311–315.

17. Knip M, Douek IF, Moore WP, et al. Safety of high-dose nicotinamide: A review. *Diabetologia* 2000;43(11):1337–1345.

18. *CFR—Code of Federal Regulations Title 21* [Internet]. [cited 2023 Aug 29], available at www.accessdata.fda.gov/scripts/cdrh/cfdocs/cfcfr/CFRSearch.cfm?fr=333.310&SearchTerm=resorcinol.

19. Zduńska K, Dana A, Kolodziejczak A, Rotsztejn H. Antioxidant properties of ferulic acid and its possible application. *Skin Pharmacol Physiol* 2018;31(6):332–336.

20. Santamaria CG, Meyer N, Schumacher A, et al. Dermal exposure to the UV filter benzophenone-3 during early pregnancy affects fetal growth and sex ratio of the progeny in mice. *Arch Toxicol* 2020;94(8):2847–2859.

21. Sunyer-Caldú A, Peiró A, Díaz M, et al. Target analysis and suspect screening of UV filters, parabens and other chemicals used in personal care products in human cord blood: Prenatal exposure by mother-fetus transfer. *Environ Int* 2023;173:107834.

22. Kowalczyk A, Wrzecińska M, Czerniawska-Piątkowska E, et al. Molecular consequences of the exposure to toxic substances for the endocrine system of females. *Biomed Pharmacother* 2022;155:113730.

23. Li H, Zheng J, Wang H, et al. Maternal cosmetics use during pregnancy and risks of adverse outcomes: A prospective cohort study. *Sci Rep* 2019;9(1):8030.

24. Couto AC, Ferreira JD, Rosa ACS, et al. Brazilian collaborative study group of infant acute leukemia. Pregnancy, maternal exposure to hair dyes and hair straightening cosmetics, and early age leukemia. *Chem Biol Interact* 2013;205(1):46–52.

25. Zhen H, Zhang F, Cheng H, et al. Association of polycyclic aromatic hydrocarbons exposure with child neurodevelopment and adult emotional disorders: A meta-analysis study. *Ecotoxicol Environ Saf* 2023;255:114770.

26. Just AC, Whyatt RM, Perzanowski MS, et al. Prenatal exposure to butylbenzyl phthalate and early eczema in an urban cohort. *Environ Health Perspect* 2012;120(10):1475–1480.

27. Marie C, Cabut S, Vendittelli F, Sauvant-Rochat MP. Changes in cosmetics use during pregnancy and risk perception by women. *Int J Environ Res Public Health* 2016;13(4):383.

16 Office Procedures during Pregnancy
Chemical Peels, Lasers, Physical Therapies

Richa Ojha Sharma

16.1 INTRODUCTION

It is not unusual for pregnant patients to approach dermatologists for treatment of skin changes that may be pre-existing or a result of pregnancy. Very often, they seek treatments for skin growths, melasma, striae and varicosities. In today's evolving times, it is no longer surprising when a pregnant woman desires cosmetic treatment for acne, pigmentation and signs of ageing. When it comes to performing office dermatology surgery or aesthetic procedures, it is crucial to adopt a cautious approach that incorporates a personalised evaluation of risks and benefits prior to planning and carrying out any procedure. This principle becomes particularly significant when dealing with pregnant patients, as the surgeon must take into account the wellbeing of both the woman and the fetus. Patient counselling acquires magnified importance when dealing with pregnant patients. All reported risks should be elaborated upon, and where there is lack of data for or against a procedure, it must be made clear to the patient. In such cases, it is best to defer the procedure to the second trimester unless absolutely urgent.

16.2 CHANGES DURING PREGNANCY

Pregnancy induces many physiological changes that should be taken into account before planning any procedure.[1,2]

1. *Circulatory changes* include an increase in blood volume, reduced haematocrit, heightened flushing and increased risk of thromboembolic episodes.
2. *There is greater melanocyte stimulation*, leading to a higher risk of post-procedure hyperpigmentation
3. *Altered wound healing* during pregnancy leads to an increased likelihood of hypertrophic scars and keloid formation.
4. *Hormonal fluctuations* during pregnancy can also result in skin manifestations such as melasma; hypertrichosis; striae; and the appearance of growths like acrochordons, angiomas, nevi and warts. These skin issues may increase in number, size or darkening during pregnancy.
5. *Moreover, pregnancy-induced immunosuppression* can be a contributing factor to multiple warts and may elevate the risk of bacterial and viral infections during and after procedures.[3]

Dermatologists must be aware of these pregnancy-related changes to provide appropriate care and management for pregnant patients undergoing skin treatments.

DOI: 10.1201/9781003449690-16   **203**

16.3   PLANNING PROCEDURES DURING PREGNANCY

The key points to be remembered when planning any procedure during pregnancy are:

1. When to treat?
2. What to treat?
3. How to treat?

16.3.1   WHEN TO TREAT

The timing of procedures is critical for the safety of the mother as well as the fetus. Procedures are avoided during the first trimester as it is the time for organogenesis and also a high-risk period for miscarriages. On the other hand, procedures done during the last trimester carry the risk of inducing preterm labour. Therefore, the second trimester—between 13 and 28 weeks—offers a window of opportunity for conducting the necessary procedures.[4]

16.3.2   WHAT TO TREAT

A biopsy or excision of a frank or suspicious malignant lesion is to be treated on priority. A friable pyogenic granuloma must also be treated immediately. Excision of non-malignant growths and cosmetic procedures are not on the priority list of treatments to be conducted during pregnancy, and since there is lack of controlled data, these procedures are better deferred until after the pregnancy. However, a judgement call can be made after due discussion with the patient, and if agreed upon, such procedures may be conducted during the second trimester.[1]

Office procedures during pregnancy can be broadly categorised into two types:

1. Minor dermatologic procedures
2. Procedures for aesthetic concerns

Table 16.1 shows the recommendations for procedures during pregnancy.

16.3.2.1   Minor Dermatologic Procedures

Procedures such as electrocautery, cryotherapy, laser treatments, intralesional steroid and minor surgical procedures are often conducted for dermatologic complaints during pregnancy such as acrochordons, seborrheic keratoses, pyogenic granulomas, haemangiomas, keloids and nevi. If a pregnant patient presents with a suspicious lesion, showing signs like bleeding, growth in size or discolouration, it is essential to perform a biopsy to confirm the suspicion, followed by the excision per guidelines. Vascular tumours such as pyogenic granulomas and glomus tumours enlarge under the hormonal effects of pregnancy. They can pose a danger of imminent bleeding and hence must be dealt with actively.

1. *Minor Surgical Procedures*
   - Biopsy, snipping, shaving and TCA cauterisation can be safely performed during pregnancy.[5]
2. *Electrocautery/Radiofrequency(RF)/Cryotherapy*
   - Electrocautery, radiofrequency and cryotherapy are safe ablative therapies for the woman and the fetus. However, the smoke plume emanating during these procedures can be mutagenic. Therefore, a smoke evacuator is preferred for reducing smoke exposure.[6] Cryotherapy may be the preferred modality of treatment of warts during pregnancy, owing to its safety.[3]
3. *Ablation Using CO_2 Laser*
   - This is considered effective and safe during pregnancy. The added benefit of coagulation during ablation minimises blood loss. However, care should be taken to minimise exposure to the smoke plume.[7]

TABLE 16.1

Recommendations and Safety Profiles for Office Procedures during Pregnancy

Type of Procedure	Name of Procedure	Recommendation
Minor dermatologic procedures	Minor surgeries	Safe
	Electrocautery/RF/Cryotherapy	Safe. Smoke evacuation advised to prevent mutagenic effects of plume
	CO_2 laser ablation	Safe. Smoke evacuation advised to prevent mutagenic effects of plume
	PDL	Safe
	Intralesional steroid injection	Not recommended
	Vitiligo surgery	Not recommended
	Liposuction/Fat grafting	Not recommended
Procedures for aesthetic concerns	Chemical peels	SA—Use should be limited to small areas
		GA—Safe
		LA—Use with caution
		TCA—Use should be limited to small areas
	Botulinum toxin	Not recommended due to paucity of safety data
	Dermal fillers	Relative contraindication
	Lasers and light	Not advised for aesthetic concerns
	PRP	Not recommended
	Sclerotherapy	Equivocal opinions. Best to delay till termination of pregnancy
	Skin-tightening treatments	Not recommended
	Thread lifts	Risky due to higher incidence of complications
	Miscellaneous	Microdermabrasion, cryotherapy and comedone extraction—Safe

4. *Pulsed Dye Laser (PDL)*
   - PDL (585 nm) may be used for treatment of vascular lesions such as pyogenic granulomas. Literature suggests a good safety profile for PDL in pregnancy except for minimal side effects like mild erythema and pain.[8]

5. *Intralesional Steroid Injections*
   - Corticosteroids are Category C drugs and carry the risk of causing hypoadrenalism, cleft lip and cleft palate in the exposed fetus. Hence, intralesional steroids for hypertrophic scars, keloids and alopecia areata are not recommended until the benefits outweigh the risk.[9]

6. *Vitiligo Surgery*
   - Since the course of vitiligo is unpredictable during pregnancy, it is not advisable to perform surgical procedures for vitiligo during this time.[3]

7. *Liposuction and Fat Grafting*
   - As there is a higher risk of fat embolism and because these procedures can compromise the nutritional supply to the fetus by impacting the fat reserves, these procedures must not be performed during gestation.[10]

16.3.2.2 Procedures for Aesthetic Concerns

A number of aesthetic concerns may arise in the course of pregnancy due to hormonal, circulatory and immunological changes. Melasma, striae distensae, varicose veins and spider angiomas may appear during pregnancy. With the increasing age of pregnant patients in current times, many women seek antiaging treatments too.

Other than the fact that complications arising from any procedure may be more difficult to treat during pregnancy, it is also to be noted that pregnant women are more prone to developing delayed healing, keloid and post-inflammatory hyperpigmentation. Hence, the treating dermatologist must proceed with extreme caution when opting for elective procedures.

16.3.2.2.1 Chemical Peels

- *Salicylic Acid (SA)*—This beta hydroxy acid is a commonly used peeling agent. However, up to 25% systemic absorption has been reported when SA is used over large surface areas.[10] It is therefore recommended that SA use be avoided or limited to small surface areas during pregnancy.
- *Glycolic Acid (GA)*—The use of this alpha hydroxy acid during pregnancy is considered safe due to minimal dermal penetration.[11]
- *Lactic Acid (LA)*—No fetal damage was observed in anecdotal reports on using LA for treating gestational acne. Additionally, LA has minimal dermal penetration. Hence, it may be used in pregnancy with caution.[12]
- *Trichloroacetic Acid (TCA)*—TCA is used safely for genital condyloma. However, while using it as a chemical peel, caution should be exercised around mucosal areas to avoid the risk of systemic absorption. Large areas must not be treated with TCA.

16.3.2.2.2 Botulinum Toxin

A literature search reveals a number of reports of the use of botulinum toxin for non-aesthetic indications such as cervical dystonia, achalasia and refractory migraine. No adverse outcomes or fetal abnormalities have been reported with such use.[13,14] Inadvertent botulinum toxin injections for cosmetic injections in pregnant patients has also been reported. Morgan et al. conducted a survey of 900 physicians and found 16 cases of injecting botulinum toxin by aesthetic physicians unaware of the pregnant status of the patients. Of these, only one patient had a miscarriage after the injection. This patient had a history of previous spontaneous abortions too.[15]

Data suggests that botulinum toxin does not get absorbed systemically in significant amounts. Moreover, the toxin molecular size inhibits it from crossing the placental barrier.[16] Additionally, the usual doses for cosmetic concerns are considered safe during pregnancy. In view of all of this evidence, Botox use for cosmetic concerns would appear to be a safe choice. However, like all other aesthetic procedures during pregnancy, the patient must be adequately cautioned regarding the paucity of completely conclusive data regarding its safety in pregnancy and the absence of any such clinical trials. Patients must be dissuaded from opting for botulinum toxin procedures until such time as clear-cut safety is established.

16.3.2.2.3 Dermal Fillers

Theoretically, dermal fillers containing hyaluronic acid (HA) should be safe, as they have the same composition as human HA. However, no studies or reports are available to safely recommend these injections. Lidocaine in fillers also carries risks, as detailed later in this chapter. Undesired effects such as bruising and infections that are seen in non-pregnant patients are also to be considered. It may be more difficult to manage such complications during pregnancy. Hence, pregnancy is considered a relative contraindication for dermal fillers.[12]

16.3.2.2.4 Laser and Light Therapy

No studies detail the use of lasers and light therapies for aesthetic concerns during pregnancy. However, various reports are available about the use of these treatments for non-aesthetic conditions. The use of CO_2 ablative and ND Yag laser for condylomas,[17,18] pulsed dye laser for urolithiasis and other lasers for acne and pyogenic granulomas[10] have shown them to be safe during pregnancy.

No safety data is available for the use of IPL for hair removal. Moreover, the benefit of any such treatment would be minimal, as hormonal stimulation during pregnancy induces hair growth.[19]

Electrolysis for hair removal is contraindicated, as there is a theoretical concern amniotic fluid is a conductor of galvanic current.[12]

In the absence of reliable safety data, lasers and light therapies must not be used for cosmetic concerns.

16.3.2.2.5 Platelet-Rich Plasma

There are no clinical studies involving the use of platelet-rich plasma (PRP) treatment for hair loss during pregnancy. With no real benefit to be attained with this treatment because telogen sets in after delivery, leading to hair loss and thinning, and the added risk of infections, PRP is best avoided during pregnancy.[3]

16.3.2.2.6 Sclerotherapy

The high incidence of varicose veins during pregnancy might lead a physician to consider sclerotherapy during pregnancy. However it is to be noted that varicosities spontaneously resolve after pregnancy. As far as safety data is concerned, a literature search reveals contradicting results. Rabe et al. disapprove of sclerosant use, as they claim that sclerosants can cross the placenta.[20] On the other hand, Abramowitz[21] and Reich-Schupke et al.[22] observed no adverse impact of sclerosant use during gestation. As such, with such contrasting views, it would be better to delay the procedure until after child birth.

16.3.2.2.7 Skin-Tightening Treatments

The use of radiofrequency and high-intensity focused ultrasound (HIFU) during pregnancy is not recommended, as there is not enough data to verify their safety.

16.3.2.2.8 Thread Lifts

Theoretically there is no risk involved with inserting absorbable sutures in the dermis for facelift and collagen generation. However, the chances of complications such as infections and a higher risk of hypertrophic scarring during pregnancy could make the procedure risky.

16.3.2.2.9 Miscellaneous

Microdermabrasion, cryotherapy and comedone extraction are considered safe. In fact, cryotherapy may be considered the first option for genital wart removal during pregnancy.[5]

16.3.3 How to Treat

Once "when to treat" and "what to treat" have been decided, "how to treat" needs to be considered. Choosing safe agents for anaesthesia, analgesia, antisepsis and antibacterial action is important during pregnancy.

16.3.3.1 Injectable Anaesthesia

Lidocaine is a Category B drug and is the most commonly used drug during pregnancy. The fetus can metabolise lidocaine that crosses the placental barrier.[23] Inadvertent arterial injection can cause fetal cardiac and central nervous system toxicity. Dermal fillers have premixed lidocaine that are far below the toxic doses. Moreover, for most dermatologic office procedures, the dose of lidocaine is well below the recommended maximum subcutaneous dosage of 4.5 mg/kg.[10]

Lidocaine used with epinephrine is preferable, as the vasoconstriction that epinephrine induces limits the absorption and spread of lidocaine.[24]

16.3.3.2 Topical Anaesthesia

Topical anaesthetics such as EMLA cream (lidocaine 2.5% + prilocaine 2.5%) are safer than injectable ones, but some case reports indicate that prilocaine in high doses carries a risk of methemoglobinemia in the fetus, because of which lidocaine-prilocaine (both Cat B) cream should be used in moderation.[25] During pregnancy, it is advisable to avoid occlusion of these creams. There can be increased risk of absorption and irritation when topical anaesthetic creams are used on mucosal surfaces as well as around the eyes. Use near periocular and mucosal surfaces should therefore be avoided.[26]

16.3.3.3 Post-Procedure Care

Most minor dermatologic procedures require application of antibiotics for a few days after the procedure. Very rarely, systemic antibiotics may be needed. Pregnancy Category A and B drugs must be chosen to ensure safety of the fetus. Penicillin and macrolide groups of antibiotics may be prescribed safely. Fluroquinolones, tetracyclines, aminoglycosides and sulphonamides must not be prescribed, as they are unsafe for the fetus.

Pre- and post-procedure antisepsis can be performed using alcohol and chlorhexidine. Povidone iodine has been shown to cause fetal hypothyroidism after percutaneous absorption and hence must be avoided. Hexachlorophene use must be avoided, as it has been reported to cause fetal central nervous system toxicity.[1]

Post-procedure analgesia may be ensured with acetaminophen for a limited period. Ibugesic must be avoided in the third trimester due to increased risk of bleeding. Salicylates are contraindicated during pregnancy due to the risk of birth defects.[4]

16.4 CONCLUSION

Based on the available evidence, minor surgical procedures, as well as a few cosmetic procedures, are deemed safe. But for many others, it is prudent to wait until termination of pregnancy. Elective procedures are better rescheduled not just because of lack of safety data but also because complications during pregnancy can be more severe and more difficult to handle than in non-pregnant women.

REFERENCES

1. Sweeney SM, Maloney ME. Pregnancy and dermatologic surgery. *Dermatol Clin.* 2006;24(2):205–214.
2. Richards KA, Stasko T. Dermatologic surgery and the pregnant patient. *Dermatol Surg.* 2002;28(3):248–256.
3. Garg AM, Mysore V. Dermatologic and cosmetic procedures in pregnancy. *J Cutan Aesthet Surg.* 2022;15(2):108–117. http://doi.org/10.4103/JCAS.JCAS_226_20.
4. Gontijo G, Gualberto GV, Brito Madureira NA. Dermatologic surgery and cosmetic procedures during pregnancy—A systematic review. *Surg Cosmet Dermatol.* 2010;2(1):39–45.
5. Manela-Azulay M, Issa MCA, Tamler C, et al. Procedimentos estéticos. In: Costa A, Alves G, Azulay L, editores. *Dermatologia e gravidez.* Rio de Janeiro: Elsevier; 2009, pp. 449–453.
6. Gatti JE, Bryant CJ, Noone RB, Murphy JB. The mutagenicity of electrocautery smoke. *Plast Reconstr Surg.* 1992;89:781–784; discussion 785–786.
7. Hsu CK, Lee JYY, Yu CH, et al. Lip verrucous carcinoma in a pregnant woman successfully treated with carbon dioxide laser surgery. *Br J Dermatol.* 2007;157(4):813–815.
8. Erceg A, Bovenschen HJ, van de Kerkhof PC, et al. Efficacy and safety of pulsed dye laser treatment for cutaneous discoid lupus erythematosus. *J Am Acad Dermatol.* 2009;60:626–632
9. Triamcinolone use during pregnancy [Internet]. *Drugs.com*; 2019. Last accessed on 2023 June 25, available at www.drugs.com/pregnancy/triamcinolone.html
10. Lee KC, Korgavkar K, Dufresne RG, et al. 2nd Safety of cosmetic dermatologic procedures during pregnancy. *Dermatol Surg.* 2013;39:1573–1586.
11. Andersen FE. Final report on the safety assessment of glycolic acid, ammonium, calcium, potassium, and sodium glycolates, methyl, ethyl, propyl, and butyl glycolates, and lactic acid, ammonium, calcium, potassium, sodium, and TEA-lactates, methyl, ethyl, isopropyl, and butyl lactates, and lauryl, myristyl, and cetyl lactates. *Int J Toxicol.* 1998;17:1–241.
12. Trivedi MK, Kroumpouzos G, Murase JE. A review of the safety of cosmetic procedures during pregnancy and lactation. *Int J Womens Dermatol.* 2017;3:6–10.
13. Wataganara T, Leelakusolvong S, Sunsaneevithayakul P, et al. Treatment of severe achalasia during pregnancy with esophagoscopic injection of botulinum toxin A: A case report. *J Perinatol.* 2009;29:637–639.

14. Bodkin CL, Maurer KB, Wszolek ZK. Botulinum toxin type A therapy during pregnancy. *Mov Disord.* 2005;20:1081–1082.
15. Morgan JC, Iyer SS, Moser ET, et al. Botulinum toxin A during pregnancy: A survey of treating physicians. *J Neurol Neurosurg Psychiatry.* 2006;77:117–119.
16. Tan M, Kim E, Koren G, Bozzo P. Botulinum toxin type A in pregnancy. *Can Fam Physician.* 2013;59:1183–1184.
17. Laser Gay C, Terzibachian JJ, Gabelle C, et al. Carbon dioxide laser vaporization of genital condyloma in pregnancy. *Gynecol Obstet Fertil.* 2003;31:214–219.
18. Buzalov S, Khristakieva E. The treatment of neglected cases of condylomata acuminata in pregnant women with the Nd: Yag laser. *Akush Ginekol (Sofiia)* 1994;34:38–39.
19. Nussbaum R, Benedetto AV. Cosmetic aspects of pregnancy. *Clin Dermatol.* 2006;24:133–141.
20. Rabe E, Pannier F. Sclerotherapy of varicose veins with polidocanol based on the guidelines of the German Society of Phlebology. *Dermatol Surg.* 2010;36:968–975.
21. Abramowtiz I. The treatment of varicose veins in pregnancy by empty vein compressive sclerotherapy. *S Afr Med J.* 1973;47:607–610.
22. Reich-Schupke S, Leiste A, Moritz R, et al. Sclerotherapy in an undetected pregnancy—a catastrophe? *Vasa.* 2012;41:243–247.
23. Kuhnert BR, Knapp DR, Kuhnert PM, et al. Maternal, fetal, and neonatal metabolism of lidocaine. *Clin Pharmacol Ther.* 1979;26:213–220.
24. Lolis M, Dunbar SW, Goldberg DJ, et al. Patient safety in procedural dermatology: Part II. Safety related to cosmetic procedures. *J Am Acad Dermatol* 2015;73:15–24.
25. Chen BK, Eichenfield LF. Pediatric anesthesia in dermatologic surgery: When hand-holding is not enough Dermatol Surg. 2001;27:1010–1018.
26. Friedman PM, Mafong EA, Friedman ES, et al. Topical anesthetics update: EMLA and beyond. *Dermatol Surg.* 2001;27:1019–1026.

17 Approach for Pregnant Women with Skin Lesions

Shalini Warman and Swati Agrawal

17.1 INTRODUCTION

Pregnancy is associated with several normal physiological skin changes and also pregnancy-specific dermatoses. Many skin and hair changes, including pigmentary, vascular, hair development, and nail and connective tissue alterations, can occur in pregnant women. It is critical to understand which dermatoses may be harmful to both the mother and the fetus. There are many skin conditions which flare in pregnancy and may require drug and dose modification for feto-maternal safety. In skin diseases like pemphigoid gestationis, pemphigus vulgaris, and systemic lupus erythematosus (SLE), there is passive transfer of maternal antibodies, which may lead to neonatal involvement. Evaluation of pigmented lesions during pregnancy might be challenging due to hormone-induced alterations in pigment synthesis. Primary care physicians and obstetricians have a crucial role to play in the identification and management of pregnant dermatoses because general dermatology may not always be easily accessible in isolated areas.

17.2 CLASSIFICATION OF SKIN DISORDERS IN PREGNANCY

Skin lesions in pregnancy may be classified as follows.[1]

1. **Physiological changes of pregnancy**
   a. *Striae gravidarum (stretch marks)*: Striae appear as pink-purple, atrophic lines or bands on the abdomen, buttocks, breasts, thighs, or arms.
   b. *Increased skin pigmentation*: There is darkening of the areola, nipple, and genital skin. The darkening of the linea alba forms the linea nigra. Melasma occurs in approximately 70% of pregnant women and is more pronounced in those with dark skin.
   c. *Hair and nail changes*: Some degree of hirsutism occurs on the face, limbs, and backin some women due to prolonged active (anagen) phase of hair growth. In the postpartum period, increased shedding of hair occurs because the scalp hair enters a prolonged resting (telogen) phase of hair growth. Faster nail growth, increased nail brittleness, appearance of transverse grooves, oncholysis, and subungual keratosis occur in pregnancy.
   d. *Vascular changes*: Changes in oestrogen production during pregnancy lead to dilation, instability, congestion, and proliferation of the blood vessels. Spider telangiectasias, palmar erythema, saphenous, vulvar, or hemorrhoidal varicosities are the common changes. Vascular changes together with an increased blood volume leads to non-pitting oedema of the face, eyelids, and extremities.
2. **Dermatological conditions modified by pregnancy**
   a. *Atopic eczema*: May worsen, improve, or stay the same.
   b. *Psoriasis*: It is likely to improve during pregnancy, though in 10–20%, it may worsen.[2] Generalised pustular psoriasis is more common in pregnancy.
   c. *Acne*: Often improves in late pregnancy.
   d. *Perioral dermatitis*.

DOI: 10.1201/9781003449690-17

  e. *Pyogenic granuloma.*

  f. *Lupus erythematosus*: Cutaneous lupus does not appear to be affected. Exacerbations of systemic lupus erythematosus can be serious and can affect the fetus (neonatal lupus).

 3. **Dermatological conditions specific to pregnancy**: These are also known as true dermatoses of pregnancy, and they occur specifically during or immediately after pregnancy and are not found in non-pregnant state. These include:

  a. Atopic eruption of pregnancy (AEP): The term encompasses atopic eczema in pregnancy, prurigo of pregnancy, and pruritic folliculitis of pregnancy.[3]

  b. Pruritic urticarial papules and plaques of pregnancy (PUPPP).

  c. Intrahepatic cholestasis of pregnancy (IHCP).

  d. Pemphigoid gestationis (PG).

  e. Impetigo herpetiformis.

AEP occurs in the first or the second trimester, and in the majority of cases, the lesions are on the flexure atopic sites. PUPP usually occurs in the third trimester, appears as vesicles or papules along the abdominal striae, and has a characteristic periumbilical sparing. IHCP is characterised by itching appearing in the third trimester in the absence of skin lesions and with raised serum bile acids. Pemphigoid gestationis is an autoimmune disease occurring in the third trimester as vesiculobullous lesions involving the umbilical region. Impetigo herpetiformis occurs in the third trimester as erythematous patches in the flexural regions.

17.3 PRECONCEPTIONAL CARE AND COUNSELLING

Behavioural counselling in the preconceptional period reduces the risk of re-infection and new incidence of sexually transmitted infections (STIs). This can thus reduce the transmission of infection to the newborn and improve the health of the woman during pregnancy and postpartum. Knowledge about safe sexual practices, cervical cancer prevention, and screening should be given. Universal preconception screening should be offered for HIV, syphilis and hepatitis B.[4] Targeted preconception screening should be offered to women who are at high risk for chlamydia, gonorrhoea, tuberculosis, and toxoplasmosis.[4] Effective and appropriate contraception should be offered to people living with HIV. Medications being used for SLE should be reviewed before and during pregnancy. Teratogenic drugs should be avoided in women planning a pregnancy. IHCP and pemphigoid gestationis may recur in subsequent pregnancies, and these women need appropriate preconceptional counselling. Oral contraceptive pills (OCPs) containing oestrogen should be used with caution and at a low dose in women with a history of IHCP. Cholestasis can develop in these women with exogeneous oestrogen use outside of pregnancy. Also, women developing cholestasis with OCP use should be monitored for IHCP during pregnancy. Women with a history of pemphigoid gestationis may experience flares with the use of oral contraceptives in the postpartum period and with menstruation in some. These women should be informed that the condition may occur earlier and may be more serious in subsequent pregnancies.

17.4 HISTORY

A detailed history may give insight into the cause and severity of illness.

17.4.1 History of Present Illness

Pregnant women with skin disease may present with a wide variety of symptoms. The key dermatological symptoms are rash, skin lesions, pain, itching, bleeding, discharge, and blisters and associated systemic symptoms like fever, malaise, weight loss, and arthralgias.

Important characteristics of rashes to be asked about are where and when it appeared, the pattern of spread, timing of rash, change in morphology of lesions, associated pain, pruritis, or any other associated symptom.

Pruritus is the main symptom of pregnancy-specific dermatological diseases but may also occur with other diseases or even physiological changes in pregnancy. The causes of pruritis in pregnancy are given in Table 17.1. The specific points in the history about pruritis are:

1. *Time of presentation*: AEP usually presents in the first trimester, whereas PUPP, PG, and ICHP manifest in the late second or third trimester.
2. *Site* (see Table 17.3).
3. *Fever*: The occurrence of pruritis with fever and rash may indicate an infective cause or a drug reaction (see Table 17.2).
4. *Presence of skin lesions*: IHCP is characterised by pruritis in the absence of skin lesions, though secondary skin lesions may be a consequence of itching.
5. *Seasonal variation or effect of weather*: Miliaria (heat rash) appears in hot weather.
6. *History of jaundice*: Yellowish discoloration of skin, urine, or stools may occur in liver disorders. Pruritis precedes jaundice in IHCP.
7. *History of insect bite*: An insect bite leads to rash.
8. *History of allergy* to soaps, cloth material, and cosmetics should also be asked.
9. *Worm infestation* may cause a rash; therefore, a history of passage of worms in stools needs to be asked.
10. *History of upper abdominal pain*: Pre-eclampsia, IHCP, acute fatty liver of pregnancy, and biliary obstruction (gallstones) may cause upper abdominal pain.

Pruritis of IHCP may be mild, but in severe cases it may cause sleep deprivation and psychological suffering in the mother. The symptom commonly occurs in the third trimester, is more severe in evening, and most commonly occurs in the palms and the soles. Excoriation marks and abrasions may occur secondary to itching. Other symptoms of cholestasis like dark and pale stools may also occur.

It is important to rule out other causes of itching.

History of fever and its onset, type of fever, and type of associated rash are important (Table 17.2).

Joint pain with rash may indicate arthritis. Rash and conjunctivitis may indicate measles or toxic shock syndrome. Fever and rash with abdominal pain may indicate typhoid fever, scarlet fever, or systemic lupus erythematosus (SLE).

17.4.2 Past History

Past medical history is important, especially about any immune compromise, valvular heart disease (warfarin-induced skin necrosis), diabetes milletus, renal disease, or splenectomy. Diabetic dermopathy may present with acanthosis nigricans, pigmented pre-tibial patches, and

---

TABLE 17.1

Causes of Pruritis in Pregnancy

Pregnancy Specific	Pregnancy Nonspecific	Systemic Causes
• Atopic eruption of pregnancy	• Xerosis	• Uraemia
• PUPPP	• Atopic dermatitis	• Polychythemia vera
• IHCP	• Allergic contact dermatitis	• Cholestasis
• Pemphigoid gestationis	• Scabies or lice	• Hyperthyroidism
• Impetigo herpetiformis		• Cutaneous T-cell lymphoma
		• HIV infection

TABLE 17.2

Differential Diagnosis of Fever with Rash

Fever with Local Rash	Fever with Generalised Rash
1. *With prominent red, hot skin*: Cellulitis, erysipelas, erythema nodosum	1. *With redness*: Drug hypersensitivity syndrome, erythema marginatum, erythroderma; infections like arbovirus, rubella
2. *With prominent blisters and erosions*: Herpes simplex, herpes zoster, impetigo	2. *With blisters and erosions*: Acute febrile neutrophilic dermatosis, bullous drug eruptions, Stevens–Johnson syndrome, varicella
3. *With pustules*: Folliculitis, furunculosis	3. *With pustules/crusts*: Acute generalised exanthematous pustulosis, eczema herpeticum, late stage of varicella
4. *With purple/black areas*: Ecthyma, meningococcal disease, necrotising fasciitis, vascular emboli	4. *With widespread purple/black areas*: Purpura fulminans, vasculitis

hyperpigmented lesions over other bony prominences. Chronic renal disease may be associated with dry skin (xerosis), generalised pruritis, and pigmented changes. Patients who had their spleen removed are prone to histoplasmosis, which may be associated with skin rash. A thorough medication history should be obtained including immunisations, use of over-the-counter preparations, past and present medications, and any history of adverse effects related to any substance. The most common drug reaction is urticaria. Drugs like corticosteroids, lithium, and anticoagulants may cause skin rash. Certain antipsychotic drugs, tetracyclines, sulpha antibiotics, antiepileptics (carbamazepine, hydantoins), and allopurinol cause erythematous maculopapular eruptions. The HIV status is to be determined. HIV is a STI and may predispose to many infectious, non-infectious, and neoplastic diseases and their cutaneous manifestations.

History of contraceptive use: In some pregnant women, chloasma may occur with history of use of combined oral contraceptives (COCs) when not protected from sunlight.[5] The skin disorders that have been found to be more prevalent in women taking COCs include erythema nodosum, accelerated systemic lupus erythematosus, porphyria cutanea tarda, herpes gestationis, spider naevus, and telangiectasia.[5] Pemphigoid gestationis may relapse with COC use.[6]

17.4.3   Social History

It should include questions regarding intravenous drug use, travel, occupational exposures, contact with animals or ill individuals, ingestion of specific foods, and sexual practices. Intravenous drug abuse causes skin, venous, and lymphatic system damage because of frequent puncture of skin and low-grade infection. This may lead to lymphedema, enlarged lymph nodes, hyperpigmentation of skin, and scarring. During travel, exposure to freshwater, marine water, insects, animals, and plants may lead to skin lesions. Fever with rash in returned travellers is most commonly due to viral infections like chikungunya, dengue, and Zika virus. Bacterial infections like meningococcemia and rickettsioses may also be associated with travel. Occupational skin diseases include contact dermatitis, and it occurs at the site of contact. Immediate red blisters or burns are caused by severe skin irritants, and eczematous skin changes are produced by weaker irritants. Proteins found in an animal's saliva, urine, or skin cells may lead to allergic dermatitis. Ringworm and hookworm infections can be passed from pets to humans and can manifest as skin rash. Contact with a cat's faeces can lead to toxoplasmosis, which can manifest as roseola, erythema multiforme, or papular urticaria. Genital herpes and syphilis are STIs and are common causes of genital ulcers. Early onset of sexual activity and pre-existing bacterial vaginosis increase the risk of genital herpes in pregnancy. Scabies may infect many members of the same family. Family history of liver dysfunctions during pregnancy in other female relatives requires inclusion because of the role of genetics in pathophysiology of IHCP.

The spouse should also be questioned about the history of any past or present STIs (urethral discharge, genital ulcers, number of sexual partners).

17.4.4 Obstetric History

The last menstrual period is to be asked about, and the gestational age as well as the obstetric score needs to be calculated. Dermatoses in pregnancy are common in late pregnancy and those with twin or multiple gestations. Atopic eruptions of pregnancy occur in the first or second trimester. IHCP and pemphigoid gestationis may recur in subsequent pregnancies with a history of prematurity or stillbirths in previous pregnancies. Pemphigoid gestationis may lead to urticarial, vesicular, or bullous lesions of the newborn. It may also lead to premature deliveries of small for gestational age fetuses.

17.4.5 Other Details of the Ongoing Pregnancy

The woman needs to be asked about her immunisation status, fetal movements, sleep, appetite, bladder and bowel habits, and diet.

17.5 EXAMINATION

- Vitals: Blood pressure is high in pre-eclampsia and its associated complications like HELLP syndrome.
- Temperature is measured: The woman may be febrile (causes of fever with rash, as discussed).
- Enlarged lymph nodes may be palpable in some viral infections like chicken pox, shingles, herpes simplex, and rubella or in systemic conditions like SLE.
- On examination, the type of skin lesion should be described (see Table 17.3).
- Any other type of skin lesion and variations may be noted.
- The most common oral mucosal changes observed in a pregnant woman are gingival hyperaemia and oedema, gingivitis, and pyogenic granuloma. The oral mucosa can be affected by impetigo herpetiformis and gestational pemphigoid in exceptional cases.[7]

TABLE 17.3
Types of Skin Lesions and Their Specific Location

Disease	Type of Skin Lesion	Location	Remarks
PUPP	Urticarial papules and plaques	Initially within abdominal striae and later spreading to extremities	Periumbilical sparing
Pemphigoid gestationis	Vesiculobullous eruptions	Starting on abdomen and later spreading to extremities	Periumbilical involvement
Atopic eruption of pregnancy	Eczematous lesions, excoriated papules and nodules	Flexural surfaces, extremities, trunk, extensor surfaces of limbs and trunk	
IHCP	No primary lesions		Secondary excoriations due to scratching
Impetigo herpetiformis	Erythematous patches with marginal grouped sterile pustules	Appear primarily in flexural regions	Centrifugal extension leads to development of erosion and crust, and later they may even become impetiginised

Skin lesions in antiphospholipid syndrome (APS) may include livido reticularis, livido vasculitis, cutaneous ulceration and necrosis, erythematous macules, purpura, and ecchymoses.[8] Iron deficiency anaemia in pregnant women leads to pallor of skin and mucous membranes, koilonychia, increased fragility of nails, angular stomatitis, filiform appearance of tongue papillae, or their atrophy. Leg ulcers may develop in sickle cell anaemia and should be kept as a differential diagnosis. The ankle region, including the lateral and medial malleoli, is the most common site of occurrence of these ulcers. Purpura in pregnancy may occur in conditions like immune thrombocytopenic purpura (ITP), thrombotic thrombocytopenic purpura (TTP), or HELLP syndrome (a complication of pre-eclampsia). Bilateral pedal oedema is a physiological condition in pregnancy, but it may also occur in pre-eclampsia (HELLP). Unilateral pedal oedema may occur in chronic lymphedema or chronic venous insufficiency and is associated with skin changes like hyperkeratosis and brown hemosiderin deposits, respectively.

Herpes simplex virus-1 (HSV-1) mostly causes oro-facial lesions and is typically found in the fifth cranial nerve (trigeminal nerve). HSV-2 causes genital herpes and is most commonly found in the lumbosacral ganglia. HSV infection may present as macular or papular lesions of the skin and the mucous membranes which progresses to vesicles and pustules. The lesions are painful and may cause local swelling of the vulva. Syphilis is characterised by sores or painless ulcers (chancres) in the primary stage and widespread muco-cutaneous lesions, patchy alopecia, and condylomata lata in the second stage. Gummas (granulomatous lesions) appear in tertiary syphilis.

- *Sterile per-speculum examination*: After a complete examination of the female external genitalia, a per-speculum examination is done. Any signs of infection (abnormal discharge, redness, bleeding on touch) should be noted. If any abnormal discharge is suspected, swabs may be taken from the posterior fornix. A Pap smear is taken if not done before (cervical cancer screening guidelines).
- *A comprehensive assessment of the sex partner* is done when STIs are suspected. General examination includes examination of the oral cavity to look for oral sores or other lesions. Examination of the external genitalia, the inguinal, and the anal region is done to look for any sores, swellings, lymph nodes, ulcers, warts, rashes (condyloma lata), and urethral or anal discharge.

17.6   INVESTIGATIONS

1. *Routine antenatal investigations at first visit/contact with the doctor*: Complete blood counts, blood group and typing, urine routine, TSH, test for syphilis (VDRL), screening for HIV-1 and 2, Australian antigen (HBsAg), and HCV screening. Screening for gestational diabetes is done by OGTT (blood sugar after 75 gm glucose load irrespective of fasting status). Neutrophilia is often observed in impetigo herpetiformis[9] and may also be observed in other skin lesions secondary to bacterial and viral infections.
2. *Routine blood tests* to be repeated at 28 weeks of gestation: Complete blood counts, TSH, urine routine, OGTT.
3. *Screening for chromosomal abnormalities*: Combined screening at 11^{+1}–13^{+6} weeks. It includes dual marker testing [Free Beta hCG (human chorionic gonadotrophin) and PAPP—A (Pregnancy-associated plasma protein A)] and fetal ultrasound for nuchal translucency and nasal bone (NT/NB) scan.
4. *Fetal anomaly scan*: Congenital septal defects, pulmonary artery stenosis, microcephaly, and hepatosplenomegaly of the fetus may be detected on prenatal ultrasound and fetal echocardiography in a rubella-infected mother.[10]
5. *Fetal growth scans*: Pemphigoid gestationis may be associated with prematurity and small-for-date babies.[11]
6. *Liver function tests*: Bile acids should be done if the pruritis is out of proportion to the examination findings. A diagnosis of IHCP is established in women with raised peak random total bile acid concentration of ≥19 micromol/L. The itch and raised bile acids resolving after birth lead to the confirmation of diagnosis. IHCP may develop as late as 15

weeks after the onset of pruritis. Therefore, liver function tests and bile acids are repeated (frequency depends on clinical conditions and gestational age) in women with persistent itching, normal bile acids, and no other apparent cause of itching.[12]

7. *Skin biopsy*: If there is any doubt about the diagnosis, the patient should be referred to general dermatology for skin biopsy and further testing. Histopathology may be required for the confirmation of diagnosis in pemphigoid gestationis and impetigo herpetiformis.

8. Low serum calcium, raised CRP, low phosphate, and low vitamin D levels are observed in impetigo herpetiformis.[9]

9. *Immunofluorescence*: Direct immunofluorescence studies are positive in pemphigoid gestationis.[9]

10. *Any other test will be guided by the clinical findings and the history*: Other dermatoses unrelated to pregnancy such as scabies, drug rashes, or viral exanthems must be ruled out. A PCR is used for the diagnosis of HSV. Screening for other sexually transmitted infections is also done in women presenting with genital herpes.[13]

17.7 TREATMENT

Treatment of specific dermatoses is dealt with in specific chapters.

17.8 ALGORITHMIC APPROACH TO DERMATOSES IN PREGNANCY

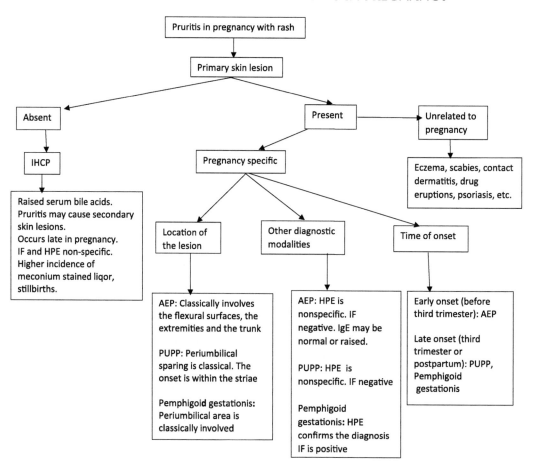

HPE: Histopathological examination, IF: Immunofluorescence

FIGURE 17.1 A diagnostic approach to pruritis with rash in pregnancy.

17.9 CONCLUSION

Temporary or permanent complications to the mother, fetus, or neonate may be caused by skin conditions that are associated with pregnancy. Early diagnosis and management of these conditions will minimise the risk and promptly mitigate the complications that arise. Any woman with pre-existing skin lesions or skin lesions complicating previous pregnancy should plan their pregnancy in consultation with an obstetrician and a dermatologist to ensure the best feto-maternal outcome.

REFERENCES

1. Tunzi M, Gray GR. Common skin conditions during pregnancy. *AM Fam Physician*. 2007;5(2):211–218.
2. Vaughan Jones S, Ambros-Rudolph C, Nelson-Piercy C. Skin disease in pregnancy. *BMJ* 2014;348:g3489.
3. Maglie R, Quintarelli L, et al. Specific dermatoses of pregnancy other than pemphigoid gestationis. *G Ital Dermatol Venereol*. 2019;154(3):286–298.
4. FOGSI. *Good Clinical Practice Recommendations on Preconception Care-India*; 2016, available at: www.fogsi.org/wp-content/uploads/2016/09/FOGSI-PCCR-Guideline-Booklet-Orange.pdf
5. Effect of contraceptives on the skin. *Aust Fam Physician*. 1988;17(10):853, 856.
6. Kroumpouzos G, Cohen LM. Specific dermatoses pregnancy: An evidence-based systematic review. *Am J Obstet Gynecol*. 2003;188(4):1083–1092.
7. Ramos-E-Silva M, Martins NR, Kroumpouzos G. Oral and vulvovaginal changes in pregnancy. *Clin Dermatol*. 2016;34(3):353–358.
8. Alegre VA, Gastineau DA, Winkelmann RK. Skin lesions associated with circulating lupus anticoagulant. *Br J Dermatol*. 1989;120(3):419–429.
9. Ting S, Nixon R. Assessment and management of itchy skin in pregnancy. *Aust J Gen Pract*. 2021;50 (12):898–903.
10. Yazigi A, De Pecoulas AE, et al. Fetal and neonatal abnormalities due to congenital rubella syndrome: A review of literature. *J Matern Fetal Neonatal Med*. 2017;30(3):274–278.
11. Ambros-Rudolph CM. Dermatoses of pregnancy—clues to diagnosis, fetal risk and therapy. *Ann Dermatol*. 2011;23(3):265–275.
12. RCOG, *Intrahepatic Cholestasis of Pregnancy*, GTG 43; 2022, available at: www.rcog.org.uk/guidance/browse-all-guidance/green-top-guidelines/intrahepatic-cholestasis-of-pregnancy-green-top-guideline-no-43/
13. Foley E, Clarke E, Beckett VA, et al. *Management of Genital Herpes in Pregnancy*. RCOG and British Association for Sexual Health and HIV; 2014, available at: www.bashhguidelines.org/media/1060/management-genital-herpes.pdf

Index

Note: Page numbers in *italics* indicate a figure and page numbers in **bold** indicate a table on the corresponding page.

*For Product Safety Concerns and Information please contact
our EU representative GPSR@taylorandfrancis.com Taylor & Francis
Verlag GmbH, Kaufingerstraße 24, 80331 München, Germany*

T - #0279 - 160425 - C234 - 254/178/11 - PB - 9781032583471 - Gloss Lamination